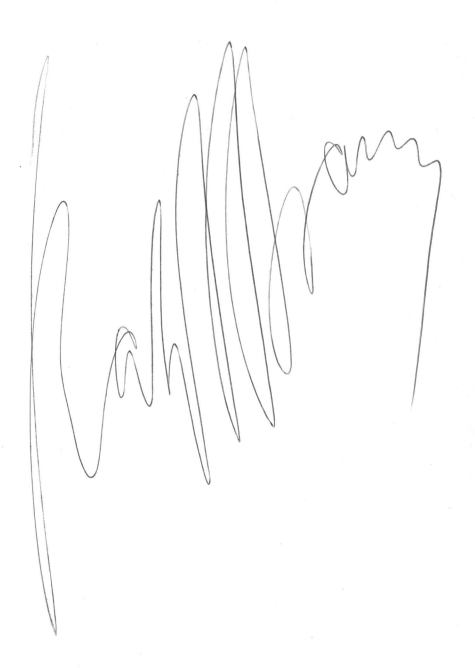

ADVANCES IN NEUROLOGY
VOLUME 5

Advances in Neurology

Advances in Neurology

Volume 5

Second Canadian-American Conference on Parkinson's Disease

*Canadian – American Conference on
Parkinson's Disease (2nd : 1973 :
Princeton, N.J.)*

Editors

Fletcher H. McDowell, M.D.
Associate Dean,
Cornell University Medical College,
New York City

André Barbeau, M.D.
University of Montreal,
Director, Department of Neurobiology,
Clinical Research Institute of Montreal

Raven Press, Publishers ▪ New York

International Standard Book Number
0–911216–63–4
Library of Congress Catalog Card Number
72–93317

Preface

It is my great pleasure to introduce the proceedings of this the Second Canadian-American Conference on Parkinson's Disease. The first conference was held in the Laurentian Mountains in Canada in 1969. The design of this conference is much the same as the original one. We hoped through the conference to bring together people who are interested in Parkinson's disease either directly or indirectly and to give them an opportunity to meet one another and exchange ideas.

The goal of the program committee (which included myself, Drs. André Barbeau, George Cotzias, Murray Goldstein, and Henry Dinsdale) was one of self-education. We selected those topics which all of us knew the least about and put together a program about them so that at least the five of us would come out wiser. In designing the program we wanted to bring into focus a number of issues related to the biochemistry of neurotransmitters and their possible role in motor disturbances in man; the bulk of the program is devoted to this. We have attempted to assemble those individuals who are foremost in investigations in this field. We also selected topics of clinical interest and concern to those of us who are treating patients with Parkinson's disease. We did not feel that review of the efficacy of particular treatments was indicated here, but we were anxious to cover clinical phenomena such as the "on-off" response to see where we stand in the understanding of this difficult problem and to find out if anyone has ideas about how to proceed further in its elucidation.

We are anxious to update, review, and publish the evidence that various analogues or metabolites of DOPA have an effect on the motor disturbance of Parkinson's disease. We also thought it was important to look at other dopaminergic systems in the central nervous system to examine the physiology of these systems and to determine if they have any relevance to Parkinson's disease. The major one on which a large amount of information is available is the neuroendocrine control system of the hypothalamus, which is in large part dopaminergic. We have invited the outstanding individuals in this field so that they will educate those of us who are not specialists in this area and provide any insight they might have about the interconnections between these systems and those governing motor phenomena.

We hope the readers of this volume will find the substance informative and helpful in providing another look at the difficult but important problem of Parkinson's disease.

Fletcher McDowell, M.D
André Barbeau, M.D.

Acknowledgments

The Second Canadian-American Conference on Parkinson's Disease was sponsored by:

The American Parkinson's Disease Association
The Medical Research Council of Canada
and
The National Institute of Neurological Diseases and Stroke.

Contents

Participants

Ellsworth Alvord, Jr.
Department of Pathology
University of Washington
Seattle, Washington 98105

Nils-Erik Andén
Department of Pharmacology
University of Goteborg
Goteborg 33, Sweden

Aaron H. Anton
Department of Anesthesiology
Case Western Reserve University
School of Medicine
Cleveland, Ohio 44106

Il Jin Bak
Planck-Institut für Hirnforschung
Deutschordenstrabe 46
6 Frankfurt A. M., Germany

André Barbeau
Department of Neurobiology
Clinical Research Institute of Montreal
Montreal, Quebec, Canada

Arthur F. Battista
Department of Neurosurgery
New York University Medical College
New York, New York 10016

M. J. Besson
Laboratory of Molecular Biology
College of Franco
11, Place Marcelin—Berthelot
Paris 5, France

Donald Borg
Brookhaven National Laboratories
Associated Universities Inc.
Upton, New York 11973

George Bartholini
Medical Research Department
Hoffmann—La Roche & Co. Ltd.
4002 Basle, Switzerland

Benjamin Boshes
Department of Neurology
Northwestern University
McGaw Medical Center
Chicago, Illinois 60611

Alan A. Boulton
Province of Saskatchewan Department of
* Health*
University Hospital
Saskatoon, Saskatchewan, Canada

Arnold Brossi
Hoffmann—La Roche Inc.
Nutley, New Jersey 07110

Gerard N. Burrow
Department of Internal Medicine
Yale University School of Medicine
New Haven, Connecticut 06510

Donald B. Calne
Royal Postgraduate Medical School
Hammersmith Hospital
London W 12, OHS, England

Arvid Carlsson
Department of Pharmacology
University of Goteborg
Goteborg 33, Sweden

Thomas N. Chase
Section on Experimental Therapeutics
National Institute of Mental Health
Bethesda, Maryland 20014

Mary Coleman
Research Institute
St. Joseph Hospital
Lancaster, Pennsylvania 17604

George C. Cotzias
Medical Department
Brookhaven National Laboratory
Associated Universities Inc.
Upton, New York 11973

James N. Davis
Department of Neurosciences
Duke University Medical Center
Durham, North Carolina 27710

John Donaldson
Department of Neurobiology
Clinical Research Institute of Montreal
Montreal, Quebec, Canada

Antoine D'Iorio
Faculty of Science and Engineering
University of Ottawa
Ottawa, Ontario, Canada

Key Dismukes
Department of Pharmacology &
* Experimental Therapeutics*
The Johns Hopkins University
* School of Medicine*
Baltimore, Maryland 21205

Roger C. Duvoisin
Department of Neurology
Columbia University
* College of Physicians & Surgeons*
New York, New York 10032

Arthur Dale Ericsson
Department of Neurology
Baylor College of Medicine
Texas Medical Center
Houston, Texas 77025

Stanley Fahn
Department of Neurology
University of Pennsylvania
* School of Medicine*
Philadelphia, Pennsylvania 19174

Lysia S. Forno
Neuropathology Laboratory
Palo Alto Veterans Hospital
Palo Alto, California 94304

Andrew G. Frantz
Columbia University
* College of Physicians & Surgeons*
New York, New York 10032

Kjell Fuxe
Department of Histology
Karolinska Institutet
Stockholm 60, Sweden

Leon Goldberg
Clinical Pharmacology Program
Emory University School of Medicine
Atlanta, Georgia 30303

Menek Goldstein
Department of Neurochemistry
New York University Medical Center
New York, New York 10016

Murray Goldstein
Director, Extramural Programs
National Institutes of Health
Bethesda, Maryland 20014

Margaret Hoehm
University of Colorado Medical Center
Denver, Colorado 80220

W. D. Horst
Research Division
Hoffman–La Roche Inc.
Nutley, New Jersey 07110

Abba J. Kastin
Endocrinology Section
Veterans Administration Hospital
and
Department of Medicine
Tulane University School of Medicine
New Orleans, Louisiana 70146

Robert Katzman
Department of Neurology
Albert Einstein College of Medicine
* of Yeshiva University*
Bronx, New York 10461

Harold L. Klawans, Jr.
Presbyterian–St. Luke's Hospital
Chicago, Illinois 60612

Irwin J. Kopin
Laboratory of Clinical Science
National Institute of Mental Health
Bethesda, Maryland 20014

Kresimir Krnjević
McGill University
Montreal 109, Quebec, Canada

Harold E. Lebovitz
Department of Medicine
Duke University Medical Center
Durham, North Carolina 27710

Aaron B. Lerner
Department of Dermatology
Yale University School of Medicine
New Haven, Connecticut 06510

Charles H. Markham
Department of Neurology
UCLA School of Medicine
Los Angeles, California 90024

Harold Mars
Mt. Sinai Hospital of Cleveland
Cleveland, Ohio 44106

Ismael Mena
Brookhaven National Laboratory
Associated Universities Inc.
Upton, New York 11973

Robert J. Mones
Department of Neurology
Mt. Sinai School of Medicine
New York, New York 10029

Manfred D. Muenter
Mayo Medical School
Rochester, Minnesota 55901

Samuel M. McCann
Department of Physiology
The University of Texas
Southwestern Medical School of Dallas
Dallas, Texas 75235

Patrick McGeer
Division of Neurological Sciences
The University of British Columbia
Kinsmen Laboratory
Vancouver 8, British Columbia, Canada

Desmond S. O'Doherty
Department of Neurology
Georgetown University Medical Center
Washington, D.C. 20007

Fletcher H. McDowell
Department of Neurology
Cornell University Medical College
New York, New York 10021

Henning Pakkenberg
Department of Neurology
Kommunehospitalet
DK 1399
Copenhagen K., Denmark

Paul Papavasiliou
Medical Department
Brookhaven National Laboratory
Associated Universities Inc.
Upton, New York 11973

George Paulson
Department of Neurology
Ohio State University Medical School
Columbus, Ohio 43221

Louis Poirier
Laboratoire de Neurobiologie
Université Laval
Faculté de Mèdecine
Cité Universitaire
Quebec 10, Ontario, Canada

Donald Reis
Department of Neurology
Cornell University Medical College
New York, New York 10021

U. K. Rinne
Department of Neurology
University of Turku
Turku 3, Finland

Eugene Roberts
Division of Neurosciences
City of Hope National Medical Center
Duarte, California 91010

Pierre Rondot
Hôpital de la Salpetrière
47 Boulevard de l'Hôpital
Paris, France

Bjorn-Erik Roos
Department of Pharmacology
University of Goteborg
Goteborg 33, Sweden

Merton Sandler
Bernhard Baron Memorial Research
    Laboratories
Department of Chemical Pathology
Queen Charlotte's Maternity Hospital
London, W6 OXG, England

Richard W. Schayer
Research Center
Rockland State Hospital
Orangeburg, New York 10962

Stuart A. Schneck
Division of Neurology
University of Colorado Medical Center
Denver, Colorado 80220

William A. Sibley
Department of Neurology
University of Arizona Medical Center
Tucson, Arizona 85724

Jean Siegfried
Kantonsspital Zürich
Neurochirurgische Universitatsklinik
8006 Zürich, Switzerland

Gerard Smith
Department of Psychiatry
The New York Hospital (Westchester
    Division)
21 Bloomingdale Road
White Plains, New York 10605

T. L. Sourkes
Departments of Psychiatry and
    Biochemistry
Allan Memorial Insitute of Psychiatry
Montreal 112, Quebec, Canada

Peter Stern
Burke Rehabilitation Center
Mamaroneck Road
White Plains, New York 10605

Richard D. Sweet
Department of Neurology
Cornell University Medical College
New York, New York 10021

Gertrude M. Tyce
Mayo Clinic and Mayo Foundation
Rochester, Minnesota 55901

Urban Ungerstedt
Department of Histology
Karolinska Institutet
Stockholm 60, Sweden

Glen R. Van Loon
Division of Special Mental Health
    Research
St. Elizabeths Hospital
National Institute of Mental Health
Washington, D.C. 20032

Melvin H. Van Woert
Department of Internal Medicine
Yale University School of Medicine
New Haven, Connecticut 06510

Martha Vogt
Institute of Animal Physiology
Babraham, Cambridge, England

Claude Wasterlain
Department of Neurology
Cornell University Medical College
New York, New York 10021

Bette F. Weiss
Department of Nutrition and Food
    Science
Massachusetts Institute of Technology
Cambridge, Massachusetts 02139

Richard J. Wurtman
Massachusetts Institute of Technology
Cambridge, Massachusetts 02139

Melvin D. Yahr
Neurological Institute
Columbia University
    College of Physicians & Surgeons
New York, New York 10032

Advances in Neurology, Vol. 5
Raven Press, New York © 1974

The Relation Between Cholinergic and Monoaminergic Activity in the Caudate Nucleus

Marthe Vogt

Institute of Animal Physiology, Babraham, Cambridge, England

ANATOMICAL CONSIDERATIONS

The striatum, comprising the caudate nucleus and the putamen, is richer in acetylcholine (ACh), choline acetyltransferase, and cholinergic terminals than any other part of the forebrain (1–4). It also contains cells that give rise to cholinergic neurons, some of which end in the pallidum and in the substantia nigra. These are particularly abundant in the monkey (5). It is now well recognized that the majority of fibers ascending from the sub-stantia nigra to the striatum are dopaminergic neurons, but there are also, according to Shute and Lewis (6), cholinergic nigrostriatal connections, some of which may be interrupted in the pallidum or the entopeduncular nucleus. The existence of nondopaminergic nigro-striatal fibers has also been suggested by observations of Fibiger, Pudritz, McGeer, and McGeer (7). These workers compared the effect of electrolytic lesions of the medial fore-brain bundle with that of intraventricular injection of 6-hydroxydopamine on two parameters: striatal tyrosine hydroxylase and formation of radioactive protein by injection of ^{14}C-leucine into one substantia nigra. The lesions diminished both hydroxylase and radioactive protein to the same extent; 6-hydroxydopamine reduced the hydroxylase to 7% of normal but the ^{14}C-protein only to 33% of control. The authors concluded that 20% of nigro-striatal fibers are nondopaminergic. Some of these may be cholinergic, although neurons containing 5-hydroxytryptamine (5-HT) or unknown transmitters may be involved. I am sure Dr. Poirier will throw more light on this question.

As far as we know, none of the cholinergic neurons are affected in Parkin-son's disease, and there is no cell loss in the striatum. If cholinergic neurons remain active when most dopaminergic axons and some tryptaminergic axons have been lost, part, at least, of the parkinsonian syndrome must be due to unchecked activity of cholinergic neurons, and this fact may be the basis for the old-established treatment with ACh antagonists. Experi-mentally, it can be shown that firing of cells can be induced in the caudate nucleus by iontophoretically applied ACh, and that this firing is suppressed by dopamine (8). However, the translation of these observations into motor effects or abnormalities still eludes us and is complicated by the fact that the responses can vary according to the site within the striatum itself. Thus, electrical stimulation of the postero-dorsal part of the cat's caudate nucleus facilitates, whereas stimulation of the antero-ventral part inhibits, cortically elicited muscle contractions (9). Furthermore, injection of L-DOPA or dopamine causes athetoid movements only if injected into the facilitating areas (10). Both regions are supplied by cholinergic and dopaminergic neurons. There is as yet no explanation of these regional differences.

EXPERIMENTS ON RELEASE

To the physiologist, the most convincing way of showing that a substance occurring in nervous tissue acts as a transmitter at a given site is to find stimuli which will release it at this site. By inserting a push-pull cannula (11) into the caudate nucleus of a cat, Mitchell and Szerb (12) obtained a release of ACh into the effluent when they stimulated certain regions of the cortex, and McLennan (13) when he stimulated the thalamic nucleus ventralis anterior.

Portig and Vogt (14, 15), looking for a method which would avoid any damage to the tissue, perfused the anterior horn of the lateral ventricle of the cat with artificial cerebrospinal fluid containing neostigmine. The perfusate, as previously found by Bhattacharya and Feldberg (16), contained ACh. Its amount tended to rise during the first hours of perfusion and later reached a steady level. As shown by MacIntosh and Oborin (17), who measured ACh release from the cerebral cortex, the height of the basal release is also determined by the depth of anesthesia: the lighter the animal, the greater its ACh production.

During perfusion of the anterior horn of the lateral ventricle, increments over the basal release of ACh were observed as a result of a variety of afferent sensory stimuli: noise, electrical stimulation of the skin of the paws or of the central ends of the sciatic nerves, stimuli which are well known to elicit evoked potentials in the caudate nucleus. A release of ACh was also seen when certain regions in the brain were stimulated, such as the substantia nigra, the nucleus centralis lateralis thalami, and (not consistently) the contralateral caudate nucleus.

Does this ACh come from the caudate nucleus? There is another gray structure, the septum, which contains ACh and borders on the anterior horn of the lateral ventricle. Yet, as shown by Krnjević and Silver (3, 4), the septum contains few cholinergic terminals, but rather many cells giving rise to cholinergic axons which end in other parts of the brain. These cells are responsible for the ACh content of the septum but cannot contribute to a release of ACh into the ventricle. The multiplicity of stimuli which gives rise to ACh release from the caudate nucleus suggests that afferent stimuli converging onto the striatum either utilize some common cholinergic pathway into the striatum or stimulate cholinergic interneurons within the striatal tissue.

Experiments with the same perfusion technique have shown that the basal release of the main dopamine metabolite homovanillic acid, like ACh, decreased with deepening anesthesia (15). It would therefore appear that cholinergic and dopaminergic activity of the striatum are positively correlated in the intact brain. Olivier et al. (5) have suggested a neuronal loop as an anatomical basis for this correlation.

The fact that there is both a cholinergic and a dopaminergic nigro-striatal pathway could be interpreted to mean that, in general, monoamines are not released unless there is simultaneous activation of a cholinergic pathway. The observation of a release of 5-HT into the anterior horn of the lateral ventricle gave us an opportunity to examine this possibility. Afferent sensory stimuli which released ACh, or stimulation of the substantia nigra, which releases ACh and dopamine, does not change the basal release of 5-HT, even if an inhibitor of monoamine oxidase is present (15). However, stimulation of one of the two most anterior nuclei of the raphe, the nucleus linearis rostralis or linearis intermedius, consistently causes an increment in the 5-HT content of the perfusate (18). There are thus tryptaminergic terminals in the gray matter bordering on the anterior horn of the lateral ventricle. Was this activity coupled with a release of ACh? To test this possibility, neostigmine was added to the perfusion fluid and ACh and 5-HT estimated in the effluent (19). The results were unambiguous: whenever the electrode was in one of the raphe nuclei, 5-HT was released but no increment in ACh appeared in the perfusate. These results do not mean that cholinergic neurons could not activate 5-HT release by impinging on cells in the raphe nuclei, but there is no suggestion that the release of 5-HT is caused by, or linked with, simultaneous release of ACh from cholinergic neurons originating in the same nuclei.

An unexpected effect of atropine (20) merits consideration: it reduces the turnover of dopamine in the brain of mice. The reduction is even more pronounced if the turnover of dopamine has been accelerated by injection of moderate doses of phenothiazines or butyrophenones. Atropine does not overcome the accelerating effect of large doses of these tranquilizers, such as chlorpromazine (100 mg/kg) or haloperidol (10 mg/kg). These effects on turnover of dopamine would be difficult to interpret if they were the result of the anti-ACh property of atropine, but might be expected if they were due to its capacity to inhibit the uptake of dopamine into neurons. Atropine shares this property with many antagonists of ACh (21), although its potency as an inhibitor of uptake into synaptosomes is rather weak. If, however, this were its mechanism of reducing the dopamine turnover, it would be just another example of the accumulation of a transmitter at the synapse reducing its rate of release.

Finally, the unusually high concentration of γ-aminobutyric acid in the substantia nigra has suggested that an inhibitory striato-nigral pathway releasing this amino acid may play a part in the control of nigro-striatal impulses (22). Any attempt at integrating the activity of cholinergic and monoaminergic neurons will also have to take this possibility into account.

REFERENCES

1. MacIntosh, F. C., *J. Physiol. (London)* 99, 436 (1941).
2. Feldberg, W., and Vogt, M., *J. Physiol. (London)* 107, 372 (1948).
3. Krnjević, K., and Silver, A., *J. Anat.* 99, 711 (1965).
4. Krnjević, K., and Silver, A., *J. Anat.* 100, 63 (1966).
5. Olivier, A., Parent, A., Simard, H., and Poirier, L. J., *Brain Res.* 18, 273 (1970).
6. Shute, C. C. D., and Lewis, P. R., *Brain* 90, 497 (1967).
7. Fibiger, H. C., Pudritz, R. E., McGeer, P. L., and McGeer, E. G., *J. Neurochem.* 19, 1697, (1972).
8. Bloom, F. E., Costa, E., and Salmoiraghi, G. C., *J. Pharmac. Exp. Ther.* 150, 244 (1965).
9. Liles, S. L., and Davis, G. D., *J. Neurophysiol.* 32, 574 (1969).
10. Cools, A. R., *Psychopharmacologia (Berlin)* 25, 229 (1972).
11. Gaddum, J. H., *J. Physiol. (London)* 155, 1P (1961).
12. Mitchell, J. F., and Szerb, J. C., *Int. Physiol. Congr.* XXII, 2 Abstr. 819 (1962).
13. McLennan, H., *J. Physiol. (London)* 174, 152 (1964).
14. Portig, P. J., and Vogt, M., *J. Physiol. (London)* 186, 131P (1966).
15. Portig, P. J., and Vogt, M., *J. Physiol. (London)* 204, 687 (1969).
16. Bhattacharya, B. K., and Feldberg, W., *Brit. J. Pharmac. Chemother.* 13, 163 (1958).
17. MacIntosh, F. C., and Oborin, P. E., *Abstr. Int. Physiol. Congr.* XIX, p. 580 (1953).
18. Holman, R. B., and Vogt, M., *J. Physiol. (London)* 223, 243 (1972).
19. Ashkenazi, R., Holman, R. B., and Vogt, M., *J. Physiol. (London)* 223, 255 (1972).
20. O'Keeffe, R., Sharman, D. F., and Vogt, M., *Brit. J. Pharmac.* 38, 287 (1970).
21. Horn, A. S., Coyle, J. T., and Snyder, H., *Molecular Pharmacol.* 7, 66 (1971).
22. Kim, J. S., Bak, I. J., Hassler, R., and Okada, Y., *Exp. Brain Res.* 14, 95 (1971).

Advances in Neurology, Vol. 5
Raven Press, New York © 1974

Dopaminergic and Cholinergic Mechanisms in Relation to Postural Tremor in the Monkey and Circling Movements in the Cat

L. J. Poirier, P. Langelier, P. Bédard, R. Boucher, L. Larochelle, A. Parent, and A. G. Roberge

Laboratoires de Neurobiologie, Faculté de Médecine, Université Laval, Québec, Canada G1K 7P4

Monkeys with lesions involving in some places the rubro-(small-celled)-olivo-cerebello-rubral loop will display postural tremor in response to harmaline, haloperidol, alpha-methyl-tyrosine (AMT), and reserpine. Under such conditions (with an intact dopaminergic nigrostriatal pathway), L-DOPA transiently abolishes tremor induced by AMT and reserpine but does not reduce harmaline- or haloperidol-induced tremor. Benztropine counteracts tremor induced by AMT, reserpine, and haloperidol but does not abolish harmaline-induced tremor (1–4). These data suggest that the above-mentioned drugs, which interfere, in one way or another, with the metabolism of dopamine (DA), cause, among other effects, a pharmacological and reversible interruption of the dopaminergic nigrostriatal mechanism. The effect of these drugs somehow duplicates the pathological or experimental destruction of the nigrostriatal pathway, a condition which represents the most characteristic disturbance associated with sustained postural tremor (5, 6). However, the effectiveness of benztropine or atropine in reducing tremor induced by lesion or haloperidol suggests that cholinergic mechanisms deprived of certain incoming influences as a consequence of the disturbance of the corresponding DA mechanism come into play in the activation of the nervous mechanisms directly responsible for the building up of the rhythmic activity associated with postural tremor. The neostriatum, with its great amount of acetylcholine and its corresponding highly rich acetylcholinesterasic striopallidal pathway (7), may represent the most important cholinergic structure involved in this type of abnormal motor activity.

In contradistinction to the above-described model of parkinsonian-like tremor which is associated with a decrease of brain DA or its inactivation, rapid and contraversive circling movements induced by L-DOPA in cats

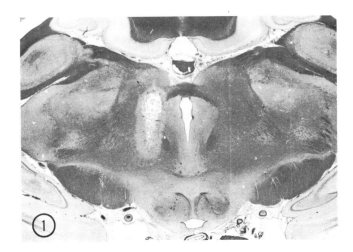

FIG. 1. Transverse section through upper midbrain showing a right dorsomedial tegmental lesion in a cat that reacted to L-DOPA by contraversive circling. Fast blue and basic fuchsin. × 3.8.

with lesions involving the midbrain dorsomedial tegmental area (Fig. 1) result from increases in brain catecholamines and, more especially, in brain DA. The latter phenomenon, which may be reproduced from day to day by administering L-DOPA (p.o. or i.p.), is duplicated by apomorphine (8) but not by amphetamine. It cannot yet be determined, however, whether the concomitant destruction of the corresponding (in reference to the lesioned side) nigrostriatal pathway contributes to increase the intensity of this type of abnormal motor activity, although it has been shown that cats with a complete interruption of the nigrostriatal fibers following lesions restricted to the area of Tsai (Fig. 2) do not display circling movements in response to L-DOPA. The fact that the L-DOPA-induced circling movements are not counteracted by cholinergic or anticholinergic drugs (Bédard and Larochelle, *unpublished data*) suggests that this type of abnormal behavior does not specifically involve a cholinergic disturbance.

On the other hand, slow and ipsiversive rotation may be induced by the administration of L-DOPA to cats with unilateral lesions involving the entopeduncular nucleus, the ventrolateral thalamic nucleus *(unpublished data),* or the mid-portion of the cerebral peduncle at midbrain level. This type of rotational behavior, which occurs with and without a concomitant involvement of the nigrostriatal pathway (8), may be compared with somewhat similar ipsiversive movements induced by the combined administration of a monoamine oxidase inhibitor plus reserpine (9) or amphetamine (10) in rats with lesions of the basal ganglia and the corresponding frontal cortex or the *pes pedunculi*. The failure of L-DOPA administered alone to induce circling movements in lesioned rats as opposed to the rapid con-

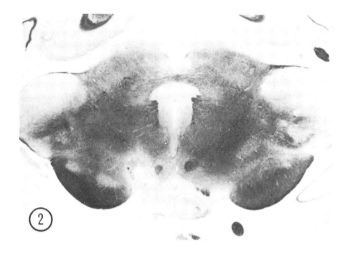

FIG. 2. Transverse section through the rostral midbrain showing a right ventromedial tegmental lesion that completely severed the corresponding nigrostriatal pathway. This cat did not display any rotation behavior following L-DOPA administered during several consecutive days. Fast blue and basic fuchsin. × 3.8.

traversive and slow ipsiversive circling movements in lesioned cats following L-DOPA is most likely related to the presence of an important decarboxylase enzymic barrier at the level of the brain capillaries in the mouse and rat (11, 12) and to the absence of such an enzymic barrier at the level of the brain capillaries in the cat as well as in the monkey (13). Actually, the administration of L-DOPA alone causes a slight increase of DA (14) and marked fluorescence of the brain capillaries (12) in the rat (Fig. 3), whereas

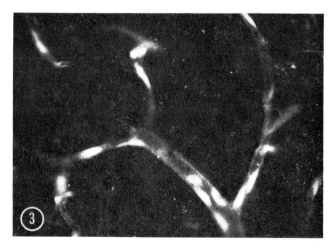

FIG. 3. Fluorescence microphotograph through the cortex of a rat administered L-DOPA 1 hr before sacrifice. Capillaries display an intense green fluorescence. × 462.

the same treatment results in a marked increase of brain DA and homovanillic acid associated with a diffuse green fluorescence of the nervous parenchyma in the cat (13). Therefore L-DOPA penetrates the nervous tissue and readily forms catecholamine and more especially DA in the cat brain but not in the rat brain.

In reference to the peculiarities of the enzymic barrier at the level of the brain capillaries, the coincidental morphological feature is of interest: in the rat most brain capillaries also display an intense cholinesterasic activity whereas in the cat they show a weak cholinesterasic activity (15). These particularities (the presence of both enzymes, decarboxylase and cholinesterase, in great amount at the level of most brain capillaries in the rat but not in the cat) may correspond to some functional interrelationship between cholinergic and dopaminergic mechanisms which, however, is different in the rat than in the cat and monkey. In the latter species, however, the capillaries, most particularly at the level of the subthalamic nucleus, display an intense cholinesterasic activity in comparison to the capillaries in other brain areas (Fig. 4). This might have some implication in the functioning of the extrapyramidal system, particularly in primates.

Postural tremor in the monkey involves an inactivation or decreased concentration of brain DA whereas rapid and contraversive circling movements in the cat are associated with an increased brain DA concentration. Anticholinergic treatment may reduce or abolish postural tremor in the monkey, but rapid circling movements in the cat are not modified by anticholinergic or cholinergic treatment. Therefore, the two types of abnormal motor activities, tremor and circling, involve entirely opposed disturbances

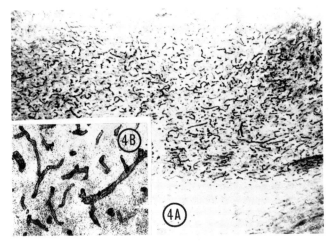

FIG. 4. Microphotographs through the subthalamic nucleus of a monkey showing the intense cholinesterasic activity within the capillaries of this structure. Thiocholine technique. × 15 (4A) and × 92 (4B).

most probably at the level of a common nervous structure, the neostriatum, in addition to disturbances in other structures peculiar to either type of motor impairment. Actually, postural tremor apparently involves cholinergic mechanisms which, as a consequence of the inactivation of the corresponding DA mechanism, are no longer influenced by the latter mechanism, and, therefore, are relatively hyperfunctioning. This is supported by the fact that L-DOPA readily counteracts AMT- and reserpine-induced tremor provided that the nigrostriatal dopaminergic pathways are intact (3, 4). Rapid and contraversive circling movements, on the other hand, are apparently related to the hyperfunctioning of as yet undetermined mechanisms which, as a consequence of a marked increase of brain DA concentration, are greatly activated. It is worth mentioning that such movements occur at a time when the excitability of the animal is greatly enhanced.

Moreover, postural tremor is probably related to a combined disturbance of the nigrostriatal dopaminergic and corresponding cerebellar mechanisms which leads to the production of an abnormal rhythmic activity at the level of the motor neurons. Rapid and contraversive circling movements imply the interruption of different nervous structures and the activation of mechanisms which are not clearly identified. Slow and ipsiversive circling, which also involves an enhancement of dopaminergic activity, apparently implies an important and concomitant disturbance along a loop which encompasses the internal pallidum (or the entopeduncular nucleus in the cat) and the thalamus and their centrifugal pathways, as well as the motor cortex and certain of its efferent descending pathways.

ACKNOWLEDGMENTS

This research was supported by grants from the Medical Research Council of Canada. The salaries of P.L., P.B., L.L., A.P., and A.G.R. were supported by awards from the Medical Research Council of Canada.

REFERENCES

1. Bédard, P., Larochelle, L., Poirier, L. J., and Sourkes, T. L., *Canad. J. Physiol. Pharmacol.* 48, 82 (1970).
2. Larochelle, L., Bédard, P., Boucher, R., and Poirier, L. J., *J. Neurol. Sci.* 11, 53 (1970).
3. Larochelle, L., Bédard, P., Poirier, L. J., and Sourkes, T. L. *Neuropharmacology* 10, 273 (1971).
4. Poirier, L. J., Bédard, P., Langelier, P., Larochelle, L., Parent, A., and Roberge, A., *Rev. Neurol.* 127, 37 (1972).
5. Poirier, L. J., *J. Neurophysiol.* 23, 534 (1960).
6. Poirier, L. J., Bouvier, G., Bédard, P., Boucher, R., Larochelle, L., Olivier, A., and Singh, P., *Rev. Neurol.* 120, 15 (1969).
7. Olivier, A., Parent, A., Simard, H., and Poirier, L. J., *Brain Res.* 18, 273 (1970).
8. Langelier, P., Boucher, R., and Poirier, L. J., *Proceed. Can. Fed. Biol. Soc.* 15, 319 (1972).
9. Andén, N. E., Dahlström, A., Fuxe, K., and Larsson, K., *Acta Pharmacol.* 24, 263 (1966).

10. Andén, N. E., Rubenson, A., Fuxe, K., and Hökfelt, T., *J. Pharm. Pharmacol.* 19, 627 (1967).
11. Bertler, A., Falck, B., and Rosengren, E., *Acta Pharmacol.* 20, 317 (1964).
12. Constantinidis, J., de la Torre, J. C., Tissot, R., and Geissbühler, F., *Psychopharmacologia* 15, 75 (1969).
13. Langelier, P., Parent, A., and Poirier, L. J., *Brain Res.* 45, 622 (1972).
14. Bartholini, G., Bates, H. M., Burkard, W. P., and Pletscher, A., *Nature* 215, 852 (1967).
15. Brightman, M. W., and Albers, R. W., *J. Neurochem.* 4, 244 (1959).

Advances in Neurology, Vol. 5
Raven Press, New York © 1974

Dopaminergic Regulation of Cholinergic Neurons in the Striatum: Relation to Parkinsonism

G. Bartholini, K. G. Lloyd, and H. Stadler

Department of Experimental Medicine, F. Hoffmann-La Roche & Co. Ltd., Basle, Switzerland

In Parkinson's disease, as well as in the parkinsonian syndrome occurring after blockade of dopamine (DA) receptors by neuroleptic drugs, some of the symptoms, e.g., rigidity and tremor, seem to be connected with the preponderance of a cholinergic function (1, 2). Thus, cholinergic drugs exacerbate and anticholinergic compounds ameliorate parkinsonism (3). These observations suggest that striatal DA and acetylcholine (ACh) neurons are in a functional balance (1). Moreover, the finding that the turnover of DA is modified by changes in cholinergic activity (4–6) indicates an interconnection between, and possibly a mutual regulation of, the two neuronal systems. However, this interregulation has not yet been demonstrated.

The influence of the dopaminergic system on cholinergic neurons has been directly investigated in the experiments reported here in which ACh liberated from the cat caudate nucleus was collected by means of an acutely or chronically implanted push-pull cannula and measured radioenzymatically (7).

Neuroleptic compounds of various chemical classes (e.g., chlorpromazine, haloperidol, and methiothepin), administered intravenously, markedly enhance the output of ACh from the caudate nucleus (Fig. 1). Neither the ACh-esterase activity nor the ACh content in the striatum is modified by these drugs indicating that the changes in ACh output reflect corresponding modifications of the transmitter turnover (2, 7).

The mechanism by which neuroleptic drugs enhance the ACh turnover seems to be secondary to the blockade of DA receptors. In fact, DA receptor-stimulating agents such as apomorphine or L-DOPA cause a reduction of striatal ACh release. Furthermore, these drugs prevent or reverse the increase of ACh induced by neuroleptic compounds. The increased liberation of striatal ACh by neuroleptic agents occurs concomitantly with the acceleration of DA turnover, which is assumed to be the consequence of blockade of DA receptors. Thus, 2 hr after administration of chlorpromazine or haloperidol, the homovanillic acid is enhanced by

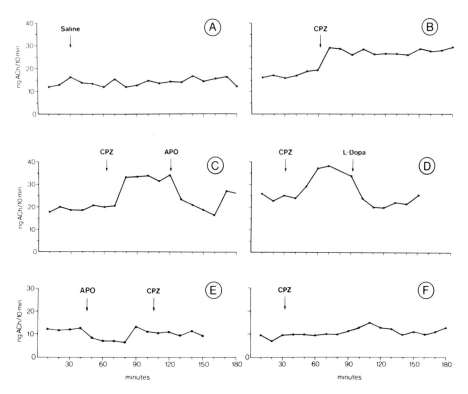

FIG. 1. Typical output of acetylcholine (ACh) into the perfusate of individual caudate nuclei (A–E) or premotor cortex (F) of different cats. Physiological saline, chlorpromazine (CPZ, 10 mg/kg), apomorphine (APO, 10 mg/kg), and/or L-DOPA (50 mg/kg) were administered intravenously. Time 0 indicates the beginning of the collection of the perfusate. Each point represents the average of duplicate determinations. For technical details see reference 7.

50% in the perfused striatum without changes in the content of DA. In contrast, promethazine, a non-neuroleptic phenothiazine, fails to increase the turnover of either DA or ACh (7, 8).

These results indicate that by blocking DA receptors neuroleptic agents remove an inhibitory influence on a striatal cholinergic system, resulting in an increase in cholinergic neuronal activity and ACh turnover. It is therefore likely that under physiological conditions this cholinergic system is tonically inhibited by a dopaminergic input.

These results represent the first biochemical evidence that neuroleptic drugs activate a striatal cholinergic system which can be assumed to be involved in the pathogenesis of parkinsonian symptoms. Based on these findings, it is suggested that impairment of dopaminergic transmission has two distinct effects: akinesia, directly related to the decreased stimulation of DA receptors, and rigidity and tremor, produced indirectly through preponderance of a cholinergic mechanism. This explains why in parkinsonian patients akinesia is ameliorated only by dopaminergic agents, mainly L-DOPA, and why dopaminergic as well as anticholinergic drugs act on rigidity and tremor (Table 1).

TABLE 1. *Possible pathogenesis of parkinsonian symptoms*

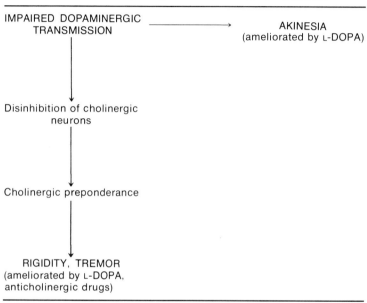

This interregulation between DA and ACh neurons is likely to occur specifically in the striatum. Thus, neuroleptic drugs do not modify the liberation of ACh from the nucleus accumbens or the septum of the cat — the areas of the limbic system with the most dense DA network — although they markedly enhance the turnover of DA in these regions (9). These drugs are also ineffective on the release of ACh from the cerebral cortex (7, 8) in which DA neurons have been recently described (10).

REFERENCES

1. Barbeau, A., *Can. Med. Assoc. J.,* 87, 802 (1962).
2. Bartholini, G., Stadler, H., and Lloyd, K. G., in: *Progress in the Treatment of Parkinsonism, Advances in Neurology, Vol. 3,* edited by D. B. Calne, Raven Press, New York (1973).
3. Duvoisin, R. G., *Arch. Neurol. Psychiat.,* 17, 124 (1967).
4. Bartholini, G., and Pletscher, A., *Experientia,* 27, 1302 (1971).
5. Andén, N. E., and Bédard, P., *J. Pharm. Pharmacol.,* 23, 460 (1971).
6. Perez-Crouet, J., Gessa, G. L., Tagliamonte, A., and Tagliamonte, P., *Fed. Proc.,* 30, 216 (1971).
7. Stadler, H., Lloyd, K. G., Gadea-Ciria, M., and Bartholini, G., *Brain Res.,* 55, 476 (1973).

8. Bartholini, G., Stadler, H., and Lloyd, K. G., in: *Frontiers in Catecholamine Research,* Pergamon Press, New York *(in press).*
9. Lloyd, K. G., Stadler, H., and Bartholini, G., in: *Frontiers in Catecholamine Research,* Pergamon Press, New York *(in press).*
10. Thierry, A. M., Stinus, L., Blanc, G., and Glowinski, J., *Brain Res.,* 50, 230 (1973).

DISCUSSION

Dr. McDowell: Are there any questions for Dr. Vogt?

Dr. Roberts: Would you say then that most of the cholinergic input to the striatum is from the thalamus and the cortex? And also what is the evidence for the indigenous nature of cholinergic neurons within the striatum and not coming from another system?

Dr. Vogt: I think there are many pathways that mostly come from systems which lie in the reticular formation and extend up into the caudate nucleus. There are also connections which are to and from the cortex and to and from the thalamic nucleus, but not everything goes by the thalamus. I think that Dr. Krnjević could answer this question better than I.

Dr. McDowell: Does anyone have any comments about Dr. Roberts' question to Dr. Vogt?

Dr. Bak: We have been unable to change choline acetylase or cholinesterase in the caudate by making lesions of any of the known major pathways into that nucleus; so that is one evidence for cholinergic interneurons.

Dr. McDowell: Are there any other comments?

Dr. A. Anton: I would like to ask Dr. Bartholini if atropine does anything to his system to prevent the increase in release of acetylcholine.

Dr. G. Bartholini: No, we injected atropine and we were unable to observe a marked effect on acetylcholine release, either with very low or tremendously high doses, for example, 25 milligrams per kilo i.v.

Dr. Anton: Was that the effect on the neuroleptic? Does atropine prevent the effects of the release caused by chlorpromazine?

Dr. Bartholini: It is known that atropine prevents or diminishes the neuroleptic-induced increase in dopamine turnover, but nothing is known of the effect of anticholinergic drugs on the neuroleptic-induced increase in the acetylcholine turnover.

Dr. Anton: The reason I asked is that we have found, at least in the periphery, that if you use tremorine, it will release norepinephrine from the heart. This is a peripheral effect, not a central one. If you administer any of the neuroleptics prior to tremorine, you get a terrific potentiation of its effect. If you administer atropine before doing this, you completely block the effect. This is why I was wondering whether there might be a similar analogous relationship with what you are seeing.

Dr. Goldstein: I would like to ask Dr. Poirier in his study of circling cats whether he measured dopamine in striatum, and whether there is a depletion of striatal dopamine.

Dr. Poirier: If I'm correct, you are asking if we measured the depletion of dopamine in recircling cats. We didn't measure it in cats with tegmental lesions. There was depletion of dopamine at the site of the lesion provided that we're not doing an experiment with DOPA. In cats with other types of lesions we find that the pre-aqueductal lesions of dopamine and ACH are similar. There is no decrease of dopamine, and the nigral cells there are intact.

I'm speaking of any type of lesion. We do not interfere in these lesions with the nigral cell pathway.

Dr. Fuxe: I would like to ask Prof. Poirier about his idea of the mechanism of the contraversive circling which is very impressive in the films. It must interfere with some pathway other than the dopamine pathway.

Dr. Poirier: We have to deal here with two types of circling. I will speak about the cat but I think what I find is also true of the rat. It takes another pharmacologic transfer, however, to reach the same conclusion because of an enzymatic barrier in the rat brain.

In the cat if we make a lesion in the area of the periaqueductal gray which involves the posterior commissure, there's an imbalance between the two sites. Then, if we give DOPA or apomorphine, we get very rapid contraversive circling.

If the nigrostriatal pathway is simultaneously involved with this area, we also observe the same type of circling, although at this moment I cannot exclude the possibility that the interruption in the nigral cell pathway might contribute to the rapidity of the circling. Most of our cats with very rapid circling movements were cats with lesions of the ventral tegmental area. We saw some cats with lesions of periaqueductal gray that had some quite rapid contraversive circling, but not as rapid as in the others.

Ipsiversive circling, as I mentioned, was observed following the same treatment repeated daily in a series of cats. The first lesions we made were also ventral and they extended more laterally and involved the tegmental region which receives corticotegmental fibers or the cerebral peduncle. From that point on we went backward and found that subthalamic lesions were also associated with ipsiversive circling.

Peduncular nucleus destruction with L-DOPA alone will lead to ipsiversive circling. We have two series of mechanisms here, but what I think is striking is that you get circling with an increase of catecholamines in the brain, especially dopamine.

For tremor, you have just the opposite effect; when you decrease the dopamine, tremor appears. Provided that the nigral cell pathway is intact, you can correct this tremor by restoring the normal level of dopamine in the brain. Tremor can be counteracted by anticholinergic treatment. We could not interfere up to now with circling either ipsiversive or contraversive with cholinergic or anticholinergic drugs.

Dr. Bak: My question is to Dr. Poirier. We did a similar experiment with the rat. When we make a lesion in the substantia nigra we get a circling movement, actually contralateral circling, but if we make a lesion in the striatum, we get ipsilateral circling movement. I think this indicates that the drug may act on the side other than the operated side.

Dr. Poirier: In my experience ipsiversive circling was always slow. We called it ipsiversive turning, and it was very slow compared to the contraversive circling, but in this case the motor system was directly involved in these animals.

Dr. Ungerstedt: At what dose was the contraversive turning elicited? Was it the same dose as would excite the normal lesioned animal or was it a much lower dose of DOPA?

Dr. Poirier: At doses from 30 milligrams up to 50 to 100 milligrams per kilo we observe contraversive circling. This would be the maximal effect and would correspond to the greater state of excitation, in general. With a similar dose the rat does not get excited whereas the cat becomes very excited. I think this can be explained by the fact that DOPA readily enters the brain and there is a marked increase of dopamine and ACh in all structures of the brain and not only the striatum in the cat.

Dr. Ungerstedt: What I was trying to get at is if you are stimulating supersensitive receptors or if you are working on intact neurons. If you are working on intact neurons, we have to accept that the cat rotates the opposite way from the rat. Since you can induce turning in the cat with a tegmental lesion or if you lesion the substantia nigra, and if you lesion the rat nigra with 6-hydroxydopamine, the rat rotates in the other direction, my feeling is that there are two systems involved: the nigralstriatal and another which might be a pallidum pathway. You can lesion either of them and induce turning. This sounds very complicated but I think I can explain it by one simple experiment.

If one produces a lesion in the substantia nigra with 6-hydroxydopamine and then gives DOPA, the rat rotates contraversively. If one superimposes a lesion by electrocoagulation in the very same site, the animal rotates ipsiversively, but on a much higher dose of DOPA. I think in order to understand the circling movements one probably has to take into account two systems. One is a dopamine system and one possibly the system leaving the globus pallidus; one would be in the afferent and the other in the efferent pathway.

Advances in Neurology, Vol. 5
Raven Press, New York © 1974

Control of Brain Serotonin by the Diet

R. J. Wurtman and J. D. Fernstrom

Laboratory of Neuroendocrine Regulation, Department of Nutrition and Food Science, Massachusetts Institute of Technology, Cambridge, Massachusetts 02139

The concentrations of tryptophan and of most other amino acids in human and rat plasma exhibit characteristic fluctuations during each 24-hr period (1, 2; Fig. 1). Among human subjects who eat at customary times, tryptophan levels are lowest between 2 and 4 A.M. and rise by 50 to 80% to attain a plateau in the late morning or early afternoon; in rats, the daily nadir and peak occur 8 to 10 hr later, a shift consistent with their nocturnal feeding. The plasma amino acid rhythms are not simply the result of the cyclic ingestion of dietary protein, inasmuch as they persist among human volunteers who eat essentially no protein for 2 weeks (1). They do disappear, however, in subjects placed on a total fast (3), which suggests that they are *not* truly circadian, but of nutritional origin (as from postprandial release of insulin and other hormones which modify tissue uptake of amino acids).

The existence of plasma amino acid rhythms suggested that the quantities of these compounds available to the brain and other tissues for synthesis of proteins and low molecular weight derivatives might also change diurnally, perhaps in response to food consumption. Such changes could influence the rates of various biosynthetic reactions. To explore the possible significance of plasma amino acid rhythms, we attempted to determine whether experimentally induced fluctuations of the same amplitude as those occurring diurnally could cause parallel changes in the rate at which a particular amino acid was incorporated into proteins or converted to a particular low molecular weight compound. The amino acid whose plasma concentration seemed most likely to influence its metabolic fate was tryptophan, the least abundant amino acid in most tissues and foods (4). Moreover, daily rhythms in the ingestion of tryptophan-containing proteins (and, presumably, in the concentration of tryptophan delivered to the liver via the portal venous circulation) generated parallel rhythms in the aggregation of hepatic polysomes (5) and in the quantity of the enzyme tyrosine transaminase in the liver (2).

As the dependent variable in our studies, we looked for changes in brain serotonin content among rats with spontaneous daily rhythms or treatment-induced fluctuations in plasma tryptophan. Three lines of evidence had suggested that the amount of tryptophan available to the brain might control serotonin synthesis: (a) a daily rhythm in brain serotonin content of rats and

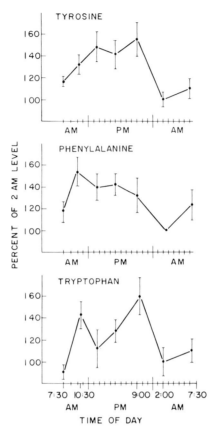

FIG. 1. Changes in plasma concentrations of tyrosine, phenylalanine, and tryptophan with time of day. Blood was taken at 7:30 and 10:30 A.M., at 1:30, 5:00, and 9:00 P.M., and at 2:00 and 7:30 A.M. Data are presented as mean ± standard error. The 2:00 A.M. mean concentrations of tyrosine, phenylalanine, and tryptophan were 12.20 ± 0.94, 8.14 ± 0.85, and 9.13 ± 1.22 μg/ml respectively.

mice (6); (b) the unusually high K_m for tryptophan shown by tryptophan hydroxylase, the catalyst of the initial step in serotonin biosynthesis* (7); and (c) the great increase of brain concentrations of serotonin and its chief metabolite, 5-hydroxyindole acetic acid (5-HIAA), caused by high doses of tryptophan (50 to 1,600 mg/kg) (4).

Initial experiments determined whether brain serotonin content could be increased by giving rats very low doses of tryptophan at a time of day when plasma and brain tryptophan and brain serotonin concentrations were known to be near their nadirs (Fig. 2). Administration of 12.5 mg/kg, i.p., of trypto-

---

* Subsequent studies using the natural pteridine cofactor indicate that this K_m might not be as high as had been believed. Still, the enzyme is almost certainly unsaturated *in vivo*.

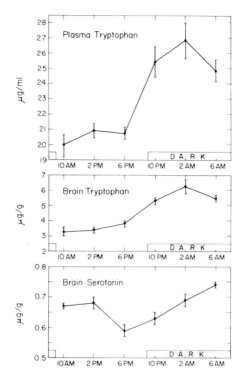

FIG. 2. Daily rhythms in plasma tryptophan, brain tryptophan, and brain 5-hydroxytrypta-mine. Groups of 10 rats kept in darkness from 9 P.M. to 9 A.M. were killed at intervals of 4 hr. Vertical bars indicate SEM.

phan to male rats weighing 150 to 200 g (less than 5% of the tryptophan that rats would ingest daily in 10 to 20 g of standard rat chow) produced peak elevations in plasma and brain tryptophan which were well within the ranges that occur nocturnally in untreated animals, and caused brain sero-tonin levels to rise by 20 to 30% ($p < 0.01$) within 1 hr of treatment (8). Doses of 25 mg/kg caused proportionately greater increases in both brain tryptophan and brain serotonin. Larger doses of tryptophan, which caused brain tryptophan concentration to rise well beyond its physiological range, produced no further increments in brain serotonin.

The increase in brain serotonin produced by the very small doses of tryp-tophan seemed to support the hypothesis that the nocturnal rise in untreated rats was related to daily rhythms in plasma and brain tryptophan (see Fig. 2). However, this substrate-induced rhythm in serotonin synthesis is not neces-sarily the *only* factor causing daily rhythms in brain serotonin; brain sero-tonin levels might also reflect rhythms in serotonin release or intraneuronal metabolism.

After small *increases* in plasma tryptophan had been shown to cause parallel changes in brain serotonin, we next set out to determine if physiological *decreases* in the plasma amino acid could depress the serotonin content.

Rats similar to those used in the previous experiments received a dose of insulin (2 IU/kg, i.p.) which is known to lower plasma concentrations of glucose and most amino acids. To our surprise, the hormone did not lower plasma tryptophan, but increased its concentration by 30 to 40% (9). This effect was independent of the route by which the insulin was administered; it was associated with a 55% fall in plasma glucose, and with major reductions in the plasma concentrations of most other amino acids, including the neutral amino acids generally believed to compete with tryptophan for uptake into the brain (10, 11). Two hr after rats received the insulin, brain tryptophan levels were elevated by 36% ($p < 0.01$), and brain serotonin by 28% ($p < 0.01$) (12).

The increase in brain serotonin observed in rats receiving insulin might have been artifactual, resulting not from increased availability of substrate, but from central reflexes activated by hypoglycemia. To determine whether physiological secretion of insulin, in *normo*glycemic rats, also increased plasma and brain tryptophan and brain serotonin, these indoles were measured in rats fasted for 15 hr and then given access to a carbohydrate diet. In a typical experiment, the animals ate an average of 5 g/hr during the first hour, and 2 g/hr during the second and third hours (9, 12). Plasma tryptophan levels were significantly elevated 1, 2, and 3 hr after food presentation; plasma tyrosine concentrations were depressed at all times studied. Brain tryptophan and serotonin were significantly elevated at 2 and 3 hr (9, 12).

Since carbohydrate consumption, by eliciting insulin secretion, raised plasma tryptophan levels and, ultimately, the concentrations of tryptophan and serotonin in the brain, we anticipated that the consumption of both carbohydrates and protein would cause an even greater rise in brain serotonin. In addition to elevating plasma tryptophan by causing insulin secretion, the tryptophan in the dietary proteins would contribute directly to plasma tryptophan; brain tryptophan and serotonin would presumably increase accordingly. However, when we gave fasted rats access to diets containing either natural proteins or synthetic mixes of amino acids, we found that the expected major increase (about 60%, $p < 0.001$) in plasma tryptophan was not accompanied by increases in brain tryptophan or serotonin (Fig. 3) (13).

It seemed possible that brain tryptophan failed to increase after protein ingestion because the plasma concentrations of other, competing amino acids increased even more than that of tryptophan. To test this hypothesis, we allowed groups of animals to eat either a synthetic diet containing carbohydrates plus all of the amino acids in the same proportions as are present in an 18% casein diet, or this diet minus five of the amino acids thought to share a common transport system with tryptophan (tyrosine, phenylalanine, leucine, isoleucine, and valine). Both diets significantly increased plasma

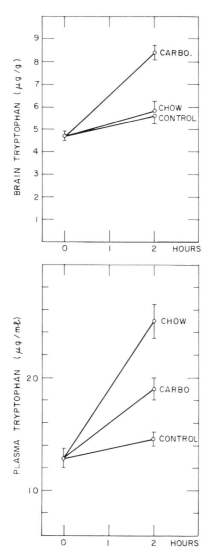

FIG. 3. Changes in brain and plasma tryptophan concentrations following the consumption of different foods. Groups of six rats were killed 1 or 2 hr after diet presentation. Vertical bars represent SEM. Two-hr plasma tryptophan levels were significantly greater in rats consuming either diet than in fasting controls (chow: $p < 0.001$; carbohydrate: $p < 0.01$). Two-hr brain tryptophan levels were significantly elevated above controls only in rats consuming the carbohydrate-plus-fat diet ($p < 0.001$) (Fernstrom, J. D., Larin, F., and Wurtman, R. J., *Life Sci.*, 13, 517, 1973).

tryptophan levels above those found in fasted controls. However, large increases in brain tryptophan, serotonin, or 5-HIAA occurred only by deleting the competing neutral amino acids from the diet (13).

When this experiment was repeated omitting aspartate and glutamate, two acidic amino acids, from the diet instead of the five neutral amino acids, plasma tryptophan concentrations again increased 70 to 80% above those of fasted controls ($p < 0.001$); however, brain tryptophan, serotonin, and 5-HIAA remained unaffected.

We postulated that brain tryptophan and 5-hydroxyindole levels did not simply reflect plasma tryptophan, but depended also upon the plasma concentrations of other neutral amino acids. This relationship was confirmed by a correlation analysis comparing brain tryptophan and the ratio of plasma tryptophan to the five competing amino acids among individual rats given diets containing various amounts of each amino acid. This analysis yielded a correlation coefficient of 0.95 ($p < 0.001$ that $r = 0$), whereas the correlation between brain tryptophan and plasma tryptophan alone was less striking ($r = 0.66$; $p < 0.001$ that $r = 0$). Similarly, the correlation coefficient for brain 5-hydroxyindoles (serotonin plus 5-HIAA) versus the plasma amino acid ratio was 0.89 ($p < 0.001$), whereas that of 5-hydroxyindoles versus tryptophan alone was only 0.58 ($p < 0.001$). The reason that brain tryptophan and serotonin appeared, in our earlier formulation, to depend upon plasma tryptophan alone was that all of the physiological manipulations tested at that time (tryptophan injections, insulin injections, carbohydrate consumption) raised the *numerator* in the plasma tryptophan: competitor ratio while either lowering the denominator or leaving it unaltered. Only when rats consumed protein were both the numerator and the denominator elevated. The effect of food consumption on 5-hydroxyindoles in rat brain may now be represented as in Fig. 4.

Tryptophan in plasma is distributed between two pools: about 10 to 20% circulates as the free amino acid, while the remainder is bound to serum albumin (14). None of the other amino acids binds appreciably to plasma proteins. Because binding in general implies storage, several investigators have suggested that the plasma free tryptophan pool determines the availability of circulating tryptophan to brain and other tissues (15).

A variety of lipid-soluble compounds which bind to albumin in the blood (e.g., hormones, drugs, fatty acids) may displace each other. Thus, for example, increasing the concentration of free fatty acids in serum *in vitro* causes free tryptophan to rise, and albumin-bound tryptophan to fall (16). In collaboration with Drs. Bertha Madras and Hamish Munro, we tested this relationship *in vivo*, by feeding rats diets that were expected to alter their serum-free fatty acid levels and then measuring the changes in free and bound tryptophan. Subsequently, we studied the response of brain tryptophan to diet-induced changes in serum-free and -bound tryptophan, to deter-

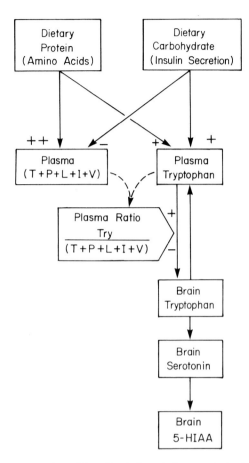

FIG. 4. Proposed sequence describing diet-induced changes in brain serotonin concentration in the rat (see text). The ratio of tryptophan to the combined levels of tyrosine, phenylalanine, leucine, isoleucine, and valine in the plasma is thought to control the tryptophan level in the brain.

mine whether the *physiological* control of brain tryptophan depends on the *total* or the *free* tryptophan concentration in the blood.

Rats were killed 1 or 2 hr after receiving a glucose load (2 g in 4 ml of water) *per os*. This caused a major elevation in *total* serum tryptophan, even though the rise was restricted to the albumin-bound fraction; as anticipated, serum-free tryptophan and serum NEFA *decreased* markedly (Table 1). Brain tryptophan concentrations *rose* significantly in these animals (17).

In other rats total tryptophan in plasma and brain were increased by insulin injection (9). This treatment altered the proportions of serum tryptophan that were free or bound to albumin in a manner similar to glucose ad-

TABLE 1. *Effect of glucose ingestion on serum and brain tryptophan*

	Control	Glucose (1 hr)	Glucose (2 hr)
Serum total tryptophan (μg/ml)	16.2 ± 0.2	19.6 ± 0.6[a]	19.9 ± 0.4[b]
Serum-free tryptophan (μg/ml)	5.5 ± 0.1	4.8 ± 0.3[c]	4.2 ± 0.2[b]
Free (% of total)	34	25	21
Serum-bound tryptophan (μg/ml)	10.7 ± 0.3	14.8 ± 0.6[a]	15.7 ± 0.5[b]
Nonesterified fatty acid (meq/liter)	1.147 ± 0.034	0.648 ± 0.077[b]	0.604 ± 0.044[b]
Brain tryptophan (μg/g)	4.16 ± 0.42	6.42 ± 0.56[a]	5.93 ± 0.72[a]

D-Glucose (2 g/4 ml tap water) was administered to three groups of 35 rats (108 to 146 g) via stomach tube. Controls received tap water via stomach tube. Serum was pooled from seven samples; all values are given as mean $\pm$ SEM. (Table taken from ref. 17.)

[a] $p < 0.01$, differs from controls.
[b] $p < 0.001$, differs from controls.
[c] $p < 0.05$, differs from controls.

ministration: *total* serum tryptophan increased, *albumin-bound* tryptophan increased, but serum-*free* tryptophan decreased.

In another experiment groups of rats were fasted overnight, and the next day, fed carbohydrates only or carbohydrates and fats. Both diets raised serum total tryptophan, albumin-bound tryptophan, and brain tryptophan (Table 2); both depressed serum-free tryptophan. Serum NEFA levels declined in both groups, but much less in the group consuming fat. Serum-free tryptophan also fell less in this group. In both dietary groups significant reductions also occurred in the blood concentration of tyrosine, one of the five competing neutral amino acids (13, 17).

The high degree of correlation between serum NEFA levels and serum-free tryptophan suggests that carbohydrates (and insulin) increase the albumin-binding of serum tryptophan by decreasing the extent to which albumin is saturated with free fatty acids and thus enhancing its affinity for tryptophan. No correlation was observed in any of these experiments between physiological changes in serum *free* tryptophan and brain tryptophan concentrations.

We have observed similar changes in serum tryptophan and free fatty acid concentrations in humans following a glucose load (18). Although *total* serum tryptophan does not increase following carbohydrate consumption, as it does in rats, neither does it decrease. However, serum-free tryptophan concentrations do decline, about 5% within 90 min, coincident with decreases in serum-free fatty acid levels. The ratio of total blood tryptophan to other neutral amino acids increases markedly in humans after carbohydrate consumption, as it does in rats. There is at present no information available

TABLE 2. *Effects of carbohydrate or carbohydrate-fat diets on serum and brain tryptophan*

		Diets	
	Fasted controls	Carbohydrate + fat	Carbohydrate
Serum total tryptophan (μg/ml)	16.5 ± 0.3	18.4 ± 0.5^a	19.1 ± 0.4^b
Serum free tryptophan (μg/ml)	6.2 ± 0.1	5.7 ± 0.2^c	3.4 ± 0.2^b
Free (% of total)	37	33	18
Serum bound tryptophan (μg/ml)	10.3 ± 0.4	12.7 ± 0.7^c	15.7 ± 0.5^b
Serum tyrosine (μg/ml)	19.5 ± 0.7	11.7 ± 0.4	14.4 ± 0.5
Nonesterified fatty acid (meq/liter)	0.831 ± 0.021	0.615 ± 0.029^b	0.301 ± 0.024^b
Brain tryptophan (μg/g)	2.24 ± 0.11	3.07 ± 0.18^b	3.45 ± 0.19^b

Groups of 22 rats weighing 170 to 200 g were deprived of food but not water at 2 P.M. and presented with one of the experimental diets at 10:30 A.M. the next day. Two hr later, the animals were decapitated and serum and brains taken for assay. Controls had free access to water and were killed throughout the experiment. Each serum value is obtained from two pooled samples. Each diet contained: dextrose, 270 g; sucrose, 221 g; dextrin, 270 g; Harper's salt mix, 40 g; vitamin mix, 10 g; and choline, 2 g; to which was added 35 g of agar in a liter of water. The fat diet had an additional 150 g of Mazola oil. All values are given as mean $\pm$ SEM. (Table taken from ref. 17.)

[a] $p < 0.01$, differs from controls.
[b] $p < 0.001$, differs from controls.
[c] $p < 0.05$, differs from controls.

concerning the effects of dietary carbohydrate on brain tryptophan or serotonin in humans.

SUMMARY

The concentrations of serotonin in rat brain, and of tryptophan in plasma and brain, normally exhibit daily rhythms largely generated by the diet. The tryptophan rhythms are in phase; the daily increase in brain tryptophan content precedes that of serotonin by several hours. The injection of a small dose of tryptophan (e.g., 12.5 mg/kg), which increases plasma and brain tryptophan significantly but not beyond their normal daily ranges, causes brain serotonin to rise within an hour. Insulin injection, or the elective consumption of a carbohydrate or carbohydrate-fat meal, *increases* plasma tryptophan levels in rats. Brain tryptophan and serotonin concentrations also rise. The plasma concentrations of most other amino acids (and of the portion of serum tryptophan not bound to albumin) fall. The consumption of a protein-containing diet induces even *larger* elevations in plasma tryptophan, but causes no changes in brain tryptophan or serotonin. Brain tryptophan and serotonin do rise if animals consume a synthetic amino acid mix lacking the neutral amino acids that compete with tryptophan for entry into the brain (tyrosine, phenylalanine, leucine, isoleucine, and valine). Insulin injection, or the consumption of carbohydrates, depresses serum-free (non-albumin-bound) tryptophan and nonesterified fatty acid (NEFA) concentrations in rats, while increasing serum albumin-bound tryptophan and brain tryptophan. In humans, glucose ingestion causes a decline in serum-free tryptophan and NEFA, but no change in serum-bound tryptophan. (The serum concentrations of other competing neutral amino acids fall markedly.) The serotonin concentration in rat brain is thus physiologically regulated by the diet, via changes in brain tryptophan. Brain tryptophan appears to reflect neither the total serum tryptophan concentration nor the smaller free pool, but rather the *ratio* of total plasma tryptophan to the sum of the competing neutral amino acids. Serotonin-containing neurons thus differ markedly from catecholaminergic neurons, in which end-product inhibition, rather than precursor availability, seems to control the rate of neurotransmitter synthesis. If, after the consumption of diets that increase brain serotonin, more of the neurotransmitter is released into synapses, then serotoninergic neurons may serve as amplifiers or sensors, providing the brain with information about peripheral metabolic state. The potency of L-DOPA and other drugs which affect the release or actions of brain serotonin may exhibit variations depending upon when and what the subject most recently ate.

ACKNOWLEDGMENT

These studies were supported in part by grants from the John A. Hartford Foundation, the National Aeronautics and Space Administration, and the United States Public Health Service (NS-10459 and AM-14228).

REFERENCES

1. Wurtman, R. J., Rose, C. M., Chou, C., and Larin, F., *New Eng. J. Med.,* 279, 171 (1968).
2. Wurtman, R. J., in: *Mammalian Protein Metabolism,* Vol. 4, edited by H. N. Munro, p. 445, Academic Press, New York (1970).
3. Marliss, E. B., Aoki, T. T., Unger, R. H., Soeldner, J. S., and Cahill, G. F., *J. Clin. Invest.,* 49, 2256 (1970).
4. Wurtman, R. J., and Fernstrom, J. D., in: *Perspectives in Neuropharmacology,* edited by S. H. Snyder, p. 145, Oxford University Press, New York (1972).
5. Fishman, B., Wurtman, R. J., and Munro, H. N., *Proc. Nat. Acad. Sci.,* 64, 677 (1969).
6. Albrecht, P., Visscher, M. B., Bittner, J. J., and Halberg, F., *Proc. Soc. Exp. Biol. Med.,* 92, 702 (1956).
7. Lovenberg, W., Jequier, E., and Sjoerdsma, A., *Advan. Pharmacol.,* 6A, 21 (1968).
8. Fernstrom, J. D., and Wurtman, R. J., *Science,* 173, 149 (1971).
9. Fernstrom, J. D., and Wurtman, R. J., *Metabolism,* 21, 337 (1972).
10. Guroff, G., and Udenfriend, S., *J. Biol. Chem.,* 237, 803 (1962).
11. Blasberg, R., and Lajtha, A., *Arch. Biochem. Biophys.,* 112, 361 (1965).
12. Fernstrom, J. D., and Wurtman, R. J., *Science,* 174, 1023 (1971).

13. Fernstrom, J. D., and Wurtman, R. J., *Science,* 178, 414 (1972).
14. McMenamy, R. H., Lund, C. C., and Oncley, J. L., *J. Clin. Invest.,* 36, 1672 (1957).
15. Knott, P. J., and Curzon, G., *Nature,* 239, 452 (1972).
16. McMenamy, R. H., and Oncley, J. L., *J. Biol. Chem.,* 233, 1436 (1958).
17. Madras, B. K., Cohen, E. L., Fernstrom, J. D., Larin, F., Munro, H. N., and Wurtman, R. J., *Nature,* 244, 34 (1973).
18. Lipsett, D., Madras, B. K., Wurtman, R. J., and Munro, H. N., *Life Sci.,* 12 (Part 2), 57 (1973).

Advances in Neurology, Vol. 5
Raven Press, New York © 1974

Serotonergic Mechanisms and Extrapyramidal Function in Man

Thomas N. Chase

Neurology Unit, National Institute of Mental Health, Bethesda, Maryland 20014

A considerable body of anatomic, pharmacologic, and neurophysiologic evidence links central serotonergic mechanisms to the regulation of such diverse functions as sleep and body temperature, as well as to the pathophysiology of human ills ranging from schizophrenia to parkinsonism. In the absence of any unifying concept sufficient to encompass all the diverse functions suggested for brain serotonin (5-HT), it nevertheless remains uncertain what role, if any, this indolealkylamine plays in the mammalian central nervous system (CNS). Increased attention to this issue arises as a consequence of recent data indicating that pharmacologic agents affecting serotonergic mechanisms are less specific than originally thought, as well as from the continuing realization that available techniques afford correlational rather than direct evidence in support of a causal relationship between 5-HT and physiologic mechanisms outside the serotonergic neuron.

An association between the activity of 5-HT-containing neuronal systems and extrapyramidal function is suggested by both preclinical and clinical observations. Unilaterally placed mesencephalic lesions in various animal species produce signs of extrapyramidal dysfunction in the contralateral extremities and reduced 5-HT levels in the ipsilateral striatum (1–3). In the primate, a relation between 5-HT-mediated function and resting tremor appears especially convincing. Tremor produced in monkeys by lesions in the ventromedial tegmentum is relieved by 5-hydroxytryptophan, the immediate precursor of 5-HT (2). 5-Hydroxytryptophan also abolishes tremor produced in lesioned monkeys by harmaline, a compound which may compete with 5-HT for available receptors (4). Conversely, *para*-chlorophenylalanine, a potent inhibitor of 5-HT synthesis, can briefly induce a fine resting tremor in the extremities of monkeys with tegmental lesions which cause hypokinesia but no tremor (4).

CLINICAL BIOCHEMICAL STUDIES

Biochemical evidence in man suggesting that serotonergic mechanisms affect extrapyramidal function derived initially from direct measurements of 5-HT levels in brain tissues at autopsy (5, 6) and later from monoamine metabolite determinations in samples of cerebrospinal fluid (CSF) obtained from the living patient. CSF levels of 5-hydroxyindoleacetic acid (5-HIAA), the principal metabolite of 5-HT, have been widely used to estimate the metabolic state of the parent amine in the CNS. Most 5-HIAA in CSF arises from central rather than peripheral metabolism, and 5-HIAA levels in ventricular or cisternal fluid tend to parallel those in the cerebral parenchyma (7). Although 5-HT-containing neuronal terminals occur in the mammalian spinal cord, recent studies in cats perfused through the spinal subarachnoid space with radioactively labeled 5-HIAA suggest that the brain contributes substantially to the lumbar CSF content of this 5-HT metabolite (8). These results are consistent with the findings of some clinical studies that 5-HIAA levels are diminished in the lumbar CSF of patients with cervical lesions which restrict the flow of CSF from above (9, 10). Moreover, it has been reported that lumbar CSF levels of 5-HIAA are not significantly reduced in patients with spinal cord transection but with no evidence of spinal fluid blockade (10). If concentrations of 5-HT and 5-HIAA in the spinal cord of man are reduced after transection, as they are in the experimental animal, then the normal 5-HIAA values in the CSF of such patients would suggest a contribution from rostral sources.

Reduced lumbar CSF levels of 5-HIAA have been reported in several, although not all, studies of parkinsonian patients (11–13). In 30 individuals with either idiopathic or postencephalitic parkinsonism, we have observed only a slight tendency for lowered 5-HIAA values (Table 1). Moreover, no relationship could be demonstrated between the degree of reduction in 5-HIAA levels and overall pretreatment parkinsonian severity ($r = 0.130$; $p > 0.05$). Although a somewhat greater diminution in 5-HIAA was found in Guamanian patients with parkinsonism-dementia, similar alterations have not been observed in any of the other extrapyramidal disorders studied (Table 1).

TABLE 1. *Levels of 5-HIAA in lumbar CSF*

Disease	Number of patients	5-HIAA level (ng/ml)*
Control	25	28 ± 1.6
Parkinsonism	30	23 ± 1.6**
Parkinsonism-dementia	16	20 ± 2.3†
Huntington's chorea	14	28 ± 3.3
Torsion dystonia	15	34 ± 2.1**
Spinocerebellar degenerations	10	29 ± 2.8
Jakob-Creutzfeldt disease	6	34 ± 6.9
Progressive supranuclear palsy	3	33 ± 8.5

* Values are the means $\pm$ SEM.
** $p < 0.05$.
† $p < 0.01$.

More recent efforts to correlate extrapyramidal function with 5-HT metabolism in man have attempted to estimate the central turnover of the amine by means of probenecid loading. Since the acute administration of probenecid inhibits 5-HIAA transport from the CSF compartment without significantly altering brain 5-HT metabolism, the probenecid-induced rise in 5-HIAA should provide an index to the rate of metabolite formation and thus to the central turnover of the parent amine (14, 15). Substantial reductions in the accumulation of 5-HIAA in lumbar CSF during probenecid treatment have been found in patients with Parkinson's disease (16) or parkinsonism-dementia but not in patients with the other extrapyramidal disorders studied (Table 2). In contrast to an earlier report (17), we ob-

TABLE 2. *Effect of probenecid on 5-HIAA levels in lumbar spinal fluid*

Disease	Number of patients	5-HIAA level (ng/ml)		
		Baseline	Treatment	Difference
Control	8	28 ± 3.1	112 ± 9.2	84 ± 8.2
Parkinsonism	20	21 ± 1.9	65 ± 6.5	43 ± 5.4*
Parkinsonism-dementia	3	12 ± 2.7	35 ± 4.0	23 ± 2.3*
Huntington's chorea	12	25 ± 2.8	111 ± 9.2	86 ± 9.3
Torsion dystonia	8	26 ± 2.2	112 ± 16	86 ± 15
Down's syndrome	6	36 ± 3.0	124 ± 13	88 ± 12

* $p < 0.001$.

served a significant inverse correlation in parkinsonian patients between the probenecid-induced rise in 5-HIAA and pretreatment severity of akinesia and rigidity (Fig. 1). No such relationship was found, however, between the accumulation of 5-HIAA during probenecid loading and the severity of parkinsonian tremor. The foregoing observations must be interpreted with caution until the validity of results from the probenecid technique receive more rigorous experimental confirmation. Nevertheless, the finding of a close association between the degree of 5-HIAA abnormality and the severity of certain parkinsonian signs supports the contention that the central metabolism of 5-HT, and thus possibly the function of 5-HT-containing neuronal systems, may relate to the pathophysiology of Parkinson's disease.

CLINICAL PHARMACOLOGIC STUDIES

Observations of the clinical effects of drugs believed to act by various means on serotonergic mechanisms provide another approach to the study of the relation of this monoamine to extrapyramidal function. It is well

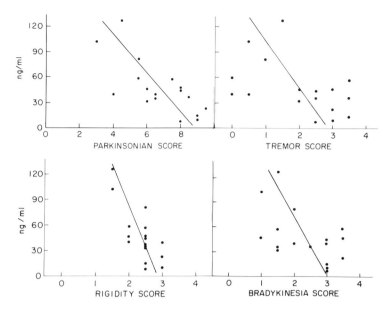

FIG. 1. Pretreatment parkinsonism severity and probenecid-induced accumulation of 5-HIAA in lumbar CSF. Tremor, rigidity, and hypokinesia were each rated on a scale of 0 (absent) to 4 (very severe) and combined to yield an overall parkinsonian score. Statistically significant correlations were found between 5-HIAA values with probenecid and overall parkinsonian severity ($p < 0.001$), rigidity ($p < 0.001$) and bradykinesia ($p < 0.05$), but not tremor ($p > 0.05$). Details of drug administration and CSF assay are as previously described (17).

known, for example, that drugs such as reserpine or tetrabenazine can induce parkinsonism but ameliorate certain hyperkinetic disorders such as Huntington's chorea. Since these agents interfere with dopamine as well as with 5-HT storage in nerve terminals, it is hardly possible to attribute their clinical effects to 5-HT depletion alone. Similar difficulties complicate the pharmacologic interpretation of reports that certain tricyclic antidepressants, such as imipramine, tend to ameliorate parkinsonian rigidity and tremor (18). Although these drugs block 5-HT uptake into neuronal tissues (19) and thus might be expected to potentiate the effects of the amine released into the synaptic cleft, they also appear to possess some central anticholinergic activity (20).

The foregoing pharmacologic observations, as well as biochemical studies on central 5-HT metabolism, nevertheless suggest that efforts to replete brain 5-HT might improve parkinsonian symptoms. In an attempt to study this possibility, seven parkinsonian patients were given L-5-hydroxytryptophan together with a peripheral inhibitor of aromatic L-amino acid decarboxylase (21). Dose levels of the 5-HT precursor were slowly increased until a definite effect on extrapyramidal function was observed.

Unexpectedly, a significant increase in akinesia and rigidity occurred in all cases (Table 3). Tremor ratings, however, showed no consistent alteration. The apparent resistance of tremor to modification by 5-hydroxytryptophan parallels the relatively poorer response of this cardinal parkinsonian sign to L-DOPA. These observations, as well as those from probenecid loading studies, are consistent with results deriving from certain animal models of Parkinson's disease (3, 4) in suggesting that neurohumoral mechanisms relating to tremor differ from those subserving rigidity and akinesia.

Although the administration of 5-hydroxytryptophan increases brain 5-HT, it is by no means certain that the central pharmacologic effects of this amino acid can be attributed to an enhancement of 5-HT-mediated function. It is known, for example, that exogenous 5-hydroxytryptophan is taken up nonspecifically in the CNS and metabolized abnormally (22). A more definitive experiment might thus be to administer L-tryptophan, the natural precursor of brain 5-HT. Although we have found, as have others (23, 24), that L-tryptophan at daily doses of up to 10 g does not modify parkinsonian signs, treatment with L-tryptophan in combination with pyridoxine reportedly exacerbates parkinsonism (24). The clinical effects of tryptophan, as well as 5-hydroxytryptophan, however, may reflect a reduction in dopamine-mediated function, since both 5-HT precursors compete with catecholamine precursors for uptake into the CNS and metabolism to the amine (25–27). On the other hand, although brain 5-HT levels are diminished in parkinsonian patients, the cerebral content of dopamine is reduced to an even greater extent (5, 6). Conceivably, an enhancement of serotonergic function relative to the activity of dopamine-mediated systems favors increased parkinsonian rigidity and akinesia.

The foregoing possibility prompted attempts to deplete selectively brain 5-HT in parkinsonian patients (Table 3). The administration of *para*-chlorophenylalanine, a relatively specific inhibitor of 5-HT synthesis, however, produced no consistent alteration in the severity of parkinsonian signs, despite a 50% reduction in CSF levels of 5-HIAA (28, 29). Although this result suggests that 5-HT-containing neuronal systems do not serve as a critical determinant of extrapyramidal function, it may only reflect the fact that the amount of 5-HT depletion attained was not sufficient to have functional significance. On the other hand, it might be argued that if the reduction in brain 5-HT which attends Parkinson's disease is responsible for any of the disease's major clinical manifestations, then further reductions in 5-HT should be expected to modify these signs.

Several lines of evidence suggest that serotonergic neurons may play a role in mediating the therapeutic or toxic effects of L-DOPA. In animals, the high-dose administration of L-DOPA significantly reduces brain 5-HT, in part due to competition between the precursors of dopamine and 5-HT for uptake and metabolism in the CNS (25, 30). Studies in rat striatal slices further indicate that some exogenous DOPA may enter central 5-HT neu-

TABLE 3. *Effect of drugs on cardinal parkinsonian signs and 5-HIAA in lumbar spinal fluid*

| | Number of patients | Average maximum dose (g/day) | Percent clinical improvement[*] | | | Percent change in 5-HIAA[*] |
			Tremor	Rigidity	Akinesia	
L-5-Hydroxytryptophan	7	0.8[**]	2.2 ± 7	-32 ± 10[†]	-42 ± 6[†]	1098 ± 295[†]
p-Chlorophenylalanine	6	4.0	7 ± 11	-0.8 ± 10	5.2 ± 3	-49 ± 8[†]

[*]Values are the means $\pm$ SEM.
[**]Given with α-methyldopahydrazine.
[†]$p < 0.02$.

rons and be decarboxylated to the amine (31). Dopamine thus formed can displace endogenously synthesized 5-HT from neuronal storage sites and be available for release from 5-HT neurons during nerve terminal depolarization (31). In an attempt to ascertain whether the acute administration of L-DOPA to man can liberate endogenous 5-HT, monoamine metabolite levels in lumbar CSF were measured in patients following a brief intravenous infusion of the amino acid (Fig. 2). Homovanillic acid values increased nearly fivefold at 8 hr after the infusion. There was also a significant rise in lumbar CSF levels of 5-HIAA at 8 and 12 hr after the infusion. Since the increase in homovanillic acid concentrations was probably insufficient to interfere with 5-HIAA transport from the CSF compartment (32), our results suggest that acute L-DOPA treatment either accelerated 5-HT turnover or released the amine from endogenous stores. The former possibility would seem unlikely in view of reports of diminished probenecid-induced accumulations of 5-HIAA in the CSF of patients receiving long-term treatment with L-DOPA (33, 34). The foregoing observations thus support the contention that therapeutic dose levels of L-DOPA significantly influence central 5-HT metabolism, and thus possibly 5-HT mediated function, in man.

The coadministration of drugs which inhibit monoamine uptake into serotonergic neurons might afford insight into the contribution of these neurons to the clinical effects of L-DOPA in parkinsonian patients. Imipramine potentiates the ability of L-DOPA to increase spontaneous motor activity in rats, but does not influence L-DOPA-induced stereotyped behavior (35, 36). Moreover, pretreatment with imipramine reportedly prevents the reduction in brain 5-HT produced by L-DOPA, without altering the rise in dopamine levels (35). These results may be attributable to imipramine's

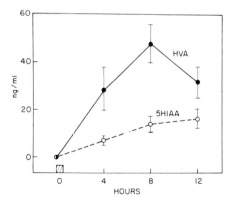

FIG. 2. Effect of L-DOPA on HVA and 5-HIAA levels in lumbar CSF. L-DOPA (1 mg/kg) was infused intravenously over a 30-min period to seven patients given L-α-methyldopahydrazine (MK 486, 150 mg p.o.) 90 min previously. Results are given as the change in mean metabolite levels ± SEM.

relatively greater ability to block monoamine transport into serotonergic than into dopaminergic neurons (19, 37), and suggest that the tricyclic antidepressant might diminish those effects of L-DOPA mediated by serotonergic neurons. We have found, however, that the addition of imipramine at daily doses of up to 300 mg for as long as 51 days to the therapeutic regimen of parkinsonian patients produces little, if any, change in the antiparkinsonian efficacy of L-DOPA. Moreover, no definite change was observed in the frequency or severity of adverse effects of L-DOPA, including dyskinesias or the on–off response. Our results thus fail to support a crucial role for the 5-HT neuron in mediating either the therapeutic or toxic effects of L-DOPA.

CONCLUSIONS

Inferences based on the results of current techniques for studying monoamines in the CNS of man must remain highly tentative in view of their uncertain validity. Nevertheless, the bulk of available information suggests an association between central 5-HT metabolism and the severity of parkinsonian akinesia and rigidity. Conceivably, the observed changes in 5-HT metabolism in parkinsonian patients reflect functional rather than structural changes in serotonergic neurons. If, for example, dopamine- and 5-HT-containing neuronal systems ordinarily operate in a balanced arrangement, it is possible that diminished dopamine-mediated function, due to degeneration of the nigrostriatal dopaminergic system, may evoke a secondary reduction in the activity of serotonergic neurons. This view is compatible with the apparent lack of consistent morphological changes in brainstem areas believed to be rich in 5-HT-containing nerve cell bodies, as well as with the ability of monoamine oxidase inhibitors to restore brain 5-HT but not dopamine to normal levels in parkinsonian patients (5). Results of studies with *para*-chlorophenylalanine or with imipramine in L-DOPA-treated parkinsonian patients cast doubt, however, on the hypothesis that the function of serotonergic systems plays a critical role either in determining the clinical severity of parkinsonian signs or in mediating the effects of L-DOPA on extrapyramidal function.

ACKNOWLEDGMENTS

Lorenz K. Y. Ng conducted the L-DOPA infusion study.

REFERENCES

1. Poirier, L. J., Sourkes, T. L., Bouvier, G., Boucher, R., and Carabin, S., *Brain* 89, 37 (1966).
2. Goldstein, M., Battista, A. F., Nakatani, S., and Anagnoste, B., *Nature* 224, 382 (1969).

3. Gumulka, W., del Angel, A. R., Samanin, R., and Valzelli, L., *Eur. J. Pharmacol.* 10, 79 (1970).
4. Battista, A. F., Goldstein, M., Nakatani, S., and Anagnoste, B., *Confin. Neurol.* 31, 135 (1969).
5. Hornykiewicz, O., in: *Biochemistry and Pharmacology of the Basal Ganglia,* edited by E. Costa, L. J. Côté, and M. D. Yahr, New York, Raven Press, 1966, p. 171.
6. Fahn, S., Libsch, L. R., and Cutler, R. W., *J. Neurol. Sci.* 14, 427 (1971).
7. Moir, A. T. B., Ashcroft, G. W., Crawford, T. B. B., Eccleston, D., and Guldberg, H. C., *Brain* 93, 357 (1970).
8. Weir, R. L., Chase, T. N., Ng, L. K. Y., and Kopin, I. J., *Brain Res.,* 52, 409 (1973).
9. Curzon, G., Gumpert, E. J. W., and Sharpe, D. M., *Nature (New Biol.)* 231, 189 (1971).
10. Post, R. M., Goodwin, F. K., Gordon, E., and Watkin, D. M., *Science* 179, 897 (1973).
11. Johansson, B., and Roos, B.-E., *Life Sci.* 6, 1449 (1967).
12. Pullar, I. A., Weddell, J. M., Ahmed, R., and Gillingham, F. J., *J. Neurol. Neurosurg. Psychiat.* 33, 851 (1970).
13. Papeschi, R., Molina-Negro, P., Sourkes, T., Hardy, J., and Bertrand, C., *Neurology* 20, 991 (1970).
14. Barkai, A., Glusman, M., and Rapport, M. M., *J. Pharmacol. Exp. Ther.* 181, 28 (1972).
15. Korf, J., Van Pragg, H. M., and Sebens, J. B., *Brain Res.* 42, 239 (1972).
16. Chase, T. N., and Ng, L. K. Y., *Arch. Neurol.* 27, 486 (1972).
17. Rinne, U. K., and Sonninen, V., *Neurology* 22, 62 (1972).
18. Strang, R. R., *Brit. Med. J.* 2, 33 (1965).
19. Carlsson, A., *J. Pharm. Pharmacol.* 22, 729 (1970).
20. Klerman, G. L., and Cole, J. O., *Pharmacol. Rev.* 17, 101 (1965).
21. Chase, T. N., Ng, L. K. Y., and Watanabe, A. M., *Neurology* 22, 479 (1972).
22. Moir, A. T. B., and Eccleston, D., *J. Neurochem.* 15, 1093 (1968).
23. Yahr, M. D., in: *L-DOPA and Parkinsonism,* edited by A. Barbeau and A. McDowell, F. A. Davis Co., Philadelphia, 1970, p. 101.
24. Hall, C. D., Weiss, E. A., Morris, C. E., and Prange, A. J., *Neurology* 22, 231 (1972).
25. Bartholini, G., DaPrada, M., and Pletscher, A., *J. Pharm. Pharmacol.* 20, 228 (1968).
26. Moir, A. T. B., *Brit. J. Pharmacol.* 43, 715 (1971).
27. Fuxe, K., Butcher, L. L., and Engel, J., *J. Pharm. Pharmacol.* 23, 420 (1971).
28. Chase, T. N., *Arch. Neurol.* 27, 354 (1972).
29. Van Woert, M. H., Ambani, L. M., and Levine, R. J., *Dis. Nerv. Syst.* 33, 777 (1972).
30. Everett, G. M., and Borcherding, J. W., *Science* 168, 849 (1970).
31. Ng, L. K. Y., Chase, T. N., Colburn, R. W., and Kopin, I. J., *Neurology* 22, 688 (1972).
32. Pullar, I. A., *J. Physiol.* 216, 201 (1971).
33. Goodwin, F. K., Dunner, D. L., and Gershon, E., *Life Sci.* 10 (Part I), 751 (1971).
34. Johansson, B., and Roos, B.-E., *Europ. J. Clin. Pharmacol.* 3, 232 (1971).
35. Friedman, E., and Gershon, S., *Europ. J. Pharmacol.* 18, 183 (1972).
36. Ross, S. B., Renyi, A. L., and Ogren, S.-O., *Life Sci.* 10 (Part I), 1267 (1971).
37. Lidbrink, P., Jonsson, G., and Fuxe, K., *Neuropharmacology* 10, 521 (1971).

DISCUSSION

Dr. McDowell: Do any of you have comments or questions for Dr. Wurtman?

Dr. Van Loon: Dr. Wurtman, you suggested that L-DOPA affects the formation of brain protein, do you have or know of any data which suggest that by this mechanism L-DOPA suppresses the formation of hypothalamic releasing hormones?

Dr. Wurtman: Let me defer that to Dr. Weiss's presentation.

Dr. Van Loon: With regard to your points about the differential effects on tryptophan and serotonin using carbohydrates and protein diets, was this simply related to the amounts of insulin secreted? Do you have measurements to show that using protein diets produced a significant amount of insulin secretion as in using the carbohydrate diet?

Dr. Wurtman: We do not have direct assays for insulin; however, it has been shown by a variety of investigators that amino acids themselves are as potent a stimulus to insulin secretion as carbohydrates. If one mixes amino acids and carbohydrates together, one would expect, if anything, to get at least as great or probably more of an insulin response, but we have not measured insulin directly.

Dr. Cotzias: I would like to know how good the evidence is that the dopamine, serotonin, and HVA in the spinal fluid come from the brain.

Dr. McDowell: Dr. Chase, will you deal with that?

Dr. Chase: The major evidence is that if you infuse either labeled 5-HIAA or HVA into the circulation very little of the labeled material comes out in spinal fluid.

Dr. Goldberg: This too is a point of ignorance, Dr. Chase, but doesn't imipramine also block catecholamine uptake? You said specifically serotonin.

Dr. Chase: It has a relatively greater influence on the uptake of various monoamines into serotonergic neurons. It is not entirely specific by any means.

Dr. Roberts: Dr. Chase, is there any evidence that serotonin neurons can inhibit dopamine neurons in another part of the brain and that the decrease in serotonin function then might be a compensatory change in response to decrement or loss of dopamine?

Dr. Chase: I do not know how to design the experiment in patients to answer your question. I think that the reduction in serotonin metabolism that we see in parkinsonian patients is probably a compensatory functional change in response to a primary effect on the dopaminergic system. But I do not know how to prove that point. In support of this concept is the fact that people have not been able to recognize lesions in areas of the brain that are known to be rich in serotonin-containing nerve cells. There is also the observation that Hornykiewicz made some years ago that if you give an

MAO inhibitor to a parkinsonian patient it restores serotonin levels, but not dopamine levels, to normal.

Dr. Klawans: A comment on serotonin in search of a role which may serve as somewhat of an answer to Dr. Roberts' question. In using amphetamine-induced stereotyped behavior which I think many people feel is related to activity of dopamine at striatal dopamine receptor sites, you can actually decrease stereotyped behavior, and even prevent it, with 5-HTP, and the resulting inhibition does correlate with brain serotonin levels. You can potentiate this behavior, that is, lower the threshold for the amount of either apomorphine or amphetamine required to produce this behavior with methysergide.

We tend to think, therefore, that 5-HTP should worsen Parkinson's disease and if anything might produce choreatic disease; at the least, it would worsen Parkinson's disease. There is some evidence for an interaction at the dopamine receptor site cells for serotonin. Dr. Wurtman, would you like to speculate that the supposed decreases of 5-hydroxyindoles reported in depressed patients may really be a dietary effect?

Dr. Wurtman: I guess it could be; one thing that tends to happen to depressed patients when they go into hospitals is they start eating, or at least their eating is monitored. There's a kind of a counterintuitive relationship between the nature of the food consumed and the change in brain serotonin. One would have expected that the more tryptophan in the food, the greater the rise in brain serotonin would be; actually, exactly the opposite occurs. I think one has to do further studies and see.

Let me make a response to the 5-HTP DOPA story. One of my associates, Loy Lytle, showed that if you give animals repeated doses of 6-hydroxy-dopamine intracisternally so that brain catecholamine levels are very low, most of the catecholamine neurons are destroyed. Then if these animals are given a dose of DOPA and the increment in brain dopamine is measured, it is not distinguishable from that in the intact normal animals.

Virtually the same thing is true, I am sure, with 5-HTP; that is, these compounds are amino acids and are taken up into virtually every cell in the head by the same transport system that takes up leucine, isoleucine, and valine. In the case of serotonergic neurons, we have a choice between forcing serotonin synthesis by giving its natural precursor tryptophan, which generates serotonin only in cells that already have it, or giving 5-HTP which produces serotonin in glia, cholinergic neurons, and the liver. Before we attribute any effect of 5-HTP to serotonergic synapses, we are obligated first to show that tryptophan has the same effect.

Dr. Sandler: I think it is a little dangerous to interpret 5-HIAA levels as some index of 5-HT turnover, because you know these data are essentially, of necessity, incomplete. When you oxidize an amine, you get an aldehyde, which can be further oxidized to its acid or reduced to an alcohol.

We know that 5-hydroxytryptophan may be increased under certain cir-

Advances in Neurology, Vol. 5
Raven Press, New York © 1974

Central Noradrenergic Neurons

Donald J. Reis

Department of Neurology, Cornell University Medical College, New York, New York 10021

THE CENTRAL NE-NEURONAL SYSTEM

Within the central nervous system, the monoamine neurotransmitter norepinephrine (NE) is almost exclusively contained within the cell bodies and processes of a specific system of neurons specialized for the synthesis, storage, and release of the neurotransmitter (1–3). These neurons, which will be referred to here as NE-neurons, are not uniformly distributed throughout the brain and spinal cord. The cell bodies of NE-neurons are concentrated in specific regions of the lower brainstem and send their axonal processes in precisely defined pathways to terminate with regional selectivity.

Present knowledge of the distribution of NE-neurons has been derived from convergent data acquired by a combination of biochemical, histological, physiological, and pharmacological methods. The most fruitful technique has been the development of specific histofluorescence for the visualization *in situ* of NE and other monoamines (1–3). By combining this method with techniques for altering the concentration of NE, commonly by electrolytic or chemical lesions, the anatomy of the system has been elaborated. The recent introduction of immunohistochemical methods for identification of NE-neurons by the use of labeled antibodies to the specific enzymes subserving catecholamine biosynthesis (4, 5) has opened an important new avenue for investigation of the NE as well as other chemically specific neuronal systems.

Three general systems of NE-neurons have been broadly distinguished on the basis of their projections (2, 3). The first is a bulbo-spinal system in which the cell bodies, localized in the medulla, send axon processes caudally into the spinal cord. The second is a group of cells with short axonal processes ramifying locally around the cell bodies in the lower brainstem. The third consists of ascending projections. On the basis of lesion studies, Ungerstedt (3) has described two principal ascending NE projections, the ventral and dorsal systems (Fig. 1).

The *ventral* ascending pathway arises from cell groups designated as A1, A2, A5, and A7 (1) in the medulla oblongata and pons. Most of these neurons are interspersed as biochemically distinctive members of nuclear

NORADRENALINE

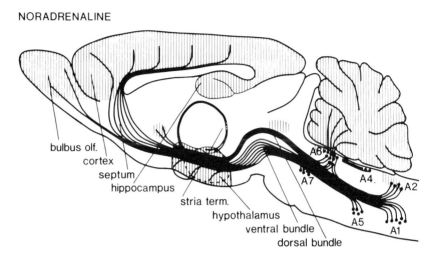

FIG. 1. The noradrenergic system of brain (from ref. 3).

groups previously considered as being relatively homogeneous by traditional staining methods. This system gives rise to NE terminals which innervate the lower brainstem, the mesencephalon, and the diencephalon, particularly the hypothalamus.

The *dorsal* NE pathway arises almost *in toto* from the nucleus of the locus coeruleus (A6). In rat, the locus coeruleus is a brainstem nucleus comprising some 1,400 medium-sized nerve cells which are mostly packed on each side of the IVth ventricle (6, 7). The majority, if not all, of the neurons of the locus coeruleus are noradrenergic. Neurons of the locus coeruleus send fibers through a descending pathway to the lower brainstem, through a lateral pathway into the cerebellum to innervate the cerebellar cortex, and through its principal ascending projection (the dorsal NE pathway) to innervate the cerebral cortex, hippocampus, and major portions of the forebrain and limbic system. There is indirect evidence that a single fiber of the locus coeruleus can send collateral branches widely ramified into the cerebellum and cerebral cortex (7). Thus, one nerve cell of the locus coeruleus innervates widely separated areas of the CNS. The extensive ramifications of NE-neurons contrasts with the discrete and focused innervation of dopaminergic neurons of the nigrostriatal system (3). The fibers of NE-neurons are unmyelinated and conduct impulses slowly (7).

THE NE-NEURON

It is generally assumed that in the brain, as in the peripheral sympathetic system, the cell body of NE-neurons is essential for the production of the proteins required for neuronal function including the enzymes required for the biosynthesis and degradation of NE, the soluble proteins released along with transmitter, the synaptic vesicles, and "structural" proteins (8). In the periphery, enzymes and vesicles as well as some NE are transported from the cell body to the periphery by axoplasmic flow. The vesicles, the enzymes tyrosine hydroxylase (TH) and dopamine-beta-hydroxylase (DBH) are believed to move at a rapid rate of flow in the peripheral sympathetic neuron (9) whereas other proteins probably move more slowly. Within the central nervous system, axoplasmic flow in the noradrenergic system has been indirectly measured (10). It has been suggested on indirect evidence that the rate of transport is about 10% of that in the periphery. Under normal circumstances, the axon terminal is capable of maintaining synthesis of the amine, and, indeed, at least in the peripheral nervous system, there is evidence that axoplasmic flow contributes negligible quantities of the amine for release (8).

As a consequence of this partial segregation of functions, NE itself is not evenly distributed within the central NE-neuron. The amine is at highest concentrations in the varicosities of the axon terminal, the site of synaptic contact with postsynaptic cells. Substantial but smaller quantities of the amine are found in the cell body (8). Very little of the amine is localized to the longer subterminal unmyelinated axon. In the peripheral adrenergic neuron, the concentration of NE in the axon terminal is about 300 times greater than that of the cell body (8). A similar concentration gradient probably exists in the brain. This fact thereby explains why NE occurs in its highest concentrations in brain areas richly innervated with NE terminals such as the hypothalamus.

In the amine-laden varicosities of the NE-neuron, most of the NE is stored within the storage granules which, by electron microscopy after specific fixation, have an electron-dense core (8). These storage granules are believed to contain most of the intraneuronal NE; they appear to protect the amines from the action of intracellular degradative enzyme and to serve as a package which is mobilized to release amine plus soluble proteins, including DBH, into the synaptic cleft in response to nerve impulse activity.

BIOSYNTHESIS OF CATECHOLAMINES

The biosynthetic pathway for the synthesis of NE is well established, as illustrated in Fig. 2 and reviewed in several recent articles (11, 12). The principal precursor for the synthesis of NE is the amino acid tyrosine. Tyrosine is transported into the brain and central adrenergic neurons by specific saturable transport mechanisms. Once it enters the cell it is hydroxylated by TH to L-DOPA. TH is viewed as the rate-limiting step in the biosynthesis of catecholamines. Its activity is dependent on the availability of oxygen and the pteridine cofactor. The pteridine cofactor, in turn, depends upon its continuous regeneration by the action of pteridine re-

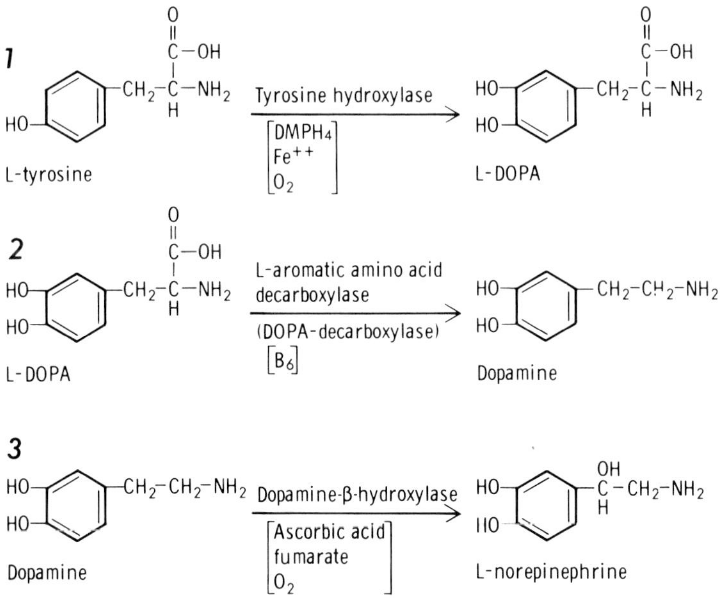

FIG. 2. Biosynthetic pathways of NE.

ductase, an enzyme which may be of importance in regulation of NE bio-synthesis (13). L-DOPA is rapidly decarboxylated by a nonspecific amino acid decarboxylase to dopamine which is then transported into the storage granules by an energy-dependent uptake process, and beta-hydroxylated to NE by DBH.

It is evident that the biosynthesis of catecholamines in the NE-neuron depends upon a series of intracellular migrations of sequentially manu-factured substrates, ultimately leading to storage of the transmitter within the vesicles. Some of the amine appears to leak back into the cytoplasm where it remains unbound.

FUNCTIONAL POOLS

On the basis of drug studies and other pieces of indirect evidence, the view has emerged that NE within the adrenergic neuron is sequestered into at least two different functional pools (14). The anatomical or molecular identity of these pools is not known. It has been proposed that newly syn-thesized NE is part of a small "available pool" which may be the physio-logically active form of the transmitter and the first released. Most of the NE within the neuron is considered to be held in a "reserve" pool, which is physiologically inactive and which can replenish the active pool. The con-cept of pools has had heuristic value but it remains a concept rather than an established fact.

RELEASE OF NE

The release of NE from nerve terminals onto the receptors in the periphery occurs in three ways (14, 15), and, presumably, similar mechanisms are operative in brain. The most physiologically important mechanism for release is initiated by nerve impulse activity. The process of excitation-release coupling has not been fully characterized for central neurons. However, the mechanisms probably depend upon the presence of calcium and other ions. The neural release of the storage granule and its contents into the extracellular space in peripheral sympathetic neurons is quantal and is believed to be by the process of exocytosis (8). In this manner the contents of the granule consisting of NE, DBH, and chromagranins are extruded into the synaptic cleft where they make contact with the postsynaptic receptor.

A second mode for NE release is by leakage of NE through the membranes of the nerve cells onto the receptors. The third mechanism is by displacement of the amine from the storage granules by drugs such as tyramine or reserpine. This is a mechanism of some pharmacological interest and may play a role in certain pathological conditions such as hepatic coma.

TURNOVER

It is now well established that measurement of the levels of NE regionally in the brain tells little of the dynamic state of the neuron. It is knowledge of the turnover of the amine which reflects the net balance between synthesis, release, and metabolism. Although changing levels of amines in tissues can reflect either selective or unbalanced changes in synthesis or degradation, under natural conditions the concentration of the amine does not fluctuate, despite wide variations in the levels of nerve impulse activity. Measurement of the turnover of the amine, therefore, is a much more sensitive index of the activity of the noradrenergic NE-neuron (15).

Several techniques have been applied for the measurement of the turnover of NE in brain including measurement of: (a) the rate of the decline of specific activity of labeled NE when administered intraventricularly; (b) the rate of fall of endogenous NE after its synthesis is blocked by administration of inhibitors of TH; and (c) the rate of synthesis of NE after introduction of labeled precursors (15).

PHYSIOLOGICAL INACTIVATION AND METABOLISM OF NE

The termination of action of NE at the receptor is of utmost physiological importance. The transmitter is rendered physiologically inactive by three principal mechanisms (14, 15). The most important is re-uptake of the transmitter into nerve endings by a stereospecific energy-dependent pump in the nerve membrane. Blockade of this pump by drugs such as imipramine will markedly facilitate the local action of the neurotransmitter. Degeneration of the nerve as a consequence of lesions will lead to the disappearance of the inactivation mechanism and may, in part, be responsible for the appearance of some denervation hypersensitivity.

A second mechanism is the metabolic inactivation of the amine itself (14, 15). Most amines leaking out of granules are inactivated intraneuronally by the action of the intracellular enzyme monoamine oxidase (MAO). Some amine, however, diffuses extraneuronally to be acted upon by the enzyme catechol-O-methyltransferase.

The third mechanism of inactivation is by diffusion of the amine away from the receptor area into the cerebrospinal fluid and thence into the bloodstream where it may be taken up into nerve terminals elsewhere, may be metabolized, or may be excreted as the amine into the urine. However, the minimal contribution of the brain to the total NE pool of the body is such as to make detection of changes of amine metabolism in the brain by examination of urine impossible. It has recently been postulated, as discussed elsewhere in this volume, that preferential metabolites of NE may be detected within the spinal fluid.

REGULATION OF SYNTHESIS OF NE

In peripheral tissues in brain, the rate of NE synthesis is largely regulated by nerve impulse activity (12, 16). With brief periods of activity, synthesis is governed at the TH step by end-product inhibition. In this manner it has been proposed that unbound NE inhibits enzyme activity possibly by some interaction with the pteridine cofactor (13). Thus, when more NE is released, tissue levels fall and the enzyme becomes less inhibited. Conversely, when nerve activity decreases, more NE is retained, thereby inhibiting the enzyme. The mechanism of end-product inhibition appears useful in the minute-to-minute regulation of NE synthesis in relation to transient fluctuations of impulse activity.

Nerve activity, however, when prolonged over hours or days may result in increased activity of several of the enzymes along the synthetic pathway (12, 16). This increase in enzyme activity is due to an increased accumulation of enzyme protein (17, 18). It is not known if the augmented accumulation reflects increased synthesis or decreased degradation of the enzyme protein. It has recently been demonstrated that a decrease in accumulation of enzyme protein may occur in central and peripheral NE-neurons in response to axonal injury (18, 19).

THE RESPONSE OF NE-NEURONS TO INJURY

Over the past few years some new insights into the processes underlying the neuronal response to axonal injury in the central nervous system have come from analysis of these reactions in NE-neurons (18, 19). The NE-neuronal system has certain distinct advantages for studying the events elicited by axonal damage with both peripheral and sympathetic nervous system. First, the cell bodies of these systems are specifically located in peripheral ganglia and within identifiable nuclei within the brain, particularly the nucleus locus coeruleus, thereby lending themselves to morphological analysis at both the light and electron microscopic levels. Secondly, the neurotransmitter, NE, produced by these cells is defined and easily measured. Third, the enzymes involved in the biosynthesis of the transmitter are known, and their activities can be assayed in reasonably small quantities of tissue. More recently, the availability of specific antibodies to most of these enzymes has permitted estimation of amounts of specific enzyme protein and the effects of lesions on the accumulation of such protein. Fourth, the cell body and processes of NE-neurons can be visualized by specific histofluorescence and, more recently, immunofluorescence techniques. Fifth, these neurons within the central nervous system have been demonstrated to sprout in response to injury (20–23), and thereby the system lends itself to an analysis of the general problem of the relationship of the reaction of the cell body to regenerative sprouting. Finally, the increasing knowledge of the function of central NE-neurons, for example, with regard to behaviors such as aggression (24) and feeding has allowed the relating of degeneration and regeneration to alterations in behavior.

ANTEROGRADE CHANGES OF CENTRAL NE-NEURONS

Axonal changes of NE-neurons in the brain have been most commonly produced by the placement of electrolytic lesions within the medial forebrain bundle. In some instances lesions of the locus coeruleus itself have been made (18). The former lesions interrupt axons ascending from the cell bodies of NE-neurons in the lower brainstem to innervate regions of the forebrain and hypothalamus. The latter accomplish the same thing by destroying the cell body. By analyzing the biochemical and histochemical changes within the degenerating axon, the anterograde reaction can be characterized. On the other hand, it is possible by studying changes within the cell bodies which lie caudal to the lesion to evaluate the nature of the retrograde reaction in the cell bodies themselves.

It is well known that the anterograde reaction in axons of central NE-neurons consists, as in the periphery, of a gradual decline in the concentration of the transmitter, and the synthetic enzymes, in the field of axonal innervation. The major difference between the anterograde response of axons of central and peripheral NE-neurons is that the rate at which the contents of the severed axon disappears centrally is considerably prolonged, taking 2 weeks to reach a nadir (17) (Fig. 3). This contrasts with the rapid

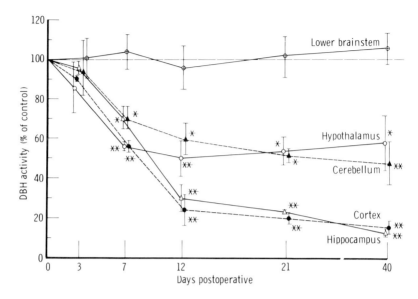

FIG. 3. The anterograde reaction of central NE-neurons. Time course of decline of DBH in different brain areas ipsilateral to a unilateral electrolytic lesion of the locus coeruleus in rat. The different magnitude of fall reflects how much of the noradrenergic innervation of a brain area is from the locus. Note the similarity of time course in different regions. Differences from unoperated control: $^*p < 0.01$; $^{**}p < 0.001$ (from ref. 18).

rate of decline of these compounds in the peripheral nervous system where the fall of transmitter enzymes occurs over 1 to 2 days.

The reason why the decline of the transmitter and its enzymes in central NE-neurons is slower than in peripheral NE systems or some central paths such as the nigrostriatal pathway is unknown. It has been suggested that it may relate to differences in the rate of axoplasmic transport between the two systems. Another possibility is that the contents of the degenerating axon are taken into astrocytes where the vesicle is transiently preserved (18).

THE RETROGRADE REACTION

The retrograde reaction of central noradrenergic neurons has been less well characterized than the response in peripheral sympathetic ganglia (see ref. 18). Recent investigations on the retrograde reaction of cells within the locus coeruleus in response to axonal injury induced by electrolytic lesions of the medial forebrain bundle, however, have begun to show certain similarities between the two reactions (18, 19). Initially, within hours after axonal damage there is an appreciable increase in the content of NE in the cell bodies of NE-neurons. This phase of "piling up" may last many days, then gradually disappear.

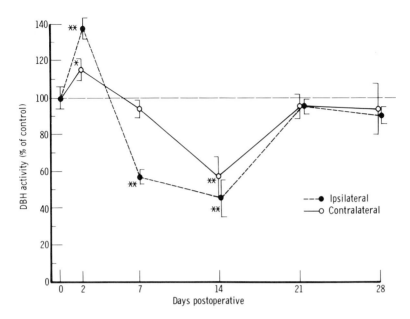

FIG. 4. The retrograde reaction of central NE-neurons. Time course of changes in DBH activity in the lower brainstem after unilateral electrolytic lesions of the medial forebrain bundle (from ref. 19). A similar reversible reduction occurs in the locus coeruleus. The reduction in enzyme activity is due to decreased accumulation of specific enzyme protein (18).

The changes of transmitter in the NE-neuron during the retrograde reaction are paralleled by a series of changes in the activities of several of the biosynthetic enzymes subserving catecholamine synthesis (18, 19) (Fig. 4). Within the first 48 hr after a lesion, there is enhanced activity of DBH. This phase is followed by a marked decline in the activity of both TH and DBH, which persists up to 2 weeks and is followed by recovery. This reversible reduction in the activity of TH and DBH is a consequence of a reduction in the accumulation of specific enzyme protein and not due to inhibition of enzyme activity by the action of endogenous inhibitors (18). Of particular interest is the fact that the reduction of enzyme protein within the cell body of neurons in the locus coeruleus resulting from damage of an axon in the hypothalamus is reflected in the collateral fibers (sustaining collaterals) projecting to the cerebellum (18, 19). The mechanism by which the injury results in reduced accumulation of these specific enzymes is unknown. It could be due either to a decrease in synthesis or to increased degradation of the enzyme.

The discovery of a reversible decrease in accumulation of the enzymes involved in the biosynthesis of the neurotransmitter in NE-neurons is of some general interest. It is generally believed that during the retrograde reaction in peripheral neurons (including neurons whose cell bodies reside within the CNS but project peripherally) there is an increase in net protein and RNA biosynthesis (24). This fact has suggested that the retrograde reaction primarily represents an anabolic event relating more to the attempts of the neuron to regenerate by sprouting than to degeneration (24, 25).

Our observations of a decrease in the accumulation of those enzymes specialized for neurotransmitter synthesis in neurons of the locus coeruleus (on the assumption that the decrease results from decreased synthesis of the enzyme) suggest that there may be a selective reordering of priorities for protein biosynthesis in the cell during the period in which it is reacting to injury. In this manner there is an increase in the production of proteins required for maintaining the neuron as a structural entity at the expense of those involved in sustaining the neuron as a cell specialized for transmission. The changes in the patterns of protein biosynthesis in regenerating neurons have also been suggested to reflect a reversion in the pattern of protein biosynthesis to that characteristic of immature nerve cells (26), i.e., nerve cells more specialized for growth.

It is of interest that during the period of the retrograde reaction in the neurons of the locus coeruleus there is little evidence of the usual morphological concomitants of the retrograde reaction, i.e., chromatolysis (18). This negative finding is of some interest because it suggests that the retrograde reaction within the central nervous system may be characterized by biochemical changes unassociated with the classical picture of cell swelling, dissolution of the Nissl substance, and nuclear eccentricity (25). If the retrograde reaction is defined as a response to injury characterized by two of three criteria—cell swelling, decreased accumulation of enzymes subserving transmitter biosynthesis, and sprouting (18)—the NE-neuron clearly demonstrates a retrograde response. This argument contradicts older views that there is no retrograde reaction in CNS because such neurons either are not so "programmed" or fail to regenerate.

SPROUTING AND REGENERATION OF CENTRAL NE-NEURONS

Within the past several years it has been recognized that central NE-neurons have a powerful regenerative capacity. The initial observations (21) demonstrated that following an electrolytic lesion of the medial forebrain bundle, the severed axonal endings developed a rich lacework of sprouts by the 7th to 19th days. The sprouts first emerge from severed axons, increase in volume and begin to fill in the interstices of the lesion, and abnormally innervate local blood vessels. The drive for sprouting in central NE-neurons appears to be so powerful that when grafts of smooth muscle are placed within the brain they rapidly become richly innervated from processes of intrinsic noradrenergic fibers (22).

Not only do central NE-neurons have the capacity to respond by sprouting in response to injury of their axons, but they may also develop collateral sprouts to innervate synapses denuded of a nonadrenergic input. For example, it has been demonstrated that partial denervation of neurons in the medial septal nucleus (20, 23) of their nonadrenergic hippocampal projection results in collateral sprouting from ascending NE fibers located in the lateral septal area. The collateral sprouts quickly occupy the abandoned synaptic sites. Indeed, the rapidity with which the NE-neuron will respond by collateral sprouting has questioned the traditional view of limited regenerative capacity of central neurons. Indeed, the drive for regeneration by sprouting of central NE-neurons is so great that it is conceivable that regeneration is limited in the central nervous system because the synaptic sites made available by degenerating axons do not remain uninnervated for the period of time which would be required for the injured axon, if situated at a distance, to regenerate to reoccupy its original synaptic site.

THE ROLE OF SUSTAINING COLLATERALS IN SIGNALLING DAMAGE TO REMOTE AXONS IN CENTRAL NORADRENERGIC NEURONS

As already noted, lesions of NE axons in hypothalamus produce reactive changes of enzyme accumulation not only in the parent cell bodies in the locus coeruleus but also in the collaterals of these same cells in cerebellum (19). This finding indicates that the whole field of innervation of a neuron shares in the induced biochemical event in the cell body, a process of *intraneuronal communication*. The biological significance of such widespread reactive impairment of neuronal function in an NE-neuron is unknown. It could reflect the reduction in the activity of the neuron during recovery from injury. More intriguing, however, is the possibility that the biochemical changes of remote terminals might be of importance in the recovery of physiological function following brain damage, i.e., the transfer of function of an activity from one brain area to another, leading thereby to "compensation." Conceivably, the NE-neuron could play a role in this mode of functional recovery since the axonal processes of NE-neurons are ubiquitously distributed and may play a role in learning.

There is also a practical implication of the phenomenon. The examination of levels of certain amines or their biosynthetic enzymes in the brain of patients with neuronal diseases, particularly lesions inflicted several days previously, may reveal abnormal levels which might be only conse quent to retrograde processes in neurons and hence transient. This could lead to unwarranted conclusions about the function of specific transmitter enzymes in specific disease processes.

ACKNOWLEDGMENTS

Portions of the research reported in this paper were supported by U.S. Public Health Service grant NS 06911 and a grant from the Harris Foundation.

REFERENCES

1. Dahlström, A., and Fuxe, K., *Acta Physiol. Scand.*, 62, Suppl. 232, 1 (1964).
2. Andén, N. E., Dahlström, A., Fuxe, K., Larsson, K., Olson, L., and Ungerstedt, U., *Acta Physiol. Scand.*, 67, 313 (1966).
3. Ungerstedt, U., *Acta Physiol. Scand.*, 82, Suppl. 367, 1 (1971).
4. Hartman, B. K., and Udenfriend, S., *Pharmacol. Rev.*, 24, 311 (1972).
5. Fuxe, K., Goldstein, M., Hökfelt, T., and Joh, T. H., *Prog. Brain Res.*, 34, 127 (1971).
6. Descarries, L., and Saucier, G., *Brain Res.*, 37, 310 (1972).
7. Hoffer, B. J., Siggins, G. R., Oliver, A. P., and Bloom, F. E., *J. Pharmacol. Exp. Ther.*, 184, 553 (1973).
8. Geffen, L. B., and Livett, B. G., *Physiol. Rev.*, 51, 98 (1971).
9. Wooten, G. F., and Coyle, J. T., *J. Neurochem.*, 20, 1361 (1973).
10. Dahlström, A., in: *Dynamics of Degeneration and Growth in Neurons*. Pergamon Press Ltd., Oxford (*in press*).
11. Molinoff, P. B., and Axelrod, J., *Ann. Rev. Biochem.*, 40, 465 (1971).
12. Cotten, M. deV. (ed.), *Regulation of Catecholamine Metabolism in the Sympathetic Nervous System*. Williams and Wilkins Co., Baltimore (1972).
13. Musacchio, J., D'Angelo, G., and McQueen, C., *Proc. Nat. Acad. Sci.*, 68, 2087 (1971).
14. Axelrod, J., and Kopin, I. J., *Prog. Brain Res.*, 31, 21 (1969).
15. Iversen, L. L., *The Uptake and Storage of Noradrenaline in Sympathetic Nerves*, Cambridge University Press, Cambridge (1967).
16. Weiner, N., *Ann. Rev. Pharmacol.*, 10, 273 (1970).
17. Joh, T. H., Geghman, C., and Reis, D. J., *Proc. Nat. Acad. Sci.* (*in press*).
18. Reis, D. J., Ross, R. A., and Joh, T. H., in: *Dynamics of Degeneration and Growth in Neurons*. Pergamon Press Ltd., Oxford (*in press*).
19. Reis, D. J., and Ross, R. A., *Brain Res.*, 57, 307 (1973).
20. Raisman, G., *Brain Res.*, 14, 25 (1969).
21. Katzman, R., Björklund, A., Owman, C., Stenevi, U., and West, K. A., *Brain Res.*, 25, 579 (1971).
22. Bjorklund, A., and Stenevi, U., *Brain Res.*, 31, 1 (1971).
23. Moore, R. Y., Björklund, A., and Stenevi, U., *Brain Res.*, 33, 13 (1971).
24. Reis, D. J., in: *Neurotransmitters*, pp. 266–297. Williams and Wilkins Co., Baltimore (1972).
25. Lieberman, A. R., *Int. Rev. Neurobiol.*, 14, 49 (1971).
26. Bråttgard, S. O., Edström, J. E., and Hyden, H., *J. Neurochem.*, 1, 316 (1957).
27. LaVelle, A., and Sechrist, J. W., *Anat. Rec.*, 166, 335 (1970).

DISCUSSION

Dr. McGeer: If one lesions the nigralstriatal bundle either electrolytically or by giving 6-hydroxydopamine, the rate of decrease of tyrosine hydroxylase and DOPA decarboxylase in the striatum is very rapid. Tyrosine hydroxylase will drop to a level near 50% in about 24 hours and then will ultimately drop to 10% or even less depending on how perfect your lesion is.

DOPA decarboxylase will not go all the way down; it will fall to 40% of the initial level but half-life is about 48 hours. In other words, the anterograde degeneration is very rapid but there is also retrograde degeneration. Tyrosine hydroxylase and DOPA decarboxylase in the substantia nigra, if you lesion the axons, will drop ultimately to zero; picnotic cells are seen, and ultimately they disappear altogether.

So why is there this difference? I presume the retrograde degeneration occurs because you have cut a main stem axon, but I do not see why the time course of the anterograde degeneration should be so different.

Dr. Reis: The anterograde changes are a fact, and there is a difference. At the moment we cannot explain why there is a difference in the time course of these changes: they just represent different characteristics of the two systems. I would interpret the retrograde changes as similar to those of any other system.

If you cut from the whole axon of any nerve cell, it is more likely to die than if you cut a collateral. Our lesions which have been placed in the posterior hypothalamus will preserve a number of collateral fibers of the system, and hence the nerve, the locus cell, will recover.

You can demonstrate this if you make lesions a little more anteriorly or rostrally in the median forebrain bundle. You may not see any change at all in the cells because the lesion has to be at a critical distance. I presume if we got near enough to the cells with our lesions we might see irreversible changes.

The substantia nigra with its projections may be a system with one major axonal trunk in which the nerve cells just cannot recover because it does not have a sustaining collateral.

Advances in Neurology, Vol. 5
Raven Press, New York © 1974

Some Aspects of Dopamine in the Central Nervous System

Arvid Carlsson

Department of Pharmacology, University of Göteborg, Göteborg, Sweden

This chapter will cover two aspects of dopamine (DA) in the central nervous system: (a) the distribution of DA and its possible nonprecursor role in regions where it occurs in low concentration, and (b) the first step in the synthesis of DA, that is, the hydroxylation of tyrosine, its regulation and response to various experimental procedures.

THE DISTRIBUTION OF DOPAMINE IN THE CENTRAL NERVOUS SYSTEM

The occurrence of DA in high concentration, that is, several micrograms per gram, in the striatum and some structures belonging to the limbic system is well established, and it is generally accepted that in these areas DA plays an independent role as a putative transmitter. On the other hand, in regions where it occurs in low concentration, its role is more difficult to define. Recent technical improvements in the quantitative analysis of DA (1, 2) have opened up new possibilities for investigation of this problem.

Recently Thierry, Stinus, Blanc, and Glowinski (3) reported some observations on the DA of the cerebral cortex. Electrolytic lesions in the locus coeruleus or microinjections of 6-hydroxydopamine in the lower brainstem caused a decrease in cortical noradrenaline (NA) but not in cortical DA, as observed 5 weeks after the lesion, indicating that the cortical DA was present in other structures than the noradrenaline-carrying ascending fiber system. On the other hand, cortical DA was uninfluenced by lesions which were assumed to destroy ascending DA-carrying fiber systems.

The question arises as to where this DA is located. It should be kept in mind that great care must be exercised in the dissection of the cortex so as to avoid contamination by small amounts of tissue from regions where the DA level is one or two orders of magnitude higher. In view of this possibility, it is somewhat disturbing that the average cortical DA levels reported by Thierry et al. show considerable variation in the control animals from one experimental series to another (from 84 to 196 ng/g). We find lower DA values in the rat cerebral cortex than Thierry et al. Moreover, they decrease in the frontal-occipital direction. In the occipital part, the level is as low as 30 ng/g. Whether DA occurs diffusely in the cortex or in some discrete areas remains to be investigated.

We tend to agree with Thierry et al. that an appreciable part of the cortical DA serves a nonprecursor role. Our reasons are the following.

In the peripheral adrenergic system or in the adrenal medulla, DA constitutes only 1 to 2% of the total catecholamines (4, 5). In the cerebral cortex, the DA/NA ratio is 0.15 in the occipital part, and even higher in the other parts. Moreover, the DA level in the cortex does not decrease appreciably after simultaneous inhibition of DA synthesis and MAO (6), in contrast to the precursor DA of the peripheral sympathoadrenal system (Carlsson and Lindqvist, *unpublished data*). Furthermore, in the spinal cord, where the DA/NA ratio is even lower than in the occipital cortex (7), the changes in DA and NA levels after transection of the spinal cord show marked differences, which are difficult to reconcile with the view that they occur in the same structure. In fact, the DA curve was remarkably similar to the striatal DA curve observed after cutting the nigrostriatal axons (14).

Finally, if all spinal DA is assumed to be precursor, calculations of spinal NA synthesis based on isotope data yield unreasonably high values (7).

Thus, a considerable part of DA in the CNS, even in low-DA regions, probably serves a nonprecursor role. At least the spinal DA appears to be located in neurons, since it disappears completely within 1 week after spinal transection below but not above the lesion.

In spite of the low levels of DA in, for example, the cerebral cortex and spinal cord, its possible functional importance as an independent transmitter in these regions cannot be disregarded.

THE FIRST STEP IN THE SYNTHESIS OF DOPAMINE; ITS REGULATION AND RESPONSE TO VARIOUS EXPERIMENTAL PROCEDURES

Methodological Aspects

Several methods are available for measuring DA synthesis and turnover rates *in vivo*. They do not always yield the same results (see below). In the present investigation, we have mainly used the technique of measuring DOPA accumulation after inhibition of the aromatic amino acid decarboxylase (6). We consider this technique more direct and convenient and perhaps also more accurate than other available *in vivo* methods.

After injection of the inhibitor of the aromatic amino acid decarboxylase NSD 1015 (3-hydroxybenzylhydrazine HCl, 100 mg/kg), DOPA and 5-hydroxytryptophan accumulate linearly for the first 30 min in rat brain. The rate of efflux of the accumulating DOPA (or 5-hydroxytryptophan) is slow, as demonstrated by the slight decrease induced by a subsequently injected inhibitor of tyrosine hydroxylase (or tryptophan hydroxylase). These observations suggest that the accumulation of DOPA (or 5-hydroxytryptophan) under these conditions is a reliable measure of the tyrosine (or tryptophan) hydroxylase activity *in vivo* (6).

Effect of Tyrosine and α-Methyltyrosine

The rate of tyrosine hydroxylation, measured as outlined above, is not influenced by injections of tyrosine causing a considerable increase in brain tyrosine levels. Thus, tyrosine hydroxylase appears to be normally saturated with its substrate, tyrosine (6).

After administration of α-methyltyrosine, a relatively specific inhibitor of tyrosine hydroxylase, the formation of DOPA (but not 5-hydroxytryptophan) is inhibited in a dose-dependent manner. This inhibition can be efficiently antagonized by the subsequent administration of tyrosine (Table 1), indicating that α-methyltyrosine inhibits the enzyme by competing with its substrate.

TABLE 1. *Rat brain tyrosine hydroxylase activity in vivo: α-methyltyrosine (α-MT) versus tyrosine, given i.p. 90 and 30 min before death, respectively*

α-MT (as methylester HCl) dose, mg/kg	α-MT alone	α-MT + tyrosine (as ethylester HCl, 500 mg/kg)
0	140 ± 13 (6)	—
25	36 ± 3 (9)	131 ± 5 (8)
50	19 ± 3 (3)	116 ± 17 (5)

From Carlsson and Lindqvist, *unpublished data.*
Data show DOPA accumulation in brain, ng/g, 30 min after NSD 1015; means ± SEM (n).

Effect of Hypoxia

The hydroxylation of tyrosine (or tryptophan) requires molecular oxygen, which may be looked upon as a second substrate of the hydroxylase. The affinity of the enzyme for O_2 does not seem sufficient for attaining saturation at normal tissue pO_2 (8, 9). Accordingly, we find that even moderate hypoxia, leaving cerebral carbohydrate metabolism and energy production intact, causes a marked inhibition of tyrosine and tryptophan hydroxylase activities (Fig. 1). Total amine levels are only slightly influenced, presumably because oxidative deamination is also inhibited. Yet this interference may be functionally relevant, because the behavioral disturbance caused by hypoxia can be significantly antagonized by L-DOPA (Fig. 2).

In our hypoxia studies, we compared several methods for measuring

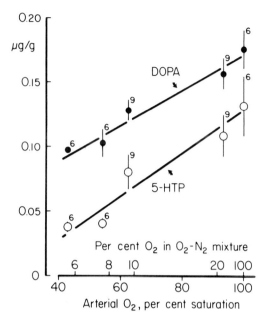

FIG. 1. Effect of hypoxia on tyrosine and tryptophan hydroxylase activities of whole rat brain *in vivo* (10). Rats received NSD 1015 (100 mg/kg, i.p.), an inhibitor of the aromatic amino acid decarboxylase, and were then immediately placed in a sealed cage, through which a gas mixture of oxygen and nitrogen in varying proportions was passed. The animals were killed after 30 min and the brains analyzed for DOPA and 5-hydroxytryptophan (5-HTP) accumulated as a result of decarboxylase inhibition. These accumulations show a linear relationship to the calculated percentage arterial O_2 saturation. (Reproduced from *J. Neurochem.*)

monoamine synthesis and turnover in the brain. Three methods gave qualitatively the same result: accumulation of DOPA after NSD 1015, of DA after monoamine oxidase inhibition by pargyline, and of homovanillic acid after blocking the efflux by probenecid. On the other hand, the accumulation of ^{3}H-DA 15 min after i.v. injection of ^{3}H-tyrosine was not significantly influenced by hypoxia. The net yield of ^{3}H-DA from ^{3}H-tyrosine may depend not only on synthesis but also on the disposition of different transmitter pools. Caution should thus be exercised in interpreting this kind of isotope data.

The turnover of DA, measured by means of synthesis inhibition, was moderately retarded by hypoxia. In contrast, the turnover of NA was accelerated; otherwise the results with NA were similar to the DA data.

Effect of Axotomy; Receptor-Mediated Feedback Control of Tyrosine Hydroxylase

If the ascending DA-carrying fiber systems are cut by a frontal hemisection of the brainstem, there is an immediate increase in tyrosine hydroxy-

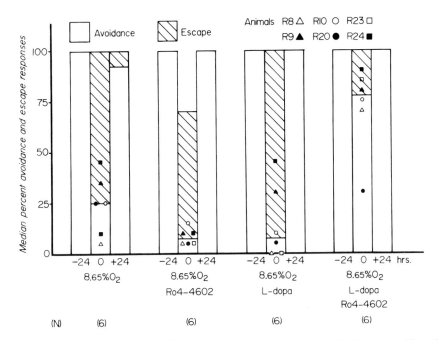

FIG. 2. Conditioned avoidance and escape responses in rats exposed to hypoxia, with and without pretreatment with L-DOPA (100 mg/kg, i.p., 30 min before trial) and/or the peripheral decarboxylase inhibitor Ro 4–4602 (50 mg/kg, i.p., 60 min before trial) (11). Shown are the median percent responses during hypoxia and during control sessions 24 hr before or after exposure to low oxygen. *Note.* Avoidance was significantly but reversibly depressed by low oxygen alone or in combination with pretreatment either with Ro 4–4602 or L-DOPA. However, combined pretreatment with these two agents significantly counteracted the hypoxia-induced depression of avoidance ($p = 0.05$). (Reproduced from *J. Pharm. Pharmacol.*)

lase activity, *in vivo*, on the side of the lesion (Fig. 3). This increase appears to be particularly pronounced in the striatal DA fiber system. Blocking DA receptors by means of haloperidol has a similar action which, however, is prevented by axotomy. Apomorphine, a DA-receptor stimulating agent, causes a decrease in tyrosine hydroxylase activity *in vivo*, both on the lesioned and on the control side; at the same time, the stimulating action of haloperidol on the activity of the enzyme is restored, and can thus be seen on both the lesioned and the intact side.

γ-Hydroxybutyric Acid

γ-Hydroxybutyric acid is known to cause an increase in striatal DA (13) in the same way as cutting DA fibers (14). It was also found to mimic axotomy in stimulating tyrosine hydroxylase activity (Table 2). This effect, which was much more pronounced in the striatal than in the limbic DA system, may be due to the same kind of feedback activation as is induced

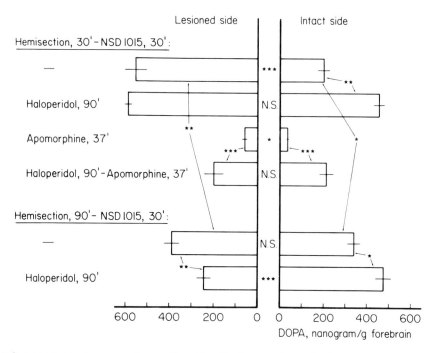

FIG. 3. Evidence for a receptor-mediated feedback control of striatal tyrosine hydroxylase activity (12). Ascending DA pathways were cut on the left side by means of a transverse hemisection of the brainstem at a level just rostral to the substantia nigra. NSD 1015 was injected to all animals either at the time of hemisection (top) or 60 min later (bottom). The animals were killed 30 min after the NSD 1015 injection. Groups of animals were pretreated as indicated with haloperidol (5 mg/kg, i.p.) or apomorphine (15 mg/kg, i.p.), 90 and 37 min before death, respectively. One group received a combination of these two drugs. Shown are the means ± SEM of DOPA accumulated in the forebrain as a result of decarboxylase inhibition. ⋯ $p < 0.001$; ⋯ $p < 0.01$; ⋅ $p < 0.05$; N.S. Not significant. *Note.* Hemisection caused a marked *in vivo* stimulation of tyrosine hydroxylase as compared to the intact side during the initial 30 min ($p < 0.001$), but not at the later 30-min period studied. Haloperidol stimulated tyrosine hydroxylase activity, but only on the intact side. Apomorphine inhibited the activity; this inhibition was significantly antagonized ($p < 0.001$) on both sides by haloperidol. Thus, the stimulating action of the receptor-blocking agent haloperidol appears to depend on the presence of an agonist (DA or apomorphine) at receptor sites. (Reproduced from *J. Pharm. Pharmacol.*)

by axotomy; γ-hydroxybutyric acid has been shown to inhibit firing in DA neurons of the substantia nigra (15).

Effect of Social Environment

The tyrosine hydroxylase activity of various brain regions was significantly reduced by isolating male mice for 6 to 8 weeks. If the isolated mice were again brought together, intense fighting was induced; these animals

TABLE 2. *Effect of γ-hydroxybutyric acid (1.5 g/kg, i.p.) on tyrosine hydroxylase activity in vivo in rat brain regions*

	Striatum	Limbic region
γ-OH-BA	1094 ± 110 (6)	656 ± 48 (3)
Control	378 ± 23 (8)	585 ± 24 (4)
Difference	716 ± 98	71 ± 49
	$p < 0.001$	N.S.

From Carlsson and Lindqvist, *unpublished data.*
Data show DOPA (ng/g) accumulated 30 min after NSD 1015, 100 mg/kg, means ± SEM (n).

had markedly elevated tyrosine hydroxylase activities in various brain regions (Modigh, *unpublished data*).

Cholinergic Control of Brain Tyrosine Hydroxylase Activity

Inhibition of cholinesterase by physostigmine (1 mg/kg, i.p.; the α-adrenergic blocking agent phentolamine was given simultaneously to prevent peripheral sympathomimetic activation) caused a significant activation of tyrosine hydroxylase in whole rat brain, suggesting that this enzyme is under some kind of cholinergic control (Carlsson and Lindqvist, *unpublished data*).

Ethanol and Diethyl Ether

Moderate doses of ethanol caused significant activation of tyrosine hydroxylase in different rat brain regions (16). In ether anesthesia, a considerable increase was found, particularly in the striatum (Kehr et al., *unpublished data*).

These effects may be related to the central stimulant properties of ethanol and ether: the stimulant action of ethanol on the motor activity of mice and rats can be efficiently prevented by pretreatment with α-methyltyrosine in moderate dosage (17). Analogous observations have been made in human subjects (18).

COMMENT

DA-carrying neuronal systems probably have a widespread distribution throughout the central nervous system. However, the majority of these systems are concentrated in a few regions, among which the striatum and some limbic structures are quantitatively most important.

The striatal DA appears to be under more rigorous feedback control than the limbic DA. As a striking illustration of this control, we consider the activation of striatal tyrosine hydroxylase by (a) axotomy, which probably

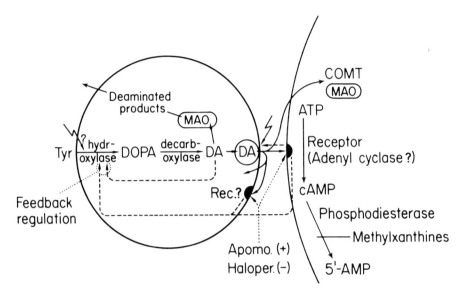

FIG. 4. Hypothetical model illustrating different mechanisms for short-term control of striatal tyrosine hydroxylase activity *in vivo*. The nerve terminal is shown to the left, the postsynaptic cell to the right. The most striking feature of striatal tyrosine hydroxylase control appears to be the receptor-mediated feedback regulation: a change in the degree of activation of postsynaptic (or hypothetical presynaptic) receptors will release a messenger capable of modulating tyrosine hydroxylase activity. The evidence for this hypothesis is derived from the interaction between axotomy, haloperidol, and apomorphine shown in Fig. 3.

The increased DA synthesis induced by axotomy, in conjunction with diminished release and metabolism, will induce a rapid increase in striatal DA. This, in turn, will result in end-product inhibition of tyrosine hydroxylase. The initial rise in tyrosine hydroxylase activity induced by axotomy (Fig. 3, top) will thus soon be balanced by end-product inhibition (Fig. 3, bottom).

The DA receptor may be adenylate cyclase, as suggested by recent observations (22).

reduces the concentration of DA at receptor sites, (b) γ-hydroxybutyric acid, which probably has a similar effect via inhibition of impulse generation, or (c) DA-receptor blocking agents. The mechanism of this apparently receptor-mediated feedback control, which appears to operate even in the absence of an impulse flow, is obscure. Some kind of chemical messenger or modulator influencing tyrosine hydroxylase activity and released by changes in postsynaptic (or, possibly, presynaptic) DA receptor activity must be postulated (see Fig. 4). Further work is needed to clarify this mechanism.

The above-mentioned paradoxical activation of striatal tyrosine hydroxylase after interruption or depression of the impulse flow raises the question of whether a supranormal impulse flow will also activate this enzyme in the striatum, as it does, for example, in the peripheral sympatho-adrenal system (4, 5). Even though direct evidence is not available, there is some support for this assumption. Thus, physostigmine (plus phentolamine) caused an increased tyrosine hydroxylase activity. This treatment was also found to cause a decrease in brain DA and NA levels and to accelerate the disappearance of brain catecholamines after inhibition of tyrosine hydroxylase (*unpublished data of this laboratory*). This is in contrast to the increase in striatal DA induced by impulse flow interruption and suggests the existence of a cholinergic mechanism, capable of increasing the firing of catecholamine-carrying fiber systems (*cf.* 19). In fact, the data of Ernst and Smelik (20), demonstrating dopaminergic stimulation by physostigmine implanted in the substantia nigra, suggest the existence of cholinergic receptors on nigral DA cells. Also, ethanol (see 21) and diethyl ether (*unpublished data*), if anything, reduce catecholamine levels in rat brain.

In the case of social stress, the data clearly support the assumption of an increase both in synthesis and turnover of catecholamines, and thus of increased firing by these neurons (Modigh, *unpublished data*).

The existence of Parkinson's disease, with specific lesions of DA-carrying neuronal systems, points to a special vulnerability of these systems. A high sensitivity to oxygen deprivation is suggested by those cases of parkinsonism in which carbon monoxide poisoning or arteriosclerosis appear to be causative factors. The question arises as to whether this phenomenon is related to the marked sensitivity of tyrosine hydroxylase to hypoxia, as referred to above. This interesting possibility merits further study.

ACKNOWLEDGMENTS

This study has been supported by grant B73–04X–155–09B from the Swedish Medical Research Council.

REFERENCES

1. Atack, C. V., and Magnusson, T., *J. Pharm. Pharmacol.* 22, 625 (1970).
2. Atack, C. V., *Brit. J. Pharmacol.*, 48, 699 (1973).
3. Thierry, A. M., Stinus, L., Blanc, G., and Glowinski, J., *Brain Res.* 50, 230 (1973).
4. Snider, S. R., and Carlsson, A., *Naunyn-Schmiedeberg's Arch. Pharmacol.* 275, 347 (1972).
5. Snider, S. R., Almgren, O., and Carlsson, A., *Naunyn-Schmiedeberg's Arch. Pharmacol.*, 278, 1 (1973).
6. Carlsson, A., Davis, J. N., Kehr, W., Lindqvist, M., and Atack, C. V., *Naunyn-Schmiedeberg's Arch. Pharmacol.* 275, 153 (1972).
7. Magnusson, T., *Naunyn-Schmiedeberg's Arch. Pharmacol. (in press)*.
8. Fisher, D. B., and Kaufman, S., *J. Neurochem.* 19, 1359 (1972).
9. Green, H., and Sawyer, J. L., *Anal. Biochem.* 15, 53 (1956).
10. Davis, J. N., and Carlsson, A., *J. Neurochem.*, 20, 913 (1973).
11. Brown, R., Davis, J. N., and Carlsson, A., *J. Pharm. Pharmacol.*, 25, 412 (1973).
12. Kehr, W., Carlsson, A., and Lindqvist, M., *J. Pharm. Pharmacol.* 24, 744 (1972).
13. Gessa, G. L., Crabai, F., Vargin, L., and Spano, P. F., *J. Neurochem.* 15, 377 (1968).
14. Andén, N.-E., Bédard, P., Fuxe, K., and Ungerstedt, U., *Experientia* 28, 300 (1972).

15. Walters, J. R., Aghajanian, G. K., and Roth, R. H., *Proc. Fifth Pharmacol. Congr.* Abstract Vol., 246, San Francisco (1972).
16. Carlsson, A., and Lindqvist, M., *J. Pharm. Pharmacol.* 25, 437 (1973).
17. Carlsson, A., Engel, J., and Svensson, T. H., *Psychopharmacologia* 26, 307 (1972).
18. Ahlenius, S., Carlsson, A., Engel, J., Svensson, T. H., and Södersten, P., *Clin. Pharmacol. Ther.,* 14, 586 (1973).
19. Corrodi, H., Fuxe, K., Hammer, W., Sjöquist, F., and Ungerstedt, U., *Life Sci.* 6, 2557 (1967).
20. Ernst, A. M., and Smelik, P. G., *Experientia* 22, 837 (1966).
21. Carlsson, A., Magnusson, T., Svensson, T. H., and Waldeck, B., *Psychopharmacologia,* 30, 27 (1973).
22. Kebabian, J. W., Petzold, G. L., and Greengard, P., *Proc. Nat. Acad. Sci.* 69, 2145 (1972).

Advances in Neurology, Vol. 5
Raven Press, New York © 1974

In Vivo Spontaneous and Evoked Release of Newly Synthesized Dopamine in the Cat Caudate Nucleus

M. J. Besson, A. Cheramy, C. Gauchy, and J. Glowinski

Groupe NB (INSERM U 114) Laboratoire de Biologie Moléculaire, Collège de France, Paris 5ᵉ, France

Various biochemical and pharmacological studies have been made to elucidate the role of the nigrostriatal dopaminergic pathway in extra-pyramidal processes. However, the transmitter release from dopaminergic (DA) terminals has been examined by only a few groups of researchers. This is mainly related to the difficulty of release studies made in deep structures of the brain. During the last few years, we have investigated various aspects of the DA release process of the surface of the caudate nucleus in the awake cat, locally anesthetized and immobilized with gallamine (Flaxedil®). First, a part of the ventricular surface of the nucleus is covered by a cup and continuously superfused with a physiological medium. Secondly, DA terminals underlying this delimited area are continuously labeled with L-3, 5-^{3}H-tyrosine contained in the superfusing fluid. Under these conditions, part of ^{3}H-DA newly synthesized from labeled tyrosine is released and can be estimated in superfusates. Finally, information about the rate of synthesis of the labeled transmitter can be simultaneously obtained by measurements of ^{3}H-H_2O quantities diffused in superfusates since ^{3}H-water is formed in DA terminals during the conversion of ^{3}H-tyrosine into ^{3}H-DOPA. Levels of ^{3}H-H_2O found in superfusates very likely underestimate the quantity of ^{3}H-DA synthesized since some of the radioactive water may be eliminated by circulatory processes. Nevertheless, the estimation of ^{3}H-H_2O in collected fractions provides an index of the first and limiting step of the ^{3}H-transmitter synthesis.

VALIDITY OF THE CUP TECHNIQUE FOR DA RELEASE STUDIES

Electrophysiological (1) and microscopic (Calas et al., *unpublished observations*) studies have revealed that superfused neuronal tissue is well preserved for many hours. Evoked potentials induced by stimulation of the substantia nigra could be recorded (1) from electrodes implanted into the cup in the superficial layer of the caudate nucleus (0.8 mm in depth). Auto-radiographic pictures indicated that ^{3}H-tyrosine was mainly localized in a superficial layer of the caudate nucleus (1 mm depth). And electron micro-scopic studies revealed that nerve terminals were well preserved. The use of purified labeled tyrosine of high specific radioactivity and of adapted tech-niques of ^{3}H-catecholamine (CA) separation by ion-exchange chroma-tography on CG-50 amberlite column and adsorption on alumina allowed reliable estimations of ^{3}H-CA quantities as low as 0.3 nC in the presence of a large amount of ^{3}H-tyrosine (40 μC).

Generally, 1 to 2 nC of ^{3}H-CA was spontaneously released in 10-min fractions. Acetylation of the ^{3}H-CA and co-chromatography indicated that ^{3}H-DA was the only labeled amine released; ^{3}H-NE was undetectable. Even after 7 to 8 hr of continuous superfusion with ^{3}H-tyrosine, ^{3}H-CA in the caudate nucleus was primarily ^{3}H-DA; ^{3}H-NE corresponded to only 2% of total ^{3}H-CA (1).

EFFECT OF NERVE ACTIVITY ON THE RELEASE OF NEWLY SYNTHESIZED ^{3}H-DA

Labeled DA was detectable in superfusates immediately after the onset of superfusion with L-3,5-^{3}H-tyrosine. The spontaneously released ^{3}H-transmitter quantities increased rapidly during the first hour and reached four to six times blank values. ^{3}H-DA spontaneous release then increased more slowly over time. Resting release of ^{3}H-DA is mainly dependent on nerve impulses. This was demonstrated in two ways. (a) The spontaneous release of newly synthesized ^{3}H-DA was immediately and markedly re-duced (60%) after the introduction of tetrodotoxin (10^{-5} g/ml) into the super-fusing medium (Fig. 1) (1). (b) The frontal transection of the nigrostriatal pathway performed with a metallic spatula (in mm A, 7; L, 1 to 7; H, −5) completely blocked the ^{3}H-transmitter release (Fig. 1) despite its persistent synthesis as revealed by the increased accumulation of ^{3}H-DA in DA termi-nals (2). Moreover, when ^{3}H-H$_2$O was estimated in serially collected frac-tions, L-3,5-^{3}H-tyrosine–^{3}H-DOPA conversion was significantly decreased (30%) 2 hr after the section of the nigrostriatal pathway (2). This result sug-gests that ^{3}H-DA synthesis in DA terminals is partly dependent on nerve activity.

Depolarization of DA nerve terminals, induced by an excess of potassium (30 mM) in the superfusing medium, markedly stimulated ^{3}H-DA release. Quantities of the ^{3}H-transmitter found in superfusates were at least 10 times those observed during spontaneous release. When potassium was added during two successive 10-min fractions, ^{3}H-DA released in the second fraction was reduced by 50% as compared to the first one. Furthermore,

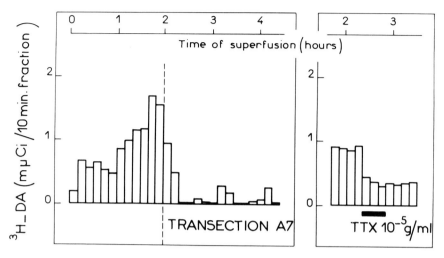

FIG. 1. Effects of transection of the nigrostriatal pathway and of tetrodotoxin (TTX) on ^{3}H-DA release. ^{3}H-DA was estimated in serially collected fractions during the continuous superfusion of a limited ventricular surface of the left caudate nucleus with L-3,5-^{3}H-tyrosine (40 μC/ml) in the awake, curarized cat. Transection was made with a metallic spatula [in mm: A, 7; L, 1 to 7; H, −5, according to the stereotaxic atlas of Jasper and Ajmone Marsan (20)]. TTX was added for 30 min into the superfusing medium.

spontaneous release of ^{3}H-DA was lower after potassium application than before introduction of the depolarizing agent. These two effects may be attributed to a rapid diminution of quantities of labeled transmitter available for release or to changes in membrane permeability (1).

In collaboration with D. Albe-Fessard, attempts have been made to estimate ^{3}H-DA release during stimulation of the pars compacta of the sub-stantia nigra. In our experimental conditions (20 Hz, 0.2 msec, 5 V), a 50% increase in ^{3}H-DA release was noted only in the fraction which followed the 10-min stimulation period. Curiously, in a few cases but not all, ^{3}H-DA release was markedly enhanced during the stimulation of the reticular forma-tion. In successful experiments, quantities of ^{3}H-DA released during stimulation and the immediate following 10-min period were approximately 250% those detected during spontaneous release (Table 1). Release of DA from DA terminals in the cat caudate nucleus has also been examined after stimulation of DA cell bodies and axons by other workers who have used different experimental approaches. Generally, the stimulation of cell bodies in the pars compacta of the substantia nigra induced an inconsistent release of DA (3–5). More constant and pronounced effects were obtained by stimu-lation of the dopaminergic pathway (4, 6). Interneuronal activation of DA neurons resulting in an increase in DA release has also been shown after stimulation of the nucleus centromedianus of the thalamus (7).

TABLE 1. *Effects of some mesencephalic stimulations on newly synthesized ^{3}H-DA release*

Structure	^{3}H-DA released in 10-min fraction		
	Before	Stimulation	After
SN	100 ± 6 (20)	107 ± 5	150 ± 20
MRF	100 ± 6 (3)	240 ± 70	255 ± 30
RN	100 (1)	345	185

The surface of the cat caudate nucleus was continuously super-fused with L-3,5-^{3}H-tyrosine (40 μC/ml) using the cup technique. Stimulation of the substantia nigra (SN), of the mesencephalic reticular formation (MRF), and of the red nucleus (RN) was made with bipolar electrodes (20 Hz, 0.2 msec, 5 V) at least 60 min after the onset of superfusion. The number of experiments is indicated in parentheses. Results are expressed as percent of ^{3}H-DA quantities measured in the 10-min fraction preceding the stimulation period.

EFFECTS OF VARIOUS DRUGS ON THE *IN VIVO* SYNTHESIS AND RELEASE OF ^{3}H-DA

Important changes in ^{3}H-DA release and synthesis have been observed with various drugs known to interact with DA metabolism in nigrostriatal DA neurons.

Inhibition of DA synthesis induced by local application of α-methyl-*para*-tyrosine (α-MpT) into the cup or after its intravenous injection rapidly reduced the spontaneous release of the labeled transmitter (Fig. 2). This effect on ^{3}H-DA release paralleled the inhibition of ^{3}H-DA synthesis which was visualized by the immediate reduction of ^{3}H-H$_2$O formation (Fig. 2) (2).

The inhibition of ^{3}H-H$_2$O output seen after α-MpT treatment indicates that labeled water is formed solely during the conversion of L-3,5-^{3}H-tyrosine into ^{3}H-DOPA in DA terminals. This was further demonstrated in the rat after complete degeneration of the nigrostriatal DA pathway; in this preparation ^{3}H-H$_2$O was no longer detectable in tissues after the microinjection of L-3,5-^{3}H-tyrosine into the striatum (8). On the other hand, it should be mentioned that ^{3}H-DA release could not be detected in superfusates after the administration of α-MpT despite the presence of high quantities of ^{3}H-DA still stored in tissues (Fig. 2) (2). The marked inhibition of ^{3}H-DA release observed immediately after the drug injection reveals the importance of the newly synthesized transmitter in DA release process. This is in agreement with other studies obtained in our laboratory which have indicated the existence of at least two DA storage forms in DA terminals (9).

In earlier experiments we demonstrated that D-amphetamine increased the release of ^{3}H-DA synthesized from L-3,5-^{3}H-tyrosine in the isolated striatum (10) or in striatal slices (11) of the rat. Similar observations were made in the awake cat preparation. D-Amphetamine locally applied in very

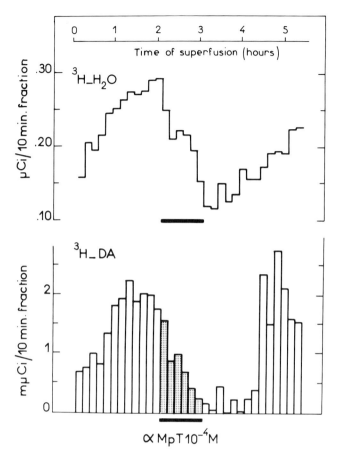

FIG. 2. Effect of α-MpT on the synthesis and release of ^{3}H-DA formed from ^{3}H-tyrosine in the cat caudate nucleus. ^{3}H-DA and ^{3}H-H$_2$O were estimated in successive fractions during the continuous superfusion of the surface of the caudate nucleus with L-3,5-^{3}H-tyrosine (40 μC/ml, 1 ml/10 min). The black horizontal bar represents the period of introduction of α-MpT into the cup.

low concentrations (10^{-6} M) increased ^{3}H-DA release by 400 to 450% (1). This effect was observed during the drug application and immediately following it. Enhancement of ^{3}H-DA release was also particularly striking after the intravenous injection of L-amphetamine (2 mg/kg) (1). Other workers have shown the effect of the local application of D-amphetamine on DA release in the cat caudate nucleus, but they used much larger concentrations of the drug (4, 12). The changes in DA release observed with small drug doses underlined the sensitivity of our experimental approach. Amphetamine may exert its effect by a direct releasing action. Both D and L-amphetamine have been shown to be potent inhibitors of the DA uptake process in rat striatal synaptosome (13); this effect, however, may be less important than the releasing action of the drug since benzotropine, another potent DA uptake inhibitor, did not act as quickly as amphetamine when added into the cup.

Inhibition of one of the main catabolic pathways of DA should affect quantities of DA available at receptor sites. This was observed after the local application or intravenous injection of various compounds known to inhibit MAO. However, some differences were seen in the effects induced by these drugs. They are certainly related to their chemical structure and to their specificity of action.

For instance, peniprazine, an MAO inhibitor (MAOI) structurally related to amphetamine, induced a marked increase in ^{3}H-DA release during its local application similar to that observed with amphetamine. In contrast, pargyline (10^{-5} M) produced a slight but long-lasting effect on the release of ^{3}H-DA. Tranylcypromine action was intermediate between those of peniprazine and pargyline. Pargyline (100 mg/kg) and tranylcypromine (10 mg/kg) also increased the ^{3}H-DA release when injected intravenously. Furthermore, in these cases, as indicated by the estimation of ^{3}H-H_2O in superfusates, the drugs gradually inhibited the *in vivo* synthesis of ^{3}H-DA from L-3,5-^{3}H-tyrosine (about 50% inhibition 2 hr after their intravenous injection). This effect is very likely related to the intraneuronal negative feedback process involved in the regulation of DA synthesis which has been demonstrated in both *in vivo* and *in vitro* studies made on the rat striatum (14).

Reversible inhibitors of MAO have also been tested. Harmine and harmaline (3,4-dihydroharmine) markedly increased ^{3}H-DA release when added to the cup. Curiously, harmine (20 mg/kg) or harmaline (20 mg/kg) was no more effective on ^{3}H-DA release when injected intravenously, whereas a marked reduction of the formation of ^{3}H-H_2O was observed as for the other MAOI. This underlines again the complexity of action of the various MAOI on DA metabolism.

Anticholinergic drugs, such as atropine and benzotropine, have been extensively used in parkinsonian therapy. These compounds have also been shown to inhibit DA uptake in striatal dopaminergic synaptosomes of the rat (15). However, benzotropine is much more active than atropine: the respective concentrations of the drugs which reduced DA uptake by 50% were 2×10^{-7} and 5×10^{-5} M. The direct application of benzotropine into the cup resulted in a progressive enhancement of the quantities of ^{3}H-DA released into superfusates (Fig. 3) (16). In less than an hour after drug application, the release of newly synthesized ^{3}H-DA was increased sevenfold as compared to spontaneous release. This effect can be attributed to an inhibition of the uptake process but also to a stimulation of ^{3}H-DA synthesis: ^{3}H-H_2O quantities formed during the conversion of L-3,5-^{3}H-tyrosine into ^{3}H-DOPA were increased by at least 70% as soon as 1 hr after the drug

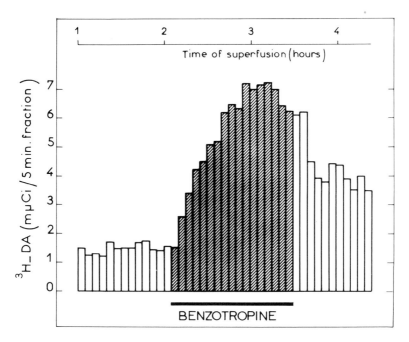

FIG. 3. Effect of benzotropine on ^{3}H-DA release. A limited ventricular surface of the left caudate nucleus was superfused with L-3,5-^{3}H-tyrosine (40 μC/ml) as described in Figs. 1 and 2. The black horizontal bar represents the period of introduction of benzotropine (10^{-6} M) into the cup. (Reproduced, with permission, from the *European Journal of Pharmacology*.)

addition (16). Atropine, although less effective than benzotropine, also stimulated ^{3}H-DA release.

It has been well established in various biochemical studies that neuroleptics of the phenothiazine or butyrophenone type markedly accelerate the turnover of DA in DA terminals. In previous studies in the rat (17), we observed that thioproperazine, a potent neuroleptic with marked cataleptic properties, was able to accelerate ^{3}H-DA synthesis and release in striatal slices only when injected before the animal sacrifice. These results supported the DA receptor blockade hypothesis postulated by various workers to explain the action of neuroleptics on DA metabolism. According to this hypothesis, the activity of DA neurons is increased by an interneuronal regulatory process induced by the blockade of DA receptors. It was of interest to investigate the effects of thioproperazine on the *in vivo* synthesis and release of ^{3}H-DA in the cat preparation. The intravenous injection of the drug (5 mg/kg) resulted in stimulation of the synthesis and release of ^{3}H-DA as indicated by the gradual increase over time of ^{3}H-H$_2$O and ^{3}H-DA quantities detected in superfusates (18). This observation provides the first direct evidence of the action of a neuroleptic on the *in vivo* DA release from DA terminals.

Another line of research was simultaneously followed in our release studies. The caudate nucleus contains numerous serotoninergic terminals and is particularly rich in acetylcholine (ACh) and in choline acetylase; serotoninergic or cholinergic neurons could interact directly with DA terminals and affect DA release.

In earlier studies made on the superfused isolated striatum of the rat (10), we observed that both serotonin (5-HT) and ACh stimulated the release of ^{3}H-DA previously synthesized from L-3,5-^{3}H-tyrosine. These findings prompted us to repeat these experiments on the *in vivo* cat preparation.

5-HT (10^{-5} M) added into the cup markedly enhanced the release of newly synthesized ^{3}H-DA. A very pronounced effect was observed with exogenous DA (10^{-5} M) (Table 2). Although 5-HT can be taken up into 5-HT neurons by a specific transport (K_m, 1.7×10^{-7} M) (15), the amine may also penetrate into DA terminals (K_m, 8×10^{-6} M) when added in concentrations similar to those used in our experiments (10^{-5} M). Both 5-HT and DA (K_m, 4×10^{-7} M) newly taken up in DA terminals may displace the newly synthesized ^{3}H-DA and favor its release. In fact, DA and to a lesser extent 5-HT effects on ^{3}H-DA release could be partially abolished by benzotropine, an inhibitor of DA uptake (Table 2). The introduction of ACh into the superfusing fluid also affected the release of ^{3}H-DA, but the effect was less pronounced than that observed with 5-HT. These data suggest possible relationships between 5-HT, ACh, and DA neuronal systems. Further

TABLE 2. *Effects of exogenous DA and 5-HT on the release of ^{3}H-DA synthesized from L-3,5-^{3}H-tyrosine*

Drugs	Before application	During application	After application
DA (10^{-5} M)	100 (3)	710	155
DA (10^{-5} M) + benzotropine (10^{-6} M)	100 (3)	200	140
5-HT (10^{-5} M)	100 (4)	210	140
5-HT (10^{-5} M) + benzotropine (10^{-6} M)	100 (2)	135	60

^{3}H-DA was estimated in successive 10-min collected fractions during the continuous superfusion of the surface of the caudate nucleus with the ^{3}H-amino acid. DA and 5-HT were added into the cup for 10 min. In experiments made in the presence of benzotropine, the drug was continuously introduced into the cup with L-3,5-^{3}H-tyrosine. The number of experiments is indicated in parentheses. Results are the mean of ^{3}H-DA quantities collected during and after the application of exogenous amines. They are expressed in percent of steady state values (quantities of ^{3}H-DA found in the fraction preceding the amines introduction into the cup).

experiments, including direct stimulation of 5-HT and ACh pathways, should be theoretically required to establish such relations definitively.

CONCLUSION

The use of a cup technique to superfuse DA terminals of a limited area of the ventricular surface of the cat caudate nucleus has been particularly fruitful in the investigation of various aspects of DA release. Continuous labeling of DA terminals with radioactive tyrosine offered various advantages. (a) ^{3}H-DA, which can be synthesized from this precursor only in DA terminals, is specifically released from these neurons. (b) The method is very sensitive since the release of the newly synthesized transmitter mainly involved in the release process is estimated. (c) Simultaneous information on ^{3}H-DA synthesis and release can be obtained over long periods in the awake, curarized animal. (d) Spontaneous release of ^{3}H-DA can be easily estimated and effects of drugs locally applied in low concentrations or injected intravenously can be demonstrated in a reproducible manner.

With this approach it could be particularly shown that changes in nerve activity resulted in marked effects on ^{3}H-DA release: the spontaneous release could be strongly diminished by tetrodotoxin and by a frontal transection of the nigrostriatal pathway. Conversely, an increased release of ^{3}H-DA could be observed after addition of potassium and stimulation of the substantia nigra and the reticular formation.

The release of newly synthesized ^{3}H-DA was increased by various drugs known to interfere with one or many processes of DA metabolism. Amphetamine and pheniprazine appeared to be powerful releasing agents. MAOI induced different effects: their potency on ^{3}H-DA release seems to depend on their chemical structure or on the route of administration. Inhibition of DA reuptake by benzotropine was followed by a progressive and marked increase in the extraneuronal quantities of the labeled transmitter. Similar observations were made after indirect activation of DA neurons with thioproperazine, a neuroleptic agent. Conversely, the inhibition of DA synthesis with α-MpT immediately suppressed the release of ^{3}H-DA. All these modifications in ^{3}H-DA release were associated with changes in the ^{3}H-transmitter synthesis. However, the estimation of the radioactive water formed during the conversion of ^{3}H-tyrosine into ^{3}H-DOPA is only an index of the labeled transmitter synthesis. At present we cannot definitively conclude that changes in ^{3}H-H$_2$O formation exactly parallel those of the synthesis of the nonlabeled transmitter since the specific activity of tyrosine in the pool involved in DA synthesis may vary under different experimental conditions. Experiments are in progress to measure simultaneously the release of nonlabeled and labeled DA. They should provide interesting and complementary information about the respective contribution of various DA storage forms in the spontaneous or evoked release of the transmitter.

The cup technique described in this chapter has recently been adapted to use in a chronic monkey preparation. Spontaneous and drug-evoked release of ^{3}H-DA could be estimated for many days in the free-moving animal (19). Experiments on the cat or monkey should in the future enable us to improve our knowledge on the rapid or long-term changes in the activity of the DA-nigrostriatal pathway occurring in various pharmacological or pathological states. We also hope to obtain new information on the inter-neuronal regulatory processes involved in the control of this DA neuronal system.

ACKNOWLEDGMENTS

This research was supported by grants of the DGRST, CNRS, INSERM, and DRME.

REFERENCES

1. Besson, M. J., Cheramy, A., Feltz, P., and Glowinski, J., *Brain Res.* 32, 407, (1971).
2. Besson, M. J., Cheramy, A., Gauchy, C., and Glowinski, J., *Naunyn—Schmiedeberg's Arch. Pharmacol.* 278, 101 (1973).
3. Vogt, M., *Br. J. Pharmac.* 37, 325 (1969).
4. Riddell, D., and Szerb, J. C., *J. Neurochem.* 18, 989 (1971).
5. Von Voigtlander, P. F., and Moore, K. E., *Neuropharmacol.* 10, 733 (1971*a*).
6. Von Voigtlander, P. F., and Moore, K. E., *Brain Res.* 35, 580 (1971*b*).
7. McLennan, H., *J. Physiol.* 174, 152 (1964).
8. Javoy, F., Agid, Y., Sotelo, C., and Glowinski, J., *Symposium on "Dynamics of Degeneration and Growth in Neurons,"* Stockholm (1973).
9. Javoy, F., and Glowinski, J., *J. Neurochem.* 18, 1305 (1971).
10. Besson, M. J., Cheramy, A., Feltz, D., and Glowinski, J., *Proc. Nat. Acad. Sci.* 62, 741 (1969*a*).
11. Besson, M. J., Cheramy, A., and Glowinski, J., *Europ. J. Pharmacol.* 7, 111 (1969*b*).
12. McKenzie, G. M., and Szerb, J. C., *J. Pharmacol. Exp. Ther.* 162, 302 (1968).
13. Coyle, J. T., and Snyder, S. M., *J. Pharmacol. Exp. Ther.* 170, 221 (1969).
14. Javoy, F., Agid, Y., Bouvet, D., and Glowinski, J., *J. Pharmacol. Exp. Ther.* 182, 454 (1972).
15. Snyder, S. H. *Biol. Psychiat.* 2, 367 (1970).
16. Cheramy, A., Gauchy, C., Glowinski, J., and Besson, M. J., *Europ. J. Pharmacol.* 21, 246 (1973).
17. Cheramy, A., Besson, M. J., and Glowinski, J., *Europ. J. Pharmacol.* 10, 206 (1970).
18. Cheramy, A., Javoy, F., Besson, M. J., Gauchy, C., and Glowinski, J., *C.I.N.P. Meeting: Striatum and Neuroleptics,* Copenhagen (1972) *in press.*
19. Bioulac, B., Gauchy, C., Cheramy, A., Besson, M. J., Glowinski, J., and Vincent, D. *Fed. Proc.,* 32, 3372 (1973).
20. Jasper, H. H., and Ajmone Marsan, C., *Stereotoxic Atlas of the Diencephalon of the Cat.* Nat. Res. Council of Canada, Ottawa (1954).

Advances in Neurology, Vol. 5
Raven Press, New York © 1974

Mechanisms Involved in the Control of Extrapyramidal Dysfunctions and in Striatal Dopamine Synthesis

M. Goldstein, B. Anagnoste, A. F. Battista, T. Miyamoto,
and K. Fuxe

Departments of Psychiatry and Neurosurgery, Neurochemistry Laboratories, New York University Medical Center, New York, New York 10016, and Department of Histology, Karolinska Institutet, 104 01 Stockholm, Sweden

In the past decade it was demonstrated that parkinsonism can result either from depletion of dopamine in the basal ganglia or from drug-induced blockade of dopamine receptors (1, 2). Evidence has also been presented that degeneration of the nigro-striatal dopamine pathway causes a supersensitivity of the dopamine receptors (3). The purpose of this chapter is to present data which will show that the activity of dopamine receptors affects the extrapyramidal dysfunction. In addition, we will report on the effects of activation and blockade of dopamine receptors and on the effects of cyclic-AMP on ^{14}C-dopamine biosynthesis in striatal slices.

THE EFFECTS OF L-DOPA AND OF AGENTS THAT STIMULATE DOPAMINE RECEPTORS ON RELIEF OF TREMOR AND ON DEVELOPMENT OF INVOLUNTARY MOVEMENTS IN EXPERIMENTAL MONKEYS

In these studies, green monkeys *(Cercopithecus sabaeus)* with ventro-medial tegmental lesions, which exhibit hypokinesia and resting tremor of the contralateral extremities, were used (4, 5). The effects of L-DOPA and of agents that stimulate dopamine receptors on the relief of tremor and on the induction of involuntary movements in monkeys are summarized in Table 1. The administration of L-DOPA in combination with 1-α-methyl-dopa hydrazine (MK 486), a DOPA decarboxylase inhibitor that acts peripherally, resulted in a transient disappearance of tremor in the extremities contralateral to the lesion, with a concomitant development of involuntary movements. Trivastal® (ET 495), an agent that stimulates dopamine receptors (6), had an effect similar to that of L-DOPA (7). Trivastal® relieved the tremor and induced involuntary movements for a longer period of time than L-DOPA. 2-Br-α-ergocryptine (CB 154), another

TABLE 1. *The effects of DOPA and of agents that stimulate dopamine receptors on tremor and on the development of involuntary movements (IM) in monkeys with VMT lesions*

Surgical lesion	Drugs* (mg/kg)	Motor impairment	Type of IM**
None	MK 486 (10) + L-DOPA (300) or ET 495 (3)	None	I
VMT	None	Hypokinesia and tremor	None
VMT	MK 486 (10) + L-DOPA (200)	Tremor stopped (1–2 hr)	I, II
VMT	ET 495 (3)	Tremor stopped (3–4 hr)	I, II
VMT	CB 154 (10)	Tremor relieved (3–24 hr)	I, II

* MK 486 was given i.p. 60 min prior to the i.p. administration of L-DOPA. CB 154 was given i.p. and ET 495 was given i.v.
** IM type I: Increased aggressiveness and restlessness, increased water intake. IM type II: Chorea-like movements (contralateral to VMT lesion), unusual posture, facial grimaces.

agent that stimulates dopamine receptors (8), also has tremor-relieving and involuntary movement-inducing activities (Goldstein, Battista, Miyamoto, and Fuxe, *unpublished data*).

THE EFFECTS OF ACTIVATION AND BLOCKADE OF DOPAMINE RECEPTORS ON DOPAMINE SYNTHESIS IN STRIATAL SLICES

In a previous study we have shown that apomorphine, an agent that stimulates dopamine receptors, inhibits the biosynthesis of ^{14}C-dopamine from ^{14}C-tyrosine more effectively in striatal slices than tyrosine hydroxylase activity *in vitro* (9). The effective inhibition of ^{14}C-dopamine biosynthesis in striatal slices by apomorphine could be due either to its accumulation in the dopamine-containing neurons and subsequent inhibition of tyrosine hydroxylase or to dopamine-receptor stimulating activity of the drug, resulting in a feedback control of dopamine biosynthesis (9).

To study further the effects of activation or blockade of dopamine receptors on presynaptic dopamine synthesis, we have investigated the effects of Trivastal® and of haloperidol on ^{14}C-dopamine synthesis from ^{14}C-tyrosine in striatal slices. Trivastal® stimulates dopamine receptors (6), but, unlike apomorphine, does not contain a catechol group and does not inhibit tyrosine hydroxylase activity *in vitro* (10). It is evident from the results presented in Table 2 that administration of Trivastal® results in an inhibition, while administration of haloperidol results in the stimulation of ^{14}C-dopamine synthesis in striatal slices. Treatment of rats with haloperidol

TABLE 2. *The effects of blockade of dopamine receptors by haloperidol and of stimulation of dopamine receptors by apomorphine or by Trivastal® on ^{14}C-dopamine synthesis in striatal slices*

Treatment*	^{14}C-Dopamine formed (ng/g/hr)	Percent change from controls
Controls	248 ± 30	
Haloperidol	390 ± 40	+57
Apomorphine	158 ± 18	−37
Trivastal®	181 ± 20	−28
Haloperidol + apomorphine**	310 ± 25	+24

* Haloperidol (10 mg/kg, i.p.), apomorphine (15 mg/kg, i.p.), Trivastal® (15 mg/kg, i.p.) were given 1 hr before the animals were sacrificed.
** Haloperidol was given (10 mg/kg, i.p.) 1 hr prior to the administration of apomorphine (15 mg/kg, i.p.). The animals were sacrificed 1 hr after the administration of apomorphine.

antagonizes the Trivastal®-induced inhibition of ^{14}C-dopamine synthesis (10). These results support the idea that a receptor-mediated feedback exists which controls the rate of dopamine synthesis (11).

THE EFFECTS OF CYCLIC AMP ON DOPAMINE SYNTHESIS IN STRIATAL SLICES AND IN OTHER REGIONS OF THE CENTRAL NERVOUS SYSTEM

The findings that agents which stimulate or block dopamine receptors affect the rate of striatal dopamine synthesis (9, 10, 11) and the recently presented evidence that a dopamine-sensitive adenylate cyclase may be the receptor for dopamine in mammalian brain (12) prompted us to investigate the effects of cyclic AMP on ^{14}C-dopamine synthesis from ^{14}C-tyrosine in slices obtained from various regions of the brain. The results of our studies have shown that dibutyryl cyclic AMP (dB-cAMP) stimulates the synthesis of ^{14}C-dopamine in striatal slices (Table 3) as well as in other regions of the brain (i.e., median eminence, cortex). In separate experiments, it was established that the cyclic nucleotide and not the butyryl moiety of dB-cAMP is effective in the stimulation of ^{14}C-dopamine synthesis. The dB-cAMP-induced stimulation of ^{14}C-dopamine synthesis was not abolished by blocking the dopamine receptors with haloperidol or by stimulating the dopamine receptors with Trivastal® (Table 3). However, this phenomenon may be dose dependent, since the results of preliminary studies indicate that the stimulation of ^{14}C-dopamine synthesis by low concentrations of dB-cAMP (5×10^{-5} M) is less effective in striatal slices obtained from haloperidol-treated rats than from the untreated controls.

The dB-cAMP-induced stimulation of ^{14}C-dopamine synthesis is antagonized by the feedback inhibition resulting from the addition of dopamine

TABLE 3. *The effect of dB-cAMP and of agents that block or stimulate dopamine receptors on ^{14}C-dopamine synthesis from ^{14}C-tyrosine in striatal slices*

Treatment	dB-cAMP (M)	^{14}C-Dopamine in striatal slices (ng/g/hr)	Percent change from control
None (control)		248 ± 28	−
Haloperidol		390 ± 44	+ 57
None	5 × 10^{-4}	580 ± 60	+135
Haloperidol	5 × 10^{-4}	690 ± 75	+176
Trivastal ®	−	181 ± 20	− 28
Trivastal ®	5 × 10^{-4}	555 ± 60	+123

Haloperidol (10 mg/kg) and Trivastal® (15 mg/kg) were given i.p. 1 hr before the animals were sacrificed.

to media in which the slices were incubated (Table 4). These findings indicate that dB-cAMP-induced stimulation occurs at the tyrosine hydroxylase step.

TABLE 4. *The effects of dopamine on cyclic AMP-induced stimulation of ^{14}C-dopamine synthesis*

Additions	^{14}C-Dopamine synthesis (ng/g/hr)	Percent inhibition or stimulation
None	275.5 ± 29.0	
Dopamine; 2 × 10^{-6}M	98.5 ± 8.5	−64
dB-cAMP; 5 × 10^{-4}M	635.0 ± 68.0	+130
dB-cAMP; 5 × 10^{-4}M + dopamine; 2 × 10^{-6}M	195.5 ± 21.5	−69 +98*

*This figure represents the percent cyclic AMP-induced stimulation when compared with incubations in the presence of dopamine.

DISCUSSION

Abnormal involuntary movements have emerged as the major dose-limiting side effect in achieving optimal therapeutic results with L-DOPA. An animal model could be very useful in studies on the mechanisms involved in the production of dyskinesias. It was reported that L-DOPA induces involuntary movements in normal squirrel monkeys (13). The findings that green monkeys with chronic denervation of the nigro-striatal pathway produced by surgical ventromedial tegmental lesions are more susceptible to development of involuntary movements by DOPA or by agents that stimulate dopamine receptors than normal monkeys (7, 14) indicate that the supersensitivity of the dopamine receptors facilitates the appearance of dyskinesias. The supersensitivity of the dopamine receptors probably also facilitates the L-amphetamine-induced involuntary movements in monkeys with ventromedial tegmental lesions (Goldstein and Battista, *unpublished data*). Since the dopamine concentration in monkeys with ventromedial tegmental lesions is reduced by approximately 80 to 90% on the lesion side in the striatum, the question has arisen whether the L-amphetamine-induced involuntary movements are due to the release of dopamine from the lesion side of the striatum. In a separate study, we have investigated the effects of the ventromedial tegmental lesion on the monoaminergic pathways in the striatum (Battista, Goldstein, and Fuxe, *unpublished data*). The results of the histochemical fluorescence analysis have shown a marked disappearance of the fluorescence in the dopamine nerve terminals of the striatum on the lesion side, but a sparse meshwork of dopamine nerve terminals remains which could have an important functional significance.

The data presented here indicate that tremor and involuntary movements are associated with a common mechanism and that extrapyramidal dysfunctions are influenced by the activity of dopamine receptors. The separation of the tremor relief from involuntary movement induction might be a prerequisite for the therapeutic usefulness of an antiparkinsonian agent. Thus, agents that mildly stimulate dopamine receptors might be therapeutically effective in parkinsonism and in other extrapyramidal disorders. Furthermore, our results suggest that agents which increase the levels of cyclic AMP in the striatum should be tested for antiparkinsonian activity.

It seems that the isolation and characterization of "dopamine receptors" might be central to the understanding of the pharmacology of the extrapyramidal system from a theoretical and therapeutic standpoint. The hypothesis that adenylate cyclase might be the receptor for dopamine in the brain (12) is a very intriguing one, but further studies are required to substantiate or deny it. We (Goldstein, Ebstein, and Ungerstedt, *unpublished data*) and others (von Voigtlander, *personal communication*) have analyzed adenylate cyclase activity in the striatum of rats following unilateral degeneration of the nigro-striatal pathway. Preliminary results of these studies do not show any difference in the adenylate cyclase activity or in the dopamine-induced stimulation of the enzyme activity on the lesion side when compared with the intact side. If adenylate cyclase is indeed the receptor for dopamine, one would expect that a supersensitive receptor on the lesion side would be more sensitive to the dopamine-induced stimulation of the enzyme activity. However, it is of considerable interest that unilateral intraneostriatal administration of dB-cAMP causes a turning of the rat toward the nontreated side, and this effect is not blocked by treatment with neuroleptics (Fuxe, Goldstein, and Ungerstedt, *unpublished data*). This suggests that cyclic AMP could modulate the activity of dopamine receptors in the striatum.

A hypothetical scheme of possible mechanisms involved in the cyclic AMP stimulation of striatal dopamine synthesis is shown in Fig. 1. The

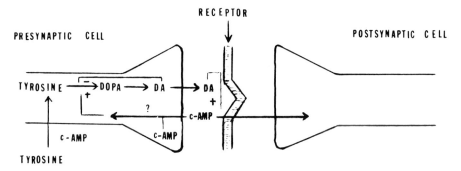

FIG. 1. The hypothetical mechanisms in cyclic AMP-induced stimulation of dopamine synthesis.

findings that cyclic AMP stimulates dopamine synthesis indicate that this chemical mediator plays an important role in the short-term regulation of the transmitter synthesis in the striatum. It is conceivable that the cyclic AMP-induced stimulation of dopamine synthesis regulates the feedback inhibition of tyrosine hydroxylase by the end products DOPA or dopamine. Since the membrane permeability of brain slices to tyrosine, dopamine, and ions might be altered by cyclic AMP (i.e., cyclic AMP may alter the state of phosphorylation of membrane proteins), it is possible that the cyclic AMP-induced stimulation of dopamine synthesis could be attributed to these changes. The specific activity of tyrosine in striatal slices was only slightly altered by cyclic AMP (10), and it seems therefore unlikely that the stimulation of ^{14}C-dopamine synthesis is due to an increased net uptake of ^{14}C-tyrosine. It is of interest to note that depolarizing agents such as K+ (15) or ouabain (16) stimulate the synthesis of catecholamines in brain slices and stimulate the formation of cyclic AMP (17). Therefore, we are now investigating whether these two effects are linked to each other. The question whether or not the cyclic AMP-induced stimulation of dopamine synthesis is influenced by changes in dopamine receptor activity must also be further clarified. The receptor involved might be located postsynaptically and cyclic AMP may mediate its activity transsynaptically, or the receptor might be located in the presynaptic cell and cyclic AMP might exert its stimulatory activity intraneuronally. Thus, the role of cyclic AMP and of other cyclic nucleotides in the receptor-mediated regulation of catecholamine synthesis deserves further investigation.

SUMMARY

The influence of dopamine receptor activity on extrapyramidal dysfunctions and on dopamine synthesis was investigated. L-DOPA or agents that stimulate dopamine receptors relieve surgically induced tremor in monkeys and concomitantly evoke involuntary movements. These results indicate that tremor and involuntary movements are associated with a common mechanism, and that the activity of the dopamine receptors influences these extrapyramidal dysfunctions. The blockade of dopamine receptors with haloperidol results in an enhancement, while the activation of dopamine receptors with Trivastal® results in an inhibition of dopamine synthesis in striatal slices. Cyclic AMP stimulates dopamine synthesis in striatal slices, and it may play a role in the regulation of catecholamine synthesis. The relationship, if any, between dopamine receptor activity and cyclic AMP-induced stimulation of dopamine synthesis is now under investigation.

ACKNOWLEDGMENTS

This work was supported by U.S. Public Health Service grant NS–06801 and National Science Foundation grant GB–27603.

REFERENCES

1. Ehringer, H., and Hornykiewicz, O., *Klin. Wschr.* 38, 1236 (1960).
2. Hornykiewicz, O., in: *Neurotransmitters,* Res. Publ. Assoc. for Research in Nervous and Mental Disease, Vol. 50, p. 390, Williams & Wilkins, Baltimore (1972).
3. Ungerstedt, U., in: *Monoamines Noyaux Gris Centraux et Syndrome de Parkinson.* (Symposium Bel Air IV, Geneva, September, 1970), p. 165, Georg & Cie, Geneva (1971).
4. Poirier, L. J., and Sourkes, T. L., *Brain* 88, 181 (1965).
5. Goldstein, M., Anagnoste, B., Battista, A. F., Owen, W. S., and Nakatani, S., *J. Neurochem.* 16, 645 (1969).
6. Corrodi, H., Fuxe, K., and Ungerstedt, U., *J. Pharm. Pharmac.* 23, 989 (1972).
7. Goldstein, M., Anagnoste, B., Battista, A. F., Ohmoto, T., and Fuxe, K., *Science* 179, 816 (1973).
8. Corrodi, H., Fuxe, K., Hökfelt, T., Lidbrink, P., and Ungerstedt, U., *J. Pharm. Pharmac.* (*in press*).
9. Goldstein, M., Freedman, L. S., and Backstrom, T., *J. Pharm. Pharmac.* 22, 715 (1970).
10. Goldstein, M., Anagnoste, B., and Shirron, C., *J. Pharm. Pharmac.* (*in press*).
11. Kehr, W., Carlsson, A., Lindqvist, M., Magnusson, T., and Atack, C., *J. Pharm. Pharmac.* 24, 744 (1972).
12. Kebabian, J. W., Petzold, G. L., and Greengard, P., *Proc. Nat. Acad. Sci.* 69, No. 8, 2145 (1972).
13. Sassin, J., Taub, S., and Weitzman, E., *Neurology* 21, 403 (1971).
14. Battista, A. F., Goldstein, M., and Ogawa, M., *Exp. Neurol.* 33, 566 (1971).
15. Harris, J. E., and Roth, R. H., *Mol. Pharmac.* 7, 593 (1971).
16. Goldstein, M., Ohi, Y., and Backstrom, T., *J. Pharmac. Exp. Therap.* 174, 77 (1970).
17. Shimizu, H., and Daly, J. W., *Europ. J. Pharmac.* 17, 240 (1972).

Advances in Neurology, Vol. 5
Raven Press, New York © 1974

The Effect of L-DOPA on Brain Poly-somes and Protein Synthesis: Probable Mediation by Intracellular Dopamine

Bette F. Weiss, Lawrence E. Roel, Hamish N. Munro, and Richard J. Wurtman

Department of Nutrition and Food Science, Massachusetts Institute of Technology, Cambridge, Massachusetts 02139

L-DOPA has now become one of the standard modes of therapy for Parkinson's disease (1, 2) and for certain dystonias of childhood (3, 4). The doses of the catechol amino acid that are administered are usually large, sometimes exceeding the combined daily oral intake of all of the aromatic amino acids found in proteins. Circulating L-DOPA apparently shares with other neutral amino acids the same transport systems that mediate their entry into brain (5, 6) and into other tissues. One such amino acid is tryptophan, whose concentration in liver cells determines the extent of polysome aggregation, and can thus rate-limit overall protein synthesis (7–9).

It had been observed that high doses of phenylalanine caused the disaggregation of brain polysomes and a coincident reduction in the free tryptophan content of brain; moreover, the polysome disaggregation could be prevented by administering tryptophan along with the phenylalanine (10). Hence, it occurred to us that L-DOPA, by competing with tryptophan for entry into the brain, might similarly disaggregate polysomes, and thereby suppress brain protein synthesis. We therefore examined the effects of exogenous L-DOPA on brain polysome aggregation in rats of various ages, and also assayed changes in the free tryptophan concentration of the brain. We found that exogenous L-DOPA did indeed cause a transient disaggregation of brain polysomes, lasting about as long after each dose as significant quantities of DOPA could be detected in the brain (11). The minimum effective DOPA dose increased with the age of the animal. In adult rats, the standard dose causing a major polysome disaggregation was approximately 500 mg/kg, or five times the usual daily human dose. Since rats generally metabolize amino acids (and most other compounds) about five times faster than humans, our rat dose was not strikingly different from the usual total daily human dose.

In contrast with the effect of exogenous phenylalanine, the polysome disaggregation caused by L-DOPA was not associated with a decrease in brain tryptophan; instead the concentration of this amino acid actually rose (11), indicating that DOPA produced its effect via a different mechanism. Subsequent studies, described below, demonstrated that dopamine was an essential intermediate in the disaggregation of brain polysomes by DOPA (12) and that the site of action of this dopamine was probably not synaptic, but rather was on a receptor present in the majority of brain cells. More recently, we have found that the administration to rats of L-5-hydroxytryptophan, the immediate precursor of serotonin, also causes polysome disaggregation, and that this effect is also mediated by a monamine, in this case serotonin, acting on an intracellular receptor. Finally, in other unpublished studies in our laboratories, evidence has been obtained that the DOPA-induced disaggregation of brain polysomes is associated with a major suppression of brain protein synthesis, in general, and specifically of vinblastine-precipitable neurotubular protein synthesis. It is not yet clear what role, if any, the actions of L-DOPA on brain protein synthesis play in the therapeutic or toxic effects of the drug.

ACTION OF L-DOPA ON BRAIN POLYRIBOSOMES

Intraperitoneal administration of L-DOPA to rats caused a marked disaggregation of whole brain polysomes (Fig. 1) (11). The minimum effective dose was age dependent: in 7- to 9-day-old rats (weighing 15 to 20 g), doses of 50 to 300 mg/kg caused polysome disaggregation that was manifested at 40 to 60 min after DOPA injection, but not at 20 or 120 min. The percent of total ribosomal RNA present as polysomes decreased from 69% in control rats to 45% after administration of L-DOPA. Older male rats (weighing 50 to 100 g) showed a similar response to L-DOPA (from 65 to 43% in 50-g rats, and from 61 to 33% in 100-g rats) but required a larger dose (500 mg/kg) (11, 12).

MECHANISM OF ACTION OF L-DOPA ON BRAIN POLYSOMES

As described above, we had originally anticipated that L-DOPA would affect polysome stability because we expected it to compete with another amino acid, L-tryptophan, for uptake into the brain. [Tryptophan availability had already been shown to control liver protein synthesis in untreated animals (7–9) and brain protein synthesis following phenylalanine administration (10).] However, intraperitoneal injections of L-DOPA were found to produce a significant elevation in brain tryptophan content associated with the polysome disaggregation (11). This indicates that the mechanism by which L-DOPA disaggregated brain polysomes differed from that of phenylalanine, and did not involve changes in brain tryptophan. Eleven other free amino acids, including methionine, were measured in rat brain after single doses of DOPA and were found not to change (11).

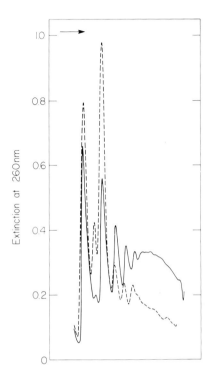

FIG. 1. Effect of L-DOPA on brain polysome profiles in 50-g male rats. Whole brains were taken 60 min after the intraperitoneal administration of 500 mg/kg L-DOPA in 0.05 N HCl, or the diluent alone. Polysomes were isolated with discontinuous sucrose gradients, and samples were spun on continuous 10 to 40% sucrose-density gradients for 70 min at 38,000 rpm. The RNA concentrations in continuous portions of the gradient were then measured with a flow cell by reading absorbance at 260 nm (11, 12). Solid line, control; dashed line, L-DOPA. The arrow indicates top of gradient.

Since disaggregation of brain polysomes was not caused by depletion of an amino acid, other aspects of brain DOPA metabolism that might mediate this disaggregation were examined (Fig. 2) (12). Administered L-DOPA is transformed by the brain to the catecholamines dopamine and norepinephrine (13, 14), and to the amino acid 3-O-methyldopa (15). The O-methylation of exogenous DOPA, catalyzed by catechol-O-methyltransferase (16, 17) had been shown to deplete the brain of S-adenosylmethionine (18). Hence, we wanted to determine if the O-methylation of exogenous L-DOPA mediated the brain polysome disaggregation, either by causing the brain to contain 3-O-methyldopa or by depleting it of S-adenosylmethionine.

To distinguish between the two major routes by which brain metabolizes exogenous L-DOPA (namely, decarboxylation to catecholamines and 3-O-methylation), two drugs were used, D-DOPA and an inhibitor of DOPA decarboxylation, Ro 4-4602 (Table 1). Administered D-DOPA is

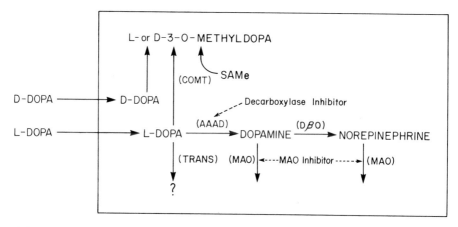

FIG. 2. Metabolism of L-DOPA and D-DOPA in rat brain. COMT, catechol-O-methyltrans-ferase; AAAD, aromatic L-amino acid decarboxylase; DβO, dopamine-β-oxidase; MAO, monoamine oxidase; TRANS, DOPA transaminase; and SAMe, S-adenosylmethionine. The decarboxylase inhibitor was Ro 4–4602; the monoamine oxidase inhibitor used was pheniprazine. From (12), reproduced with permission of the publisher; copyright 1972 by the American Association for the Advancement of Science.

taken up by the brain, and, like L-DOPA, changed to 3-O-methyldopa by catechol-O-methyltransferase (16, 17), thus depleting brain S-adenosyl-methionine (18). However, unlike L-DOPA, D-DOPA is not decarboxylated to dopamine because it is not a substrate for the enzyme aromatic L-amino acid decarboxylase (AAAD) (19). Administering a decarboxylase inhibitor before giving L-DOPA accomplishes essentially the same thing as giving D-DOPA; in other words, it permits 3-O-methylation to occur, but prevents the elevation of brain catecholamines.

Sixty min after 50-g male rats were given L-DOPA alone (500 mg/kg), brain polysomes were disaggregated maximally. At this time, the brain DOPA concentration was elevated, but had passed its peak; as expected, the brain also contained large amounts of 3-O-methyldopa, and its S-ade-nosylmethionine content was significantly depleted. Brain dopamine con-centration was four times control values, and brain norepinephrine was slightly but not significantly elevated.

Administration of large doses of 3-O-methyldopa itself failed to affect brain polysomes (Table 1). S-Adenosylmethionine depletion was also shown not to mediate L-DOPA-induced polysome disaggregation, inasmuch as doses of D-DOPA sufficient to produce concentrations of brain DOPA and 3-O-methyldopa similar to those following L-DOPA, and to deplete the brain of S-adenosylmethionine, did not affect brain polysomes. Unlike L-DOPA, D-DOPA did not elevate brain dopamine concentrations. If the conversion of exogenous L-DOPA to brain dopamine was inhibited by pre-treatment of the rats with the AAAD inhibitor Ro 4-4602, brain polysomes

TABLE 1. *Effects of L-DOPA and related drugs on brain polysome profiles and DOPA metabolism of 50-g male rats*

Treatment	Route of administration	Dose (mg/kg)	Time after injection (min)	Polysomes (percent of profile)	DOPA (μg/g)	3-O-Methyl-dopa (μg/g)	S-Adenosyl-methionine (percent of control)[a]	Dopamine (ng/g)	Norepinephrine (ng/g)
Control	i.p.	0	60	65	<0.1	<0.1			
L-DOPA	i.p.	500	40		18.7[b]	0.5[b]			
			60	43[b]	6.8[b]	1.2[c]			
3-O-Methyldopa	i.p.	500	60	60	0.3[d]	4.6[d]			
			120	65	0.3[b]	11.8[b]			
Control	i.p.	0	60		<0.1	<0.1	100	505	300
L-DOPA	i.p.	500	60	61	9.5[b]	3.4[b]	32[b]	2,230[c]	330
D-DOPA	i.p.	500	60	65	10.7[b]	2.9[b]	27[b]	640	310
Ro 4-4602	i.p.	800	90		2.9[d]	0.1	45[c]	346[c]	188[b]
Ro 4-4602 plus L-DOPA	i.p.	800 / 500	90 / 60	60	40.2[b]	4.3[b]	39[c]	298[c]	200[b]
Control	i.p.	0	60	73	<0.1			508	305
L-DOPA	i.p.	100	60	75	2.3[b]			780[d]	348
Pheniprazine	i.p.	10	180	62	<0.1			779	398[d]
Pheniprazine plus L-DOPA	i.p.	10 / 100	180 / 60	32[b]	1.2[b]			2,890[b]	618[c]
Pheniprazine plus L-DOPA	i.p.	10 / 500	180 / 60	41[c]	17.0[b]			30,000[b]	801[b]
		(micrograms per rat)							
Control	i.c.	0	45	60	<0.1	<0.1	100	470	289
Dopamine	i.c.	100	15	59	<0.1	<0.1	92	6,020[d]	308
			45	58	<0.1	<0.1	86	903	212[d]
Norepi-nephrine	i.c.	100	15	57	<0.1	<0.1	94	555	20,800[b]
			45	54	<0.1	<0.1	82	593	10,200[b]

[a] Control brains contained an average of 13.4 μg of S-adenosylmethionine per gram.
[b] $p < 0.001$ differs from control group (p evaluated by Student's t-test).
[c] $p < 0.01$ differs from control group.
[d] $p < 0.05$ differs from control group.

remained aggregated (i.e., even though brain S-adenosylmethionine was depleted, 3-O-methyldopa was formed, and brain DOPA concentrations were four times greater than in rats receiving the same dose of L-DOPA alone and in which brain polysomes were disaggregated). These observations indicated that the synthesis of catecholamines (most likely dopamine, the brain concentration of which was increased much more than norepinephrine) mediated the effect of L-DOPA on brain polysomes.

When dopamine and norepinephrine were injected directly into the cerebrospinal fluid intracisternally, in doses sufficient to elevate brain catecholamine concentrations to post-L-DOPA levels, brain polysomes did not disaggregate. This lack of effect (which was shared by intraperitoneal apomorphine; Fig. 3) suggested that the dopamine had to enter the majority of brain cells, neurons, and glia in order for extensive polysome disaggregation to occur. It also indicated that the levels of action of the dopamine might be not synaptic, but intracellular. In other studies from our laboratory, it has been shown that almost all of the brain dopamine formed after L-DOPA is administered is localized *outside* cells that normally produce catechol-

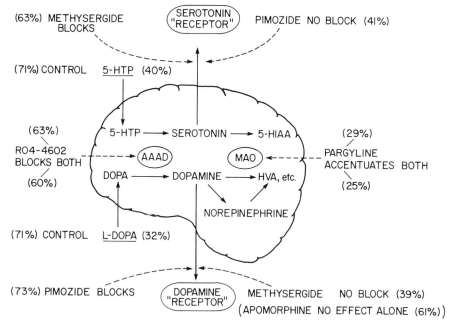

FIG. 3. Synthesis of biogenic amines from L-DOPA and L-5-hydroxytryptophan in rat brain: Effects of pretreatment with related drugs on brain polysomes. 5-HTP, L-5-hydroxytryptophan; AAAD, aromatic L-amino acid decarboxylase; MAO, monoamine oxidase; 5-HIAA, 5-hydroxyindoleacetic acid; and HVA, homovanillic acid. Ro 4–4602 inhibits AAAD. Pargyline inhibits MAO. Pimozide blocks dopamine receptors. Apomorphine stimulates dopamine receptors. Methysergide blocks serotonin receptors. The percent of total rRNA present as polysomes 60 min after L-DOPA or L-5-HTP administration is indicated beside each drug. Apomorphine was given alone, 60 min before autopsy.

amines. If L-DOPA is administered systemically to animals pretreated with sufficient intracisternal 6-hydroxydopamine to deplete brain dopamine and norephinephrine (presumably by destroying catecholamine nerve terminals), the peak concentrations of dopamine found in the brain are indistinguishable from those in intact animals(20).

In order to potentiate the elevation in brain dopamine and norepinephrine levels following L-DOPA administration, animals were pretreated with an inhibitor of monoamine oxidase, pheniprazine. Inhibition of catecholamine deamination *potentiated* the disaggregation of brain polysomes by L-DOPA; a dose (100 mg/kg) which alone did not disaggregate polysomes in 50-g rats now had this effect (Table 1). The brain dopamine level after 100 mg/kg L-DOPA in these monoamine oxidase-inhibitor-treated rats was equivalent to that found in other animals treated with 500 mg/kg of L-DOPA alone, although the concentration of DOPA in brain was low, providing additional evidence that catecholamine (probably dopamine) synthesis in the majority of brain cells mediates the brain polysome disaggregation that follows L-DOPA. The mechanism by which dopamine disaggregates brain polysomes is unknown, but is under investigation by our laboratory. As described below, it appears to involve a specific intracellular receptor.

ACTION OF L-DOPA ON BRAIN PROTEIN SYNTHESIS *IN VIVO*

Studies were undertaken to determine if the changes in polysome aggregation induced by L-DOPA were coincident with changes in the actual *in vivo* synthesis of brain proteins. In four separate experiments, male rats, weighing 50 g, were injected intraperitoneally with 500 mg/kg L-DOPA or its diluent; 45 min later they received intracisternally 1.5 μC of either uniformly labeled ^{14}C-leucine or ^{14}C-lysine. Animals were killed 7, 15, or 30 min after receiving the radioactive amino acid, and their brains assayed for isotopically labeled proteins. In each experiment there was a significant decrease in the incorporation of amino acids into trichloroacetic acid-precipitable brain protein among L-DOPA-injected rats compared to controls (Fig. 4). At the intervals after L-DOPA that the rats received the radioactive amino acids and were sacrificed, brain polysomes were, as expected, disaggregated. Thus there was a correlation between the state of polysome aggregation and the rate at which amino acid was incorporated into brain proteins. Subsequent experiments have shown an inhibitory effect of L-DOPA on the synthesis of "neurotubular" protein (i.e., vinblastine-precipitable soluble brain protein).

ACTION OF L-5-HYDROXYTRYPTOPHAN ON BRAIN POLYRIBOSOMES

Recently we compared the action of L-5-hydroxytryptophan (5-HTP), the amino acid precursor of serotonin, on brain polysomes with that of

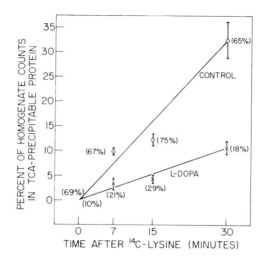

FIG. 4. Correlation of brain polysome disaggregation in rats after L-DOPA with decreased *in vivo* protein synthesis. Forty-five min after 500 mg/kg L-DOPA in 0.05 N HCl (or the diluent alone) was injected intraperitoneally, 50-g male rats received 1.5 μC of uniformly labeled ^{14}C-lysine intracisternally. They were killed after 7, 15, or 30 min. The percent of homogenate counts found in the trichloroacetic acid-precipitable protein fraction was compared in controls and L-DOPA-treated rats, as was the percent of rRNA present as polysomes.

L-DOPA (Fig. 3). Like L-DOPA, 500 mg/kg 5-HTP intraperitoneally significantly disaggregated brain polysomes after 1 hr in 50-g male rats. Pretreatment with pargyline, an inhibitor of monoamine oxidase, potentiated the disaggregations caused by both L-DOPA and 5-HTP. Just as inhibition of amine synthesis after L-DOPA prevented polysome disaggregation, this effect of 5-HTP on brain polysomes was also blocked in rats pretreated with Ro 4-4602, the inhibitor of aromatic L-amino acid decarboxylase. Thus the polysome aggregation produced by both hydroxylated amino acids appears to be mediated by their corresponding biogenic amine products. Unlike L-DOPA and 5-HTP, phenylalanine was found not to require decarboxylation in order to disaggregate polysomes: disaggregation continues to occur after treatment with Ro 4–4602, indicating that the amino acid, and not its monoamine product, mediates this effect.

EFFECT OF AMINE RECEPTOR BLOCKERS ON L-DOPA- AND 5-HTP-INDUCED POLYSOME DISAGGREGATION

The specificity of the effects of L-DOPA and 5-HTP on brain polysomes was examined by the use of drugs that block amine receptors (Fig. 3). Pretreatment of rats with the dopamine receptor blocker pimozide blocked the effect of L-DOPA on brain polysomes. However, methysergide, a serotonin receptor blocker, did not interfere with the disaggregation after L-DOPA.

In contrast, the effect of 5-HTP on brain polysomes was blocked by methysergide but not by pimozide. Although additional data are needed before conclusions can be drawn, these observations suggest the participation of specific dopaminergic and serotonergic receptors in the effects of L-DOPA and 5-HTP on brain protein synthesis. If, as we have postulated, the exogenous amino acids and the monoamines produced from them work intracellularly, it is curious that specific receptors should exist within cells (e.g., glia) that are not thought normally to contain the monoamines that stimulate these receptors. Perhaps both the dopamine and the serotonin are interacting with a "receptor" for some other endogenous amine.

CONCLUSION

Administration to rats of L-DOPA or 5-HTP results in a profound disaggregation of whole-brain polyribosomes and a concurrent decrease in brain protein synthesis *in vivo*. These effects are dependent upon the decarboxylation of the amino acids to form the corresponding amines dopamine and serotonin. The experiments described above pose several important questions that we are presently trying to answer. First, how do the dopamine and serotonin synthesized intracellularly from L-DOPA and 5-HTP affect brain polysomes, and do these changes mimic a physiological action of a biogenic amine or brain protein synthesis? Second, do the amines, as postulated, act via an intracellular mechanism or is their effect on polysomes also mediated by synapses? If the former, how does one explain the existence of dopamine or serotonin receptors related to polysome function within the great majority of brain cells, which probably never normally contain these amines? Finally, do the effects of L-DOPA on brain protein synthesis participate in the therapeutic or toxic effects of this drug in the treatment of brain disease?

ACKNOWLEDGMENTS

This work was supported by U.S. Public Health Service grants NS-10459 and AM-15364.

REFERENCES

1. Cotzias, G. C., Papavasiliou, P. S., and Gellene, R., *N. Engl. J. Med.* 280, 337 (1969).
2. Yahr, M. D., Duvoisin, R. C., Shear, M. J., Barrett, R. E., and Hoehn, M. M., *Arch. Neurol.* 21, 343 (1969).
3. Barbeau, A., *Neurology* 20, 96 (1970).
4. Eldridge, R., *Neurology* 20, 1 (1970).
5. Blasberg, R., and Lajtha, A., *Brain Res.* 1, 86 (1966).
6. Blasberg, R. G., *Prog. Brain Res.* 29, 245 (1968).
7. Sidransky, H., Bongiorno, M., Sarma, D. R. S., and Verney, E., *Biochim. Biophys. Acta* 87, 525 (1967).
8. Baliga, B. S., Pronczuk, A. W., and Munro, H. N., *J. Mol. Biol.* 34, 199 (1968).

9. Pronczuk, A. W., Baliga, B. S., Triant, J. W., and Munro, H. N., *Biochim. Biophys. Acta* 157, 204 (1968).
10. Aoki, K., and Siegel, F. L., *Science* 168, 129 (1970).
11. Weiss, B. F., Munro, H. N., and Wurtman, R. J., *Science* 173, 833 (1971).
12. Weiss, B. F., Munro, H. N., Ordonez, L. A., and Wurtman, R. J., *Science* 177, 613 (1972).
13. Carlsson, A., Lindqvist, M., Magnusson, T., and Waldeck, B. *Science* 127, 471 (1958).
14. Chalmers, J. P., Baldessarini, R. J., and Wurtman, R. J., *Proc. Nat. Acad. Sci.* 68, 662 (1971).
15. Bartholini, G., and Pletscher, A., *J. Phamacol. Exp. Ther.* 161, 14 (1968).
16. Axelrod, J. A., and Tomchick, R., *J. Biol. Chem.* 233, 702 (1958).
17. Wurtman, R. J., Chou, C., and Rose, C., *J. Pharmacol. Exp. Ther.* 174, 351 (1970).
18. Wurtman, R. J., Rose, C. M., Matthysse, S., Stephenson, J., and Baldessarini, R., *Science* 169: 395 (1970).
19. Lovenberg, W., Weissbach, H., and Udenfriend, S., *J. Biol. Chem.* 237, 89 (1962).
20. Lytle, L. D., Hurko, O., Romero, J. A., Cottman, K., Leehey, D., and Wurtman, R. J., *J. Neural. Transmission* 33, 63 (1972).

DISCUSSION

Dr. McDowell: Dr. Carlsson, I presume that the changes in tyrosine hydroxylase related to hypoxia are always reversible. That is, if you increase the oxygen levels, the activity of the enzyme goes back up; is that so?

Dr. Carlsson: Yes, so far all the changes we have seen are reversible but we are continuing these studies and cannot be sure.

Dr. Cotzias: I have two questions. I'd like to ask Dr. Carlsson whether he has considered the effect of oxygen tension on monoamine oxidase, which also has a great sensitivity to oxygen as a second substrate and to its presence *in vitro* and *in vivo*.

My second question is to Dr. Weiss. What is the effect of apomorphine on disaggregation of polyribosomes?

Dr. Weiss: Apomorphine, as I mentioned, in whatever dose I gave, and I gave quite a range and for various times, had absolutely no effect on polysomes. That is why I thought that just by stimulating dopamine receptors using this drug we would not find changes in polysomes.

Dr. McDowell: Dr. Carlsson, would you respond?

Dr. Carlsson: Yes. This question of Dr. Cotzias' is, of course, very important. We believe that monoamine oxidase is inhibited to about the same extent as the tyrosine hydroxylases because these very pronounced decreases in synthesis do not cause any considerable decrease in amine levels. The only explanation that we can find is that MAO is inhibited at the same time. In further support of this, 5-hydroxyindoleacetic acid levels in the brain are reduced by hypoxia.

Dr. Burrows: Dr. Goldstein, there is growing evidence that cyclic AMP-dependent protein kinase may be the substance that mediates cyclic AMP; do you think that phosphorylation of the receptor could play a role?

Dr. Goldstein: I think the postulation may be that the membrane proteins may play a role; I do not know exactly which is the receptor. However, another role of cyclic AMP might be induction of protein synthesis, but we do not think these short-term experiments reveal this, and we do not deal with the role of tyrosine hydroxylase synthesis.

Dr. Goldberg: Dr. Weiss, I'm curious about the rather large dose of L-DOPA, 500 milligrams per kilo, that you give. If you gave this to a dog, the blood pressure would rise to approximately 500 millimeters of mercury.

Dr. Weiss: I did not go into this but the dose response varies greatly with the age of the animal. With a very young rat you get an effect with 50 milligrams per kilo, but the adult needs 500 milligrams per kilo. Presumably, from what I have heard, the metabolic rate of the rat is such that this is not such a massive dose.

Dr. Smith: A question for Dr. Carlsson and Dr. Goldstein. Both of you suggested that a preterminal receptor site is a possibility. I wonder if you have any evidence for such a thing, or does it remain a theoretical question?

Dr. Carlsson: As far as I am concerned this is purely hypothetical. I would be happy if it did not exist: I think the story is more exciting that way.

Dr. Reis: Dr. Carlsson, on your graphs showing the change of tyrosine hydroxylase activity with a reduction of oxygen you did not reach an asymptote at 100%. Do you think that if you increase the oxygen content more, you would increase the tyrosine hydroxylase activity?

Dr. Carlsson: Yes, on the basis of the *in vitro* data on isolated enzymes, this is probably so. You do not reach saturation even at PO_2 corresponding to 20% as in the air. More than 20% would give a higher than normal hydroxylation rate, but since we have not pursued this, we have no significant evidence on this point.

Dr. Kopin: Going back to the question of the presynaptic receptor, there is evidence that there are presynaptic receptors in tissue culture. If one takes a sympathetic ganglion and allows it to grow in culture, you can get an axonal sprout. These axonal sprouts, of course, are only presynaptic; there are no postsynaptic sites. Under these conditions one can demonstrate that phenoxybenzamine will enhance release of radioactive norepinephrine which has been taken up and which has been stimulated to release by an electrical field, or high potassium.

This I think must be a presynaptic action because there are no postsynaptic sites and there is no inhibition of uptake to account for it.

Dr. Vogt: Dr. Besson, you showed a delayed release of radioactive dopamine after stimulating the substantia nigra; did you use a monoamine oxidase inhibitor in these experiments?

Dr. Besson: No, in these experiments we measured only the release of dopamine, but we did not use a monoamine oxidase inhibitor. It is a simple spontaneous release of dopamine without inhibitor of the main processes.

Dr. Vogt: I am surprised that they survived so long. I cannot explain your delay unless it was caused by the stimulating cells or terminals which are away from the surface.

Dr. McDowell: Dr. Siegfried has some comments.

Dr. Siegfried: The morphological evidence of the presence of dopamine in the living human brain can be confirmed by biopsies and histofluorescent studies of brain specimens. In a series of 20 patients who underwent a stereotactic operation, we performed a small biopsy of the head of the caudate nucleus, and Dr. J. Constantinidis did histofluorescent examinations. In this series, we had 13 patients suffering from Parkinson's disease and seven with other affections (essential tremor, pain syndrome). Among the parkinsonian patients, six were not treated with L-DOPA at the time of the operation, four were under treatment with L-DOPA alone, showing an optimal clinical result without any side effects, and three were under treatment with L-DOPA and the decarboxylase inhibitor Ro 4–4602. The figure below shows the caudate nucleus in a case of essential tremor (a), Parkinson's disease without L-DOPA (b), with L-DOPA (c), and with L-DOPA

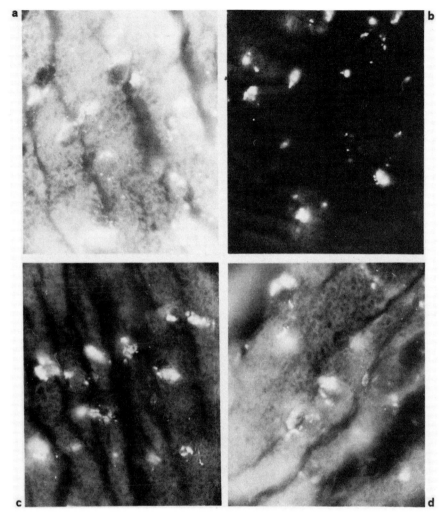

FIG. 1. Histofluorescent study of the human caudate nucleus (method of Falck and Hillarp). (By courtesy of Dr. J. Constantinidis.)

plus decarboxylase inhibitor (d). Essential tremor is not related to a dopamine deficiency in the caudate nucleus. The treatment of Parkinson's disease with L-DOPA or, better, with L-DOPA plus decarboxylase inhibitor partially restores the content of dopamine in the caudate nucleus.

Advances in Neurology, Vol. 5
Raven Press, New York © 1974

Dynamics of Brain Histamine

Key Dismukes and Solomon H. Snyder

Departments of Pharmacology and Experimental Therapeutics and Psychiatry and Behavioral Sciences, Johns Hopkins University School of Medicine, Baltimore, Maryland 21205

Knowledge of histamine's presence in the brain is at least as ancient as that of other biogenic amines. Abel and Kubota (1) identified histamine in the pituitary more than half a century ago. In 1943 Kwiatkowski (2) found that in the brain proper histamine is concentrated more in gray than in white matter, and in 1952 Harris, Jacobson, and Kahlson (3) determined that the hypothalamus contains considerably higher concentrations than does any other brain region. Nevertheless, histamine has never received the attention given other biogenic amines. One difficulty has been that brain levels of histamine are very low (~ 50 ng/g), and only recently has a sensitive biochemical assay which allows rapid determination of large numbers of samples become available.

The enzymatic-isotopic assay developed by Taylor and Snyder (4) uses the enzyme histamine methyltransferase to transfer a tritiated methyl group from the donor S-adenosylmethionine to molecules of histamine. The resulting ^{3}H-methylhistamine is separated from the labeled S-adenosylmethionine by extraction into chloroform. The chloroform is evaporated, and the residue is taken up into scintillation fluor and counted. The radioactivity observed is linearly proportional to the amount of histamine present in the samples over the range 0 to 20 ng. This simple technique allows the measurement of as little as 10 picograms of histamine and the use of tissues as small as is convenient to homogenize.

Several lines of evidence indicate that histamine has some function in the brain separate from its roles in the rest of the body. First of all, it is distributed in a nonuniform pattern similar to that of norepinephrine and serotonin (5). Levels of histamine are highest in the hypothalamus and successively lower as we pass upward to the thalamus, midbrain, and then cerebrum (Table 1). The concentrations of histamine in cerebellum, medulla, and pons are less than one-tenth of that found in the hypothalamus. Histamine is synthesized from histidine by the enzyme histidine decarboxylase. The regional activity of this enzyme closely parallels the distribution of histamine. In contrast, histidine levels are fairly uniform throughout the brain.

Subcellular distribution can give clues to a neurochemical's function. An

DYNAMICS OF BRAIN HISTAMINE

TABLE 1. *Regional distribution of histamine in the rat brain*

Brain region	Histamine (ng/g)	Histidine (μg/g)	Histidine decarboxylase (nmole/hr/g protein)	Histamine methyl transferase (μmole/hr/g protein)
Hypothalamus	550 ± 40	25.4 ± 2.1	28.8 ± 2.4	1.05 ± 0.09
Thalamus-midbrain	75 ± 4	13.5 ± 0.9	12.6 ± 0.9	0.91 ± 0.06
Corpus striatum	56 ± 4	19.7 ± 1.1	10.4 ± 0.8	0.92 ± 0.05
Hippocampus	50 ± 6	21.8 ± 1.9	6.8 ± 0.4	0.83 ± 0.05
Cerebral cortex	39 ± 5	9.4 ± 1.5	6.3 ± 0.4	0.83 ± 0.05
Medulla-pons	25 ± 4	16.3 ± 1.6	4.7 ± 0.4	0.47 ± 0.03
Cerebellum	26 ± 5	18.7 ± 0.6	3.3 ± 0.2	0.32 ± 0.02

Rats were killed by decapitation, their brains dissected and frozen until assayed, by the method of Snyder and Taylor (5). Numbers quoted are the mean ± SEM of five to 10 determinations.

important criterion for putative neurotransmitters is that they be localized in synaptic endings, along with synthesizing enzymes. When brain tissue is homogenized in isotonic sucrose, nerve endings pinch off, forming "synaptosomes," membranous sacs containing synaptic vesicles, mitochondria, and cytoplasm (6). These synaptosomes can then be separated from other subcellular fractions by differential and sucrose gradient centrifugation. Support for the candidacy of several putative neurotransmitters—among them acetylcholine, norepinephrine, and serotonin—has been obtained by using these subcellular fractionization techniques to demonstrate localization in nerve endings.

Several workers have observed a particulate localization of brain histamine (7–11). In our laboratory studies of the subcellular localization of brain histamine in ongoing work, we homogenized rat hypothalami in isotonic sucrose and used differential centrifugation to obtain four fractions of cellular fragments: a nuclear pellet (P1), a crude mitochondrial pellet (P2), a crude microsomal pellet (P3), and the supernatant (S). The peak of endogenous histamine distribution occurred in P2, the crude fraction into which synaptosomes also sediment. This P2 pellet was lysed to disrupt synaptosomes and recentrifuged to obtain two fractions; one enriched in synaptic vesicles, the other in membrane fragments. Two-thirds of the histamine was associated with the vesicular fraction.

Further differentiation was obtained in experiments in which the P2 pellet was lysed and layered on a discontinuous sucrose gradient. Six layers, of increasing density, were used; 25% of the histamine appeared in the second layer; 49% in the third. Electron microscopy revealed that this second layer contained many small (500 Å) translucent vesicles with a few larger (1,000 Å) dense-core vesicles. However, in the third fraction, which contained the peak of histamine distribution, the dense-core vesicles predominated. In this context it is interesting to note that in the supraoptic nucleus of the hypothalamus which contains one of the highest levels of hypothalamic histamine, dense-core particles of this sort have been suggested to be associated with neuroscretory granules.

RELEASE OF HISTAMINE FROM BRAIN TISSUE

Since histamine is at least in the right place to be a neurotransmitter, we might ask if it can be released from neurons by depolarization. This question was examined by Taylor and Snyder (12). Using the very sensitive enzymatic-isotopic assay, it was possible to measure the endogenous histamine released from brain slices as they were incubated under various conditions. They found a temperature-dependent spontaneous efflux of histamine which was considerably augmented when potassium was added to the medium to cause neural depolarization. The potassium-induced release of histamine could be blocked by EDTA, which chelates calcium ions. In these experiments the release of histidine was also measured for comparison. There was a spontaneous efflux of histidine, but in contrast to histamine it was not temperature dependent nor was it altered by any of the experimental conditions.

TURNOVER OF HISTAMINE

Another way of getting information about what a neurochemical does is to look at its turnover, and at the conditions which alter turnover. Histidine decarboxylase can be inhibited by Brocresine (4 bromo-3-hydroxy benzyl-oxyamine dihydrogen phosphate) or by α-hydrazino histidine. When rats are injected interperitioneally with either of these drugs, brain histamine falls rapidly, reaching a maximum depletion within about 20 min (13). This response of brain histamine to inhibition of synthesis is so fast that it might actually represent the rate of delivery of the inhibitor to the brain, rather than the turnover rate of histamine. Accordingly, these experiments have been repeated, using tail-vein injections of Brocresine or α-hydrazino histidine. Both drugs maximally reduce brain histamine within about 1 min. From the slopes of the depletion curves shown in Fig. 1 we can estimate the half-life of histamine to be around 30 sec, which is comparable to that quoted for the half-life of acetylcholine, and in marked contrast to the much longer time reported for other biogenic amines.

Another way of looking at turnover is to inject the labeled precursor of a neurochemical, and watch the appearance of radioactivity in the neurochemical pool over time. In a series of experiments, purified ^{3}H-histidine was injected into a lateral ventricle and the time course of its disappearance and the appearance of ^{3}H-histamine and ^{3}H-methylhistamine was followed in several brain regions (Fig. 2). Activity of ^{3}H-histidine falls in a biphasic manner, rapidly at first, then in a slower exponential decay. ^{3}H-histamine is rapidly formed, peaking in about 45 min, then decaying more slowly, at a

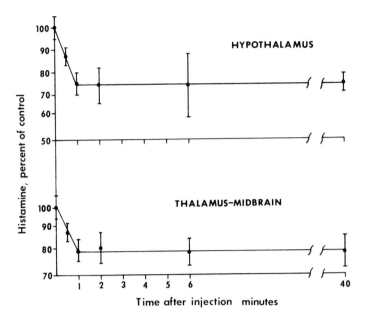

FIG. 1. Depletion of histamine in two rat brain regions produced by injecting Brocresine, 300 mg/kg, intraperitoneally at time zero. Four to eight rats were used for each time point, representing mean ± SEM.

rate paralleling the disappearance of ^{3}H-histidine. The ratios of ^{3}H-histamine to ^{3}H-histidine in the three regions examined were in the same order as the levels of endogenous histamine: hypothalamus > thalamus-midbrain > telencephalon. In other words, regions with highest levels of endogenous histamine also have the greatest histamine-forming capacity.

Ring N-methylation is a major pathway of brain histamine metabolism (14). In these experiments the time course of ^{3}H-methylhistamine activity closely followed that of ^{3}H-histamine although its peak was only about one-third of the latter.

Taylor and Snyder (15) reported that prolonged exposure of mice to cold (4°C) or restraint led to reduction of histamine in the telencephalon and diencephalon. Presumably the stress increased histamine utilization beyond the rate at which it could be synthesized. Subsequently, it was found that when the same stress was applied before and after intraventricular injection of ^{3}H-histidine, almost three times as much ^{3}H-histamine was formed, with its peak occurring 30 min earlier than in unstressed controls.

It is desirable to have more than one independent method for measuring half-life. The inhibition of synthesis technique might conceivably lead to erroneous values if the inhibitor itself altered turnover. The time course of appearance of ^{3}H-histamine in the isotopic studies above is a function of the half-life of endogenous histamine, as well as its rate of synthesis and the level of ^{3}H-histidine in the precursor pool. If it were possible to separate the

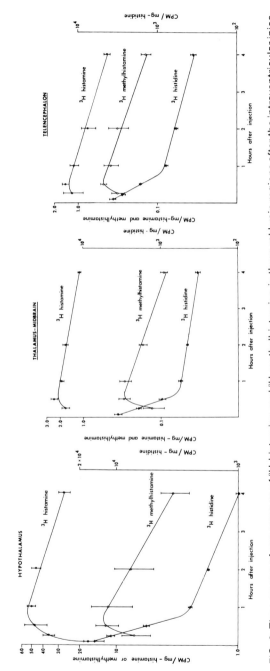

FIG. 2. Time course of appearance of ³H-histamine and ³H-methylhistamine in three rat brain regions after the intraventricular injection of 20 μC of ³H-histidine (20 μl). Each value is the mean ± SEM of six to eight determinations, in CPM/mg tissue.

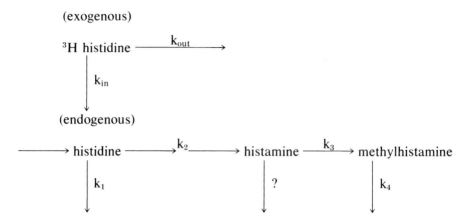

FIG. 3. Proposed model for the disposition of ^{3}H-histidine injected intraventricularly, and the subsequent formation of ^{3}H-histamine.

contribution of each of these three factors, then we would have a second independent measure of histamine half-life. To this end a model was developed to relate the ^{3}H-histidine and ^{3}H-histamine curves of Fig. 2 to the parameters and constants involved. The basic assumptions of this model (illustrated in Fig. 3) are: 1. The biphasic shape of the ^{3}H-histidine curve indicates the existence of two kinetic pools. 2. ^{3}H-histidine uniformly labels the endogenous histidine pool, precursor to the histamine pool. 3. Endogenous histamine lies within a single kinetic pool. 4. Endogenous histidine and endogenous histamine are in equilibrium; i.e., rate of synthesis equals rate of catabolism.

The mathematics of this model are described in detail elsewhere. Differential equations were set up and integrated to yield one equation describing levels of ^{3}H-histidine; another, of ^{3}H-histamine, as a function of time and the kinetic constants. Ranges of values of these constants were then tried in the equation to obtain a fit of the theoretical curves to the experimental data. In this manner a value of <1 min was obtained for the half-life of histamine, in good agreement with the inhibition of synthesis method.

ARE THERE TWO KINETIC POOLS OF HISTAMINE IN THE BRAIN?

In none of the experiments with inhibitors of histamine synthesis could brain histamine be depleted by more than about one-third. Doses of Brocresine and of α-hydrazino histidine up to the lethal range were tried, as well as multiple doses and ventricular injections, without achieving any greater reduction. This suggests that the brain's histamine might lie in two kinetic pools. The rapid 20 to 30% depletion of histamine following inhibition of synthesis would represent a small, quickly turning over pool, and the virtually flat second phase (Fig. 1) would represent a second pool turning

TABLE 2. *Comparison of reduction of endogenous histamine with reduction of ^{3}H-histamine caused by Brocresine*

Brain region		Percent of ^{3}H-histamine activity[a]			
		1 hr after Brocresine		3 hr after Brocresine	
		Endogenous HA	^{3}H-HA	Endogenous HA	^{3}H-HA
Hypothalamus	control	100 ± 5	100 ± 2	100 ± 5	100 ± 6
	Brocresine	77 ± 7	78 ± 7	73 ± 10	73 ± 9
Midbrain	control	100 ± 11	100 ± 14	100 ± 5	100 ± 8
	Brocresine	84 ± 6	89 ± 11	82 ± 7	75 ± 6
Telencephalon	control	100 ± 12	100 ± 12	100 ± 12	100 ± 8
	Brocresine	93 ± 6	107 ± 15	104 ± 9	114 ± 8

Rats were injected intraventricularly with 20 μC of ^{3}H-histidine (20μl). One hr later one group received 300 mg/kg of Brocresine, intraperitoneally. They were killed 1 or 3 hr after the Brocresine injection and the activity of ^{3}H-histamine determined. Other rats, killed at the same length of time after ^{3}H-histidine injection, received saline injection instead of Brocresine.

[a] ± SEM, with saline controls chosen as 100%.

over so slowly that no significant reduction is achieved in the several hours during which inhibition is maintained by the drug. On the other hand, other explanations are possible. For instance, *in vivo* the drug may not achieve the nearly complete inhibition of synthesis it does *in vitro* (15).

To examine the question the following experiment was devised. ^{3}H-histidine was injected into lateral ventricles, as described above. One hr later, when ^{3}H-histamine levels had peaked and begun to slowly decline, an i.p. injection of Brocresine was given. One or 3 hr after the i.p. injection, the rats were killed and brain levels of ^{3}H-histamine were determined. The rationale was that if there were two kinetic pools of histamine, then ^{3}H-histamine must be formed entirely within the fast one, because there would not be appreciable turnover in the slow pool in a few hours. Therefore, if the 20 to 30% Brocresine reduction of brain histamine represents complete depletion of a fast pool, ^{3}H-histamine activity should be drastically reduced. On the other hand, if there is only one, rapidly turning over pool, ^{3}H-histamine should be lowered to only the same extent as endogenous histamine. Our results (Table 2) indicate that this latter alternative is the correct one. Reduction of ^{3}H-histamine paralleled that of endogenous histamine in each brain region at 1 and at 3 hr after Brocresine administration. This result also increases our confidence that the ^{3}H formed in this procedure labels the endogenous pool of histamine almost exclusively.

SUMMARY

It may be instructive to compare the kinetic constants of brain histamine with those of more familiar biogenic amines (see Table 3).

TABLE 3. *Comparison of brain histamine kinetic constants with those reported by other authors for several putative neurotransmitters*

Neurochemical	% of total pool	Endogenous levels (nmole/g)	Turnover rate (nmole/min/g)	K (min^{-1})
Histamine				
hypothalamus	100	5.00 ± 0.50	7.0 ± 0.2	1.4 ± 0.5
cortex	100	0.52 ± 0.05	0.73 ± 0.07	1.4 ± 0.5
striatum	100	0.45 ± 0.04	0.63 ± 0.06[4]	1.4 ± 0.5[4]
whole brain	100	0.46 ± 0.04	0.64 ± 0.06[4]	1.4 ± 0.5[4]
Norepinephrine				
cortex[1]	77	1.41	0.0052	0.0038
	23	0.42	0.029	0.07
whole brain[2]	100	2.5 ± 0.18	0.0070 ± 0.0015	0.0028 ± 0.0006
Dopamine				
striatum[1]	77	50.4	0.25	0.0056
	23	15.0	1.14	0.076
whole brain[2]	100	7.5 ± 0.2	0.054 ± 0.008	0.0072 ± 0.0010
Serotonin				
whole brain[2]	100	2.84 ± 0.20	0.038	0.0135
Acetylcholine				
whole brain[3]	100	25.0	50.0	2.0

[1] Adapted from: Glowinski.
[2] Adapted from: Costa.
[3] Adapted from: Schuberth.
[4] Assumed.

The extremely short half-life of histamine in the brain distinguishes it from other biogenic amines. Dopamine, norepinephrine, and serotonin are generally reported to have half-lives in the range 2 to 4 hr. The two catecholamines have also been reported to have small pools turning over much faster (5 to 10 min) although there has been some argument over the interpretation of these results. Our value for the half-life of histamine is quite similar to that reported for acetylcholine.

The regional levels of histamine are generally considerably lower than those of the other amines quoted in Table 3. However, because of its extremely short half-life, the number of molecules of histamine synthesized per unit time is greater than that of any putative transmitter except acetylcholine. Turnover rate is one of the kinetic parameters most closely scrutinized in studying the dynamic state of neurochemicals, particularly if they are putative neurotransmitters. Characterizing the dynamic behavior of a neurochemical has been a means of getting clues as to its cellular function, which is so hard to ascertain directly.

If we let ourselves imagine that histamine really is a central neurotransmitter, then we can speculate on the meaning of these numbers. For instance, if we postulate that neurons of different chemical types secrete transmitters at roughly the same rate, then histaminergic cells would be more than 10 times as numerous as those using other amines. Contrariwise, if the density of histaminergic neurons were about the same as catecholaminergic ones, then histaminergic cells must release transmitters at 10 times the catecholamine rate. All of this should not be taken very seriously, except to point out that the values of these kinetic constants make very definite statements about how a neurochemical may be used.

The brain has frustrated efforts to elucidate which are its neurotransmitters. Of a growing list of candidates only acetylcholine has been shown to fulfill in the central nervous system the rigorous criteria established for neurotransmitters in the periphery. The biogenic amines norepinephrine, dopamine, and serotonin have received a tremendous amount of attention as putative neurotransmitters, although the evidence for their candidacy is largely of an indirect, biochemical nature. In this review we have pointed out that these same biochemical measures would also apply to histamine. It is unevenly distributed throughout the brain. It is localized to synaptic endings, along with its synthesizing enzymes. It is released from brain slices by depolarization. It is also distinguished from histamine outside the brain by extremely rapid turnover which can be altered by behavioral stress.

These facts make it seem worthwhile to explore the physiological, and perhaps behavioral, role of histamine in the brain. At the same time it is wise to remember that the role of neurotransmitter is not the only interesting function a neurochemical may play.

REFERENCES

1. Abel, J. J., and Kubota, S., *J. Pharmacol. Exp. Ther.*, 13, 243 (1919).
2. Kwiatkowski, H., *J. Physiol.*, 102, 32 (1943).
3. Harris, G. W., Jacobson, D., and Kahlson, G., in: *Ciba Foundation Colloquia*, p. 186, Churchill Press, London (1952).
4. Taylor, K. M., and Snyder, S. H., *J. Neurochem.*, 19, 1343 (1971).
5. Snyder, S. H., and Taylor, K. M., in: *Perspectives in Neuropharmacology*, edited by S. H. Snyder, p. 43, Oxford University Press, Oxford (1972).
6. Whittaker, V. P., *Prog. Biophys. Molec. Biol.*, 15, 39 (1965).
7. Kataoka, K., and DeRobertis, E., *J. Pharmacol. Exptl. Ther.*, 156, 114 (1966).
8. Michaelson, I. A., and Coffman, P. Z., *Biochem. Pharmacol.*, 16, 2085 (1967).
9. Carlini, E. A., and Green, J. P., *Brit. J. Pharmacol.*, 20, 264 (1963).
10. Kuhar, M. J., Taylor, K. M., and Snyder, S. H., *J. Neurochem.*, 18, 1515 (1971).
11. Snyder, S. H., Brown, B., and Kuhar, M. J., *J. Neurochem. (in press)*.
12. Taylor, K. M., and Snyder, S. H., *J. Neurochem. (in press)*.
13. Taylor, K. M., and Snyder, S. H., *J. Pharmacol. Exptl. Ther.*, 179, 619 (1971).
14. Reilly, M. A., and Schayer, R. W., *Brit. J. Pharmacol.*, 38, 478 (1970).
15. Taylor, K. M., and Snyder, S. H., *J. Neurochem.*, 19, 341 (1972).

Advances in Neurology, Vol. 5
Raven Press, New York © 1974

Evidence for a Specific Function of Histamine in Brain

Richard W. Schayer

Research Center, Rockland State Hospital, Orangeburg, New York 10962

Histamine has been under consideration for a function in brain mainly because it, and enzymes which catalyze its formation and catabolism, are present in brain. Further, it can affect neural tissues in various ways. These and other aspects of research on brain histamine through early 1969 have been well reviewed by Green (1).

There is no literature known to me which relates histamine to Parkinson's disease. However, if the general role of brain histamine can be clarified, some relationship may become discernible. Accordingly, I shall present four points of evidence obtained by my group which suggest that histamine does have a function specific for the brain.

ABSENCE OF DEMONSTRABLE INDUCIBILITY OF BRAIN HISTIDINE DECARBOXYLASE

Histidine decarboxylase activity can be increased in animal tissues by subjecting them to a variety of systemic stressors; for instance released catecholamines are the common inducers in stress (2, 3). The enzyme is also activated locally by irritants, such as injected turpentine (4). Bacterial endotoxins are the strongest known inducers, presumably because they release catecholamines as well as cause widespread local irritation to the cells which phagocytize them (4, 5). However, neither endotoxin nor norepinephrine, injected systemically or directly into brain, produced any detectable effect on histamine formation in mouse brain *in vivo*. A variety of other substances, including psychoactive drugs, have also failed to produce a significant effect (6). This evidence, being negative, is weak. Brain histidine decarboxylase may respond to its own type of activator, or local activation in some small region may occur but be obscured by the presence of larger amounts of unaffected tissue.

EFFECT OF INHIBITORS OF PROTEIN SYNTHESIS ON BASAL HISTIDINE DECARBOXYLASE ACTIVITIES OF VARIOUS MOUSE TISSUES

Data in Table 1 show that treatment of normal mice with inhibitors of protein synthesis markedly reduces histidine decarboxylase activity in the

TABLE 1. *Effect of protein synthesis inhibitors on histidine decarboxylase (HD)*
activity of mouse tissues

Experimental	Tissue	Group	n	HD*
1. Saline or puromycin, 1.5 mg, i.p., at	Liver	Sal	4	100
0, 1, 2, and 3 hr, sacrificed at 4 hr		puromyc	4	28
	Lung	Sal	4	100
		puromyc	4	28
2. Similar to (1) but tenuazonic acid	Lung	Sal	4	100
(TZA) used, 1.5 mg, 4 × i.p.		TZA	4	27
3. Similar to (1) and (2), TZA, 1.5 mg,	Skin	Sal	5	100
and cycloheximide, 0.75 mg,		TZA	5	87
4 × i.p.		cyclohex	5	96
4. Similar to 1–3, same timing and	Brain	Sal	6	100
doses, 4 × i.p.		puromyc	4	115
		TZA	4	100
		cyclohex	4	101
5. Sal and cyclohex, 0.2 mg or 0.4 mg,	Brain	Sal	5	100
inj. i.c., 1 × 4 hr before sacrifice		cycl. 0.2	5	89
		cycl. 0.4	5	83
6. Sal or cyclohex, 0.2 mg, i.c., at 0, 2,	Brain	Sal	5	100
and 4 hr, sacrificed at 6 hr		cycl 3 ×	5	87

* Mean of controls arbitrarily set at 100.

liver and lung (which contain an inducible form of enzyme, not associated with mast cells) but fails to affect the skin enzyme (largely found in mast cells) or that in brain. Evidently, the inducible form of histidine decarboxylase is dependent on new protein synthesis; since the basal level of activity drops to roughly one-fourth of the initial value during 4-hr treatment with protein-synthesis inhibitors (4), the half-life is relatively short, approximately 2 hr. Brain and mast cell histidine decarboxylase appear to have a much longer half-life. In this test, brain enzyme behaves similarly to that of mast cells.

DURATION OF BINDING OF ENDOGENOUSLY FORMED HISTAMINE BY BRAIN AND BY MAST CELLS

The only physiological study on histamine turnover in brain, that is, one in which the precursor, ^{14}C-L-histidine, was given systemically, showed that after intravenous injection of mice with ^{14}C-L-histidine, ^{14}C-histamine was maximal at the earliest time tested, 10 min, but became undetectable at some time between 250 and 1,250 min (7).

Exogenous histamine probably does not enter the brain; in normal mice sacrificed 2.5 min after intravenous injection of ^{14}C-histamine, the concentration of the latter in brain was only 2.0% of blood ^{14}C-histamine. Since brain is said to contain roughly 2% blood, all the ^{14}C-histamine could be in blood perfusing the brain (7).

In rats injected intracisternally with ^{14}C-L-histidine,[14]C-histamine levels of major regions dropped rapidly from a maximum at 10 min, and at 24 hr were virtually undetectable (8); clearly, brain does not retain the histamine it forms for prolonged periods.

In contrast, mast cells firmly bind the ^{14}C-histamine formed within them for many days (9). For example, in mice pretreated with saline (controls) or a histidine decarboxylase inhibitor, decaborane, then injected subcutaneously with ^{14}C-L-histidine 2.0 μ and sacrificed 3 days later, the abdominal skin of controls contained 11,300 ± 1,250 d.p.m. ^{14}C-histamine per gram skin, while for the test group the value was 2,200 ± 370 (10). In a second experiment, mice were pretreated with saline or α-hydrazino-histidine (a histidine decarboxylase inhibitor), then injected subcutaneously with ^{14}C-L-histidine 5.0 μC and sacrificed 4 days later. Abdominal skin contained 29,800 ± 1,180 d.p.m. ^{14}C-histamine per gram skin, whereas the value for the test group was 2,600 ± 180 (11). In these and other similar experiments, normal skin, in which histamine is largely in mast cells, retained newly formed ^{14}C-histamine for prolonged periods. Data from the test groups show that the low values were probably due to histidine decarboxylase inhibition, and not to disruption of mast cells, reduction of available ^{14}C-L-histidine, or other possible mechanisms.

PARALLELISM BETWEEN RATES OF HISTAMINE FORMATION AND CATABOLISM IN VARIOUS TISSUES

Using major brain regions of three species (mice, rats, and guinea pigs), we determined activities of histidine decarboxylase (a measure of the rate of histamine formation) and of histamine-methylating enzyme (a measure of the rate of histamine destruction). When these data are expressed as activities relative to midbrain = 100 and ratios of the two enzymes calculated, relative activities of both enzymes in the three species are (with one exception) midbrain > cerebrum > medulla > cerebellum. Only the value of guinea pig cerebellum histamine-methylating enzyme was aberrant; however, since it was matched by an unusually high value for histidine decarboxylase, the ratio for this tissue was close to that of mouse cerebellum. Ratios for rat brain regions were somewhat different, but in rats values for both enzymes were low; in rat cerebellum, activities were too low to warrant calculation of a ratio. Obviously, comparison of activities of two enzymes, assayed by quite different procedures, can produce only a rough approximation of the *in vivo* situation. But since a thorough investigation of histamine formation and catabolism in a number of other tissues of mice and rats revealed no relationship whatsoever (12, 13), the data of Table 2 are consonant with the possibility that newly formed histamine in brain may act at,

TABLE 2. *Relative activities of histidine decarboxylase (HD) and histamine-methylating enzyme (HME) in brain regions (relative to midbrain = 100)*

	Mice			Rats			Guinea pigs		
	HD	HME	R*	HD	HME	R*	HD	HME	R*
Midbrain	100	100	1.00	100	100	1.00	100	100	1.00
Cerebrum	51	86	0.59	55	73	0.75	59	95	0.62
Medulla	32	76	0.42	26	36	0.72	31	83	0.37
Cerebellum	8	55	0.15	Low	Low	—	26	124	0.21

*R = HD/HME.

or near, its site of formation and then be destroyed to a large extent by methylation. The extremely low levels of endogenous histamine in most brain regions support this concept. If this view is correct, the participation of a catabolic enzyme in modifying or terminating the action of newly formed histamine may be unique for brain, and may be evidence that histamine has a specific function in brain.

ACKNOWLEDGMENTS

This work was supported by National Institutes of Health grant AM-10155. Rockland State Hospital is an institution of the New York State Department of Mental Hygiene. Data of Tables 1 and 2 are reproduced with permission of the *Journal of Pharmacology and Experimental Therapeutics*, the *British Journal of Pharmacology*, and the *Journal of Neurochemistry*.

REFERENCES

1. Green, J. P., in: *Handbook of Neurochemistry*, Vol. 2, p. 221, Plenum Press, New York (1970).
2. Schayer, R. W., *Science* 131, 226 (1960).
3. Schayer, R. W., *Am. J. Physiol.* 202, 66 (1962).
4. Schayer, R. W., and Reilly, M. A., *Am. J. Physiol.* 215, 472 (1968).
5. Schayer, R. W., *Am. J. Physiol.* 198, 1187 (1960).
6. Schayer, R. W., and Reilly, M. A., *Arch. Int. de Pharmacodynamie et de Therap.* 203, 123 (1973).
7. Schayer, R. W., and Reilly, M. A., *J. Neurochem.* 17, 1649 (1970).
8. Schayer, R. W. and Reilly, M. A., *J. Pharmacol. Exp. Therap.* 184, 33 (1973).
9. Schayer, R. W., *Ann. N.Y. Acad. Sci.* 103, 164 (1963).
10. Schayer, R. W., and Reilly, M. A., *J. Pharmacol. Exp. Therap.* 177, 177 (1971).
11. Reilly, M. A., and Schayer, R. W., *Brit. J. Pharmacol. Chemother.* 34, 551 (1968).
12. Reilly, M. A., and Schayer, R. W., *Brit. J. Pharmacol.* 38, 478 (1970).
13. Reilly, M. A., and Schayer, R. W., *Brit. J. Pharmacol.* 43, 349 (1971).

DISCUSSION

Mr. McGeer: I would like to ask Dr. Dismukes if the basis for suggesting histamine as a neurotransmitter was its high concentration (40%) in the P2 fraction. The P3 fraction had only 15%, but the RSA was almost three times as high and I would like to ask why that should be so?

Dr. Dismukes: I am not at all certain about the meaning of relative specific activities when talking about amino acids. It may be better to talk about relative specific activities of enzymes. It simply reflects a difference of distribution of protein, the total amount of protein that falls in each segment.

I do not think there is much relationship between the protein distribution and the histamine distribution, so perhaps we should not use that figure.

Dr. McDowell: Are there other questions for Dr. Dismukes?

Dr. Roberts: We recently got into this field because we wanted to study the metabolism of metesol acetic acid. Try as we might, by injecting very high specific activities of radioactive histidine into brains of frogs and mice, we could not get a single count from histamine. This does not correlate with some of the other experiments. When you get extremely low levels as with histamine, you should be very concerned about your chemistry and the possible small trace impurities in the original isotope that is used, and possibly exchange of tritium. ^{14}C does not present this problem; therefore I am a little worried because, as I see what was presented here, there is no cogent evidence yet in the literature that histamine is formed from histidine in brain.

With regard to the enzyme histidine decarboxylase, I am not so sure that it is a specific enzyme. It has a very high K_M as far as I can tell. Histidine levels of the brain are very low, but I do not know the distribution of histidine, so even that does not support a cogent picture that this enzyme is really there and acting rapidly on the histidine that becomes available to it.

Lastly, could your hydrazino histidine merely be replacing histidine or a decarboxylated product? After all, the hydrazino group gives it a few extra properties that histidine itself does not have and what you are seeing is not the result of the inhibition of the decarboxylase but an actual displacement of histamine by the hydrazino histidine.

Dr. Dismukes: First, you must be very, very careful when working with tritiated histidine as a control as you suggest. We do purify it first, and follow the rate of tritium exchange on the columns which we use to separate tritiated histamine from tritiated histidine. I think the best information on this is Schayer's work using ^{14}C-histidine. I see no problems there.

Regarding the distribution of histidine, it is fairly uniform, as you would expect for an amino acid of this sort, and it is about one hundred times the highest level of histamine.

As for the inhibitors there is a problem here. We have used more than one inhibitor: the fairly specific inhibitor alpha-hydrazinol-histidine and the less specific one SD1055 (known by the trade name of Brocresine) which probably works by the same mechanism, competing for the pyridoxal phosphate site.

Dr. Roberts: The chemistry usually is not very good, as in the final stage of the actual isolation of pure histamine that is done on a column. Rarely do you have actual proof that you have pure histamine which you are measuring.

Dr. Dismukes: Have you looked at Dr. Schayer's work where he used an entirely different technique?

Dr. Roberts: I just want to leave here with some feeling that there is a definitive piece of evidence that histamine is made from histidine in brain. I will be satisfied if you have it.

Dr. Schayer: I have worried about that too, going back to the first experiment. As a consequence, for years we have used an isotope dilution technique in which, I agree, I am very frightened about measuring a thousandth of a microgram of radioactive histamine. We add 40 milligrams of nonisotopic histamine, extract that, wash it, and convert it to the benzene sulfanile derivative which is a crystalline compound. We can recrystallize that to constant activity using different solvents, different absorbents, etc., and when it is constant I think that is about all you can do. Earlier we made a picrate and got that to constant activity, removed the picric acid, sublimed it, and got the three basic histamines with the same specific activity.

Furthermore, we used ^{14}C-histidine which has no problems like the tritium-labeled histidine. Finally, the histidine decarboxylase inhibitors do knock this way down, and in the physiological experiments where histidine was given i.p. we could find it in all the tissues except cerebellum, which is a good blank.

Dr. Roberts: Just one last comment. The time courses of these experiments and the rate of histidine leaving the brain, even when histidine is put into the brain, are such that it could be that histidine acts returning via the circulation to be a possible precursor of histamine rather than the histidine that you put in yourself.

We are finding that a number of histamine and histidine derivatives do get through the blood-brain barrier. Has this possibility been eliminated?

Dr. Schayer: Yes, in the physiological experiment we did, the ^{14}C-histamine in brain as percentage of ^{14}C-histamine in blood came out to be about 1.8 to 1.9. According to the literature, brain contains roughly 2% blood so that blood histamine apparently is not getting into the brain. Everything could be accounted for by a derivative.

Dr. McDowell: Are there any other comments?

Dr. McCann: I was wondering if there is any information as to exactly where the histamine is located in the hypothalamus since the concentration is highest there. That might give a clue as to its function. Also, was the increased turnover of histamine observed in stress situations in the hypothalamic histamine? That was not clear from the slide.

Dr. Dismukes: A much more detailed map of brain histamine has been made by Edgar Feller and Ken Taylor using a monkey brain. They have examined about a hundred nuclei, and the supraoptic nucleus, the periventricular nucleus, and the mammillary bodies have the highest concentration. The median eminence is rather surprisingly low in comparison.

The experiment on stress examined just the hypothalamus, not the whole brain. We have not looked at the effects of stress on histamine concentration in other brain regions.

Advances in Neurology, Vol. 5
Raven Press, New York © 1974

Effect of L-DOPA on the Synthesis and Excretion of Tyramine

Alan A. Boulton and P. H. Wu

Psychiatric Research Unit, University Hospital, Saskatoon, Saskatchewan, Canada

In the unconjugated form, urinary p-tyramine has been shown in the human to be predominantly of endogenous origin (1–3). In approximately 60% of patients suffering with Parkinson's disease it is excreted in above-normal amounts (1, 3, 4). This is quite the reverse of the situation with respect to dopamine, which has been shown to be excreted in decreased quantities (5). A group of 28 parkinsonian patients were admitted to University Hospital, Saskatoon, and maintained for 2 weeks without chemotherapy of any kind. At the end of this period, a 24-hr urine specimen was collected and the EEG assessed as previously described (1, 6). L-DOPA was then administered, on an increasing dose schedule, over a 4- to 6-week period until an optimum dose (usually between 1.5 and 6 g daily), as assessed clinically, was achieved. At this time, and before termination in those cases that did not respond, a second EEG assessment and urine collection were made. The changes in the EEG have been described elsewhere (6). Briefly, it was noticed that L-DOPA produced a 'normalization' of the EEG record and that the coefficient of variation (CV scores) and the mean integrated amptitude (MIA), as obtained after integration (7, 8), correlated significantly with changes on the Columbia Scale of Disability (9), with tremor, and with a decrease in the urinary p-tyramine (1, 6). These correlations were even more significant in postsurgical cases.

The effect of L-DOPA treatment on urinary unconjugated p-tyramine and tryptamine is shown in Table 1. In all patients tyramine decreased from an above-normal (range 75–2,910 µg/g creatinine) to a below-normal value (range 21–555 µg/g creatinine). In those 'normal' subjects (ingesting, respectively, 2, 2, and 3 g of L-DOPA daily for 3 weeks), a decrease was not observed (1). Neither in patients nor in the three control subjects was there a change in the excretion of tryptamine. By observing the change in urinary tyramine excretion, it was possible to split the parkinsonian population into two groups. Group A (17 of 28) had initially high urinary p-tyramine values (range 174–2,910 µg/g creatinine), and these reduced during L-DOPA treatment to low values (range 21–416 µg/g creatinine). Group B (11 of 28) had initially low excretion values, and either exhibited no change or even a

TABLE 1. Effect of L-DOPA ingestion on the urinary excretion of unconjugated p-tyramine and tryptamine in parkinsonism

Group	p-Tyramine[a]		Tryptamine[b]	
	Before	During	Before	During
Control population	312 ± 162 (n = 31)	—	83 ± 36 (n = 16)	—
Parkinsonian population	500 ± 725 (n = 28)	152 ± 120 (n = 28)	72 ± 44 (n = 27)	66 ± 36 (n = 27)
Group A[c]	726 ± 820 (n = 17)	125 ± 108 (n = 17)	70 ± 33 (n = 16)	61 ± 22 (n = 16)
Group B[c]	161 ± 54.5 (n = 11)	192 ± 132 (n = 11)	72 ± 56 (n = 11)	76 ± 43 (n = 11)

[a] Results, corrected for recovery, are expressed at μg/g creatinine, mean ± standard deviation. Assessed photodensitometrically as its 1-nitroso-2-naphthol fluorophore after chromatographic separation (11).
[b] Analyzed according to the procedure described by Udenfriend (12).
[c] See text for details.

slight increase (range 77–555 μg/g creatinine). It is difficult to explain why tyramine should decrease and tryptamine remain unchanged in parkinsonian patients consuming L-DOPA. L-Aromatic amino acid decarboxylase, as purified from mammalian kidney (10), is extremely efficient in converting DOPA to dopamine. If, therefore, it were simply a case of enzyme saturation as a consequence of the high circulating levels of L-DOPA, one would expect a decrease in tryptamine as well as tyramine. Alternatively the explanation may relate to the recent discovery of dopamine dehydroxylation (13–15).

After intraventricular injections of tyrosine and dopamine to rats pretreated with pargyline, the phenolic amines tyramine, octopamine, and synephrine have been isolated as their dimethylaminonaphthalene-5-sulfonyl (DNS) derivatives (see references 13 and 14 for complete details). After intraperitoneal injections of these substrates (suitably labeled with ^{14}C or ^{3}H), we were able to locate, in the case of ^{14}C-dopamine, small numbers of counts associated with tyramine in several tissues (kidney, spleen, lung, and liver). We were unable to find any tyramine following injection of tyrosine even after relatively large doses (1 mC supplemented with 1 mg cold tyrosine).

Prior to an analysis of the formation of tyramine and octopamine in regions of the rat brain, we investigated the amounts of these amines remaining in whole brain at various times following intraventricular injection of ^{14}C-tyrosine and ^{14}C-dopamine. In the case of tyrosine, tyramine was maximally present at 15 min but octopamine was still increasing after 120 min. Tyramine and octopamine, as formed from dopamine, exhibited a maximum

TABLE 2. *Distribution of ^{3}H-p-tyramine and ^{3}H-octopamine in the presence of pargyline, in regions of the rat brain 60 min after an intraventricular injection of ^{3}H-p-tyramine*

Region	Total radioactivity (dpm × 10^{-6}/g)	DNS-*p*-tyramine[a] (dpm × 10^{-4}/g)	DNS-octopamine[a] (dpm × 10^{-4}/g)
Hypothalamus	6.15 ± 0.08	26.8 ± 0.2	234.5 ± 2.9
Caudate nucleus	3.35 ± 0.15	119.7 ± 17.9	15.6 ± 1.1
Brainstem	3.36 ± 0.36	15.7 ± 1.4	129.3 ± 8.4
Cerebellum	2.07 ± 0.08	10.0 ± 1.0	92.6 ± 9.2
'Rest'	1.54 ± 0.02	20.1 ± 1.0	57.3 ± 5.5

Each value mean ± mean deviation of two experiments.
[a] Not corrected for recovery.

in the 60- to 120-min period. Such an observation in view of the reported distribution of dopamine-β-hydroxylase (16) suggests that these phenolic amines produced from their different precursors might possess different functions.

The regional distribution of *p*-tyramine and octopamine, in the presence of pargyline, 1 hr after an intraventricular injection of 5 μC of purified ^{3}H-*p*-tyramine (specific activity 7.3 C/mmole), is listed in Table 2. With the exception of the caudate nucleus, the bulk of the radioactivity in the other regions is associated with octopamine. This finding agrees with those reported by Anagnoste and Goldstein (17) and Steinberg and Smith (18).

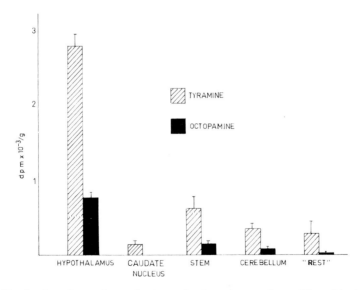

FIG. 1. Distribution of tyramine and octopamine in various regions of the rat brain 15 min after an intraventricular injection of ^{14}C-L-tyrosine-U. Each value mean ± mean deviation of three experiments, not corrected for recovery. Recovery of tyramine and octopamine as their DNS derivatives was approximately 24% and 60%, respectively.

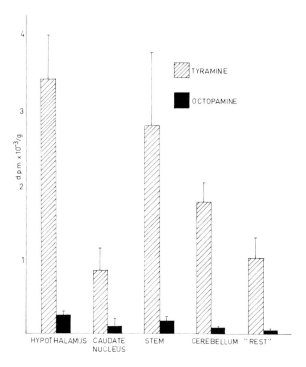

FIG. 2. Distribution of tyramine and octopamine in various regions of the rat brain 60 min after an intraventricular injection of ^{14}C-dopamine. Each value mean ± mean deviation of four experiments, not corrected for recovery.

The amount of ^{14}C-tyramine and ^{14}C-octopamine, expressed in disintegrations per minute per gram (d.p.m.) of tissue, found in various regions of the rat brain at 15 and 60 min, respectively, following intraventricular injections of 10 μC ^{14}C-tyrosine (specific activity 410 mC/mmole) and 4.6 μC purified ^{14}C-dopamine (specific activity 55 mC/mmole) are shown in Figs. 1 and 2. It can be seen that after an injection of tyrosine the greatest concentrations of tyramine and octopamine are found in the hypothalamus; in the case of dopamine both the hypothalamus and the brainstem retain the greatest concentrations, although significant quantities of tyramine are also found in the cerebellum, 'rest,' and caudate nucleus.

By investigating the disappearance from whole brain and from certain regions of ^{3}H-tyramine and ^{3}H-octopamine after intraventricular injections, both in the presence and absence of pargyline, it was possible to show that, in some instances, in some regions in the absence of pargyline, there was a linear loss of amine. In most cases, however, the loss of amine was non-linear and nonexponential. In all cases the clearance rate (half-life) was much faster than with either the catecholamines or 5-hydroxytryptamine.

In an attempt to discover whether the treatment of rats with L-DOPA had any effect on the amount of tyramine and/or octopamine, rats were

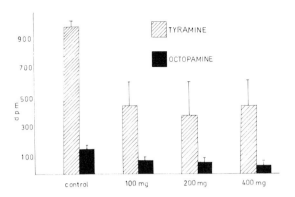

FIG. 3. Effect of chronic L-DOPA injections on the formation of tyramine and octopamine from tyrosine in rat brain. Each value mean ± standard deviation of seven experiments, not corrected for recovery.

treated with L-DOPA in both an acute and a chronic situation. Briefly, L-DOPA (50, 100, or 200 mg) suspended in Krebs-Ringer solution containing 4 drops of the detergent Tween 80 per 10 ml, at pH 7.2, was injected i.p. to rats at 10:00 A.M. At 2:15 P.M. pargyline (75 mg/kg) was injected i.p., and at 3:00 P.M. ^{14}C-tyrosine (10 μC) was injected into the left lateral ventricle. Fifteen min later the rats were sacrificed, and the whole brain phenolicamines, tyramine, and octopamine were isolated, dansylated, and separated as previously described (14). The same procedure was followed in the chronic experiments except that the rats were injected twice daily, at 10:00 A.M. and 3:00 P.M., for 7 days. On the eighth day the rats were injected at 10:00 A.M. and sacrificed at 3:15 P.M. in the case of tyrosine or 4:00 P.M. in the case of dopamine. The amounts of tyramine and octopamine formed from tyrosine at the different injected L-DOPA levels are shown in Figs. 3 and 4. It can be seen that substantial inhibition occurred for both tyramine

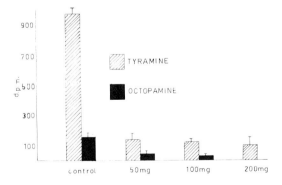

FIG. 4. Effect of an injection of L-DOPA on the formation of tyramine and octopamine from tyrosine in rat brain. Each value mean ± mean deviation of four experiments, not corrected for recovery.

and octopamine amounting to 55 and 47% at a dose level of 100 mg/day; 61 and 55% at 200 mg/day, 54 and 68% at 400 mg/day in the case of chronic treatment; and 86 and 76% at a dose of 50 mg, 88 and 83% at 100 mg, and 89.5 and 100% at 200 mg, respectively, in the case of an acute treatment. There was no significant change in the amount of tyramine and octopamine synthesized from dopamine after chronic injections of L-DOPA.

ACKNOWLEDGMENTS

We thank the Psychiatric Services Branch, Province of Saskatchewan, the Medical Research Council of Canada, and Hoffman-LaRoche (Canada) for financial support, Dr. G. L. Marjerrison for his EEG data, Mrs. Lillian Dyck for information on the peripheral dehydroxylation of dopamine, and Dr. A. H. Rajput for urine samples from his patients.

REFERENCES

1. Boulton, A. A., and Marjerrison, G. L. *Nature* 236, 76 (1972).
2. Boulton, A. A., Marjerrison, G. L., and Majer, J. R. *J. Acad. Med. Sci.* (USSR) 5, 68 (1971).
3. Boulton, A. A. *Prog. Neurogenet.* 1, 437 (1969).
4. Smith, I., and Kellow, A. H. *Nature* 221, 1261 (1969).
5. Barbeau, A., Murphy, G. F., and Sourkes, T. L. *Science* 133, 1706 (1961).
6. Marjerrison, G. L., Boulton, A. A., and Rajput, A. *Dis. Nerv. Syst.* 33, 164 (1972).
7. Goldstein, L., Sugerman, A. A., Stolberg, H., Murphee, H. B., and Pfeiffer, C. C. *EEG Clin. Neurophysiol.* 19, 350 (1965).
8. Marjerrison, G. L., Krause, A. E., and Keogh, R. P. *EEG Clin. Neurophysiol.* 24, 35 (1968).
9. Yahr, M. D., Duvoisin, R. C., Schear, M. J., Bassett, R. E., and Hoehn, M. M. *Arch. Neurol.* 21, 343 (1969).
10. Christenson, J. G., Dairman, W., and Udenfriend, S. *Arch. Biochem. Biophys.* 141, 356 (1970).
11. Boulton, A. A. *Meth. Biochem. Anal.* 16, 328 (1968).
12. Udenfriend, S. *Fluorescence Assay in Biology and Medicine,* p. 164, Academic Press, New York (1962).
13. Boulton, A. A., and Quan, L. *Can. J. Biochem.* 48, 287 (1970).
14. Boulton, A. A., and Wu, P. H. *Can. J. Biochem.* 50, 261 (1972).
15. Boulton, A. A., and Wu, P. H. *Can. J. Biochem.* 51, 418 (1973).
16. Glowinski, J., and Iverson, L. *J. Neurochem.* 13, 655 (1966).
17. Anagnoste, B., and Goldstein, M. *Life Sci.* 6, 1535 (1967).
18. Steinberg, M. I., and Smith, C. M. *J. Pharm. Exp. Therap.* 173, 176 (1970).

DISCUSSION

Dr. Sandler: We thought we might try to confirm the data of Boulton and his colleagues and of Smith and Kellow in human parkinsonism about tyramine excretion, but unfortunately we just could not. I suppose there may be differences in population. What we did find (and, Dr. Boulton, you know you should have looked at this conjugative story because some rather intriguing things emerged) was that there was a significant increase of conjugated tyramine in our parkinsonian population. In one experiment we gave the patients lactose on one day and tyramine on another day, both orally. In those receiving lactose, in particular, you can see quite a significant increase in conjugated tyramine 3-hour urine collection periods.

After an oral tyramine load, there was a slower rise in conjugated tyramine in the parkinsonian patients than in the normal population that we studied, and this difference reached significance at 6 to 9 hours.

These data are a bit difficult to interpret, but we think we are probably dealing with a gut stagnation phenomenon. Some of these patients were on anticholinesterase drugs, others were not. We thought that it may well be a cholinesterase-anticholinesterase phenomenon but there was no difference between the two groups of parkinsonian patients; if anything, there was more conjugation of tyramine in patients who were not on cholinesterase drugs.

There are indications in the literature that there may be some degree of malabsorption in parkinsonism but this is as far as one can go in trying to interpret these data at the present time.

Dr. McDowell: Are there any questions or comments?

Dr. Carlsson: I wonder whether Dr. Boulton did not after all have a model in mind subconsciously because he said that DOPA would inhibit the formation of tyramine and octopamine. My question is, couldn't it be instead that you release the tyramine and octopamine by means of the dopamine formed? We know from studies where you administer radioactive tyramine and get octopamine formed in the adrenergic nerves that after you give another amine it is surprising how easily dopamine and octopamine are released from the stores.

Advances in Neurology, Vol. 5
Raven Press, New York © 1974

Disinhibition as an Organizing Principle in the Nervous System—The Role of Gamma-Aminobutyric Acid

Eugene Roberts

Division of Neurosciences, City of Hope National Medical Center, Duarte, California 91010

All normal or adaptive activity in nervous systems is a result of the co-ordinated dynamic interplay of excitation and inhibition within and between neuronal subsystems. A basic inadequacy in this interplay could lead to an abnormal (disease) process such as is found in Parkinson's disease, Huntington's chorea, schizophrenia, epilepsy, depression, manic-depressive disorder, hyperkinetic behavior in children, psychosomatic disorders, and so on.

HOW THE NERVOUS SYSTEM MAY BE PUT TOGETHER

Wherever one looks at nervous systems as a whole or at functional sub-units, one is impressed by the absence of permissivity and democracy. All of the neurons are not firing independently of each other, nor is the activity of the systems the result of a statistical consensus. Instead, it seems that a nervous system and its subunits consist largely of poised, genetically pre-programmed circuits which are released for action by neurons (command neurons) that are strategically located at junctions in neuronal hierarchies dealing with both sensory input and effector output. In some instances it has been possible to identify a hierarchy of controls within a neuronal population. A command neuron seems to be in control of the whole unit, a ganglion, for example; and its activity is the key to the activity of the ganglion.

In a hierarchical segmental system, such as has been found in crustacea and analyzed in the case of the system involved in control of swimmeret movement in the crayfish (1, 2), the activity of a command neuron of a particular segment is controlled to a considerable extent by the neuronal activities of the segments above it in the hierarchy, with the head ganglion or brain exerting the highest level of control. If the communication between the segments is interrupted by cutting the connectives, then command neurons within each particular segment assume control of the activity of the segment. From considerable experimental evidence, it appears that segmental command neurons, like the circuits they control, are largely inhibited from above, and that a decrease in inhibition allows command neurons to fire, thereby releasing the preprogrammed circuits over whose activity they preside. A striking instance of this is the release of the highly coordinated stereotypical sexual behavior of the male praying mantis when his head is bitten off by the female (3). Although similar patterns of relationships are discernible in the higher nervous systems of vertebrate forms, the order of complexity is greatly increased. An example of this in humans may be the stereotypical postural effects and paranoia produced by overdoses of amphetamines (4). Paranoid thinking may be a complicated, but stereotypical, genetically preprogrammed process that can be evoked by skillful demagogues as well as by drugs.

In behavioral sequences, innate or learned, genetically preprogrammed circuits may be *released* to function at varying rates and in various combinations by inhibition of neurons which are tonically holding in check pacemaker cells with capacity for spontaneous activity. If the pacemaker neurons are triggering a circuit related to the regulation of a vital function such as heart action or respiration, the inhibitory neurons might act in such a way as to vary the rate of the discharge of the pacemaker neuron. On the other hand, if a behavioral sequence involves the voluntary movement of a limb muscle, the pacemaker neuron might be held in complete check by the tonic action of inhibitory neurons and might be allowed to discharge in a graded manner related only to demand. A detailed discussion of the above concepts has been published (5), particularly with reference to the etiology of schizophrenia. In this view, excitatory input to pacemaker neurons would have only a modulatory role. Thus, disinhibition appears to be one of the major organizing principles in nervous system function. The importance of its role was succinctly stated by Maynard (6) just before his untimely death: "Most patterned neural activity can be expressed as a time series of instructions telling specific units (a) when to fire and/or (b) when to be silent. The relative importance of these two instructions in determining the pattern depends upon the 'initial' or intrinsic activity of the system. If all or most elements are quiescent, then the instruction, 'fire' is necessary; if most elements are intrinsically active, then the instruction, 'quiet' is paramount. *Disinhibition* will be most evident in the latter case where it may either (a) act as a switch, turning on a specific coherent pattern which is otherwise actively and continuously inhibited, or (b) play a role in the organization of sequential and alternating discharges among separate groups of elements.

"In the stomatogastric ganglion of crabs and lobsters disinhibition is important in the organization of patterned activity controlling sequential contractions of the muscles of the pyloric stomach (7). All known chemical synapses among the 14 identified neurons involved in the pyloric patterns are inhibitory. Electrical junctions are present and are important in producing synchrony when two or more elements must discharge together, but alternation and sequencing result solely from inhibition and disinhibition.

In this system, however, genesis of the output pattern requires not only disinhibition but also slow, intrinsic pacemaker activity in appropriately connected elements. In addition, direct excitation via chemical excitatory synapses from modulating interneurons is important in turning on overall system activity and perhaps in modulating parameters within the pattern.

"If the situation observed in the stomatogastric ganglion can be generalized to larger and more complex neural systems, then one must conclude that disinhibition, while of critical importance in the organization of patterned activity and perhaps of major importance in certain situations, is but one of several organizing principles. It is important to determine exactly where and how disinhibition interacts with these other principles."

When one deals with whole neuronal systems in intact organisms, the situation becomes quite complex. For instance, the overall effect of inhibition at the synaptic level may be either activation or inhibition of the system. Thus, inhibition of inhibitory neurons may lead to disinhibition or excitation of the system as a whole; inhibition of excitatory neurons may lead to inhibition of the system; inhibition of excitatory neurons that act on inhibitory neurons may lead to disinhibition or excitation, and so on. It is important to realize that the overall physiological or behavioral effects of an excitatory or inhibitory synapse depend on the circuit of which it is a part. The Purkinje cells of the cerebellar cortex, which convey the output of that structure, make only inhibitory connections with neurons in a number of deeper structures. The activity of the Purkinje cells is modified by powerful inhibitory synapses formed by presynaptic endings of basket cells on their somas. Therefore, basket cell activity has a disinhibiting or activating effect on the activity of those cells that receive an input from the Purkinje cells. Gamma-aminobutyric acid (GABA) probably is the transmitter substance employed by both the Purkinje and basket cells. Motor neurons of the spinal cord which employ acetylcholine as transmitter, in addition to their primary excitatory effect on muscles, send excitatory collateral fibers to inhibitory interneurons that lie in ventral regions of the cord. These neurons, in turn, may inhibit the same motor neurons that excite them as well as other motor neurons in the vicinity. Thus, release of an excitatory transmitter may result in physiological inhibition. Similarly, behavioral inhibition or depression must not be equated in a one-to-one way with synaptic inhibition.

THE SYSTEM OF NEURONS UTILIZING GABA IS A MAJOR INHIBITORY SYSTEM IN THE CENTRAL NERVOUS SYSTEM

A consideration of the biochemical, pharmacological, and physiological data currently available about nervous system function suggested that a major neural system exerting tonic inhibition on pacesetter neurons could be the system of inhibitory neurons utilizing GABA as transmitter (8, 9). GABA neurons are present ubiquitously in the central nervous system

(CNS) of vertebrate species, and on a quantitative basis GABA is much more extensively and relatively more evenly distributed throughout the various brain regions than the neuronal systems that employ other known neural transmitters such as acetylcholine, the catecholamines, or serotonin (5).

I would like to summarize briefly some current knowledge about the GABA system, a subject with which my colleagues and I have been concerned for over 20 years. The first report of the presence of GABA in uniquely large concentrations in the vertebrate CNS was made in 1950 (10). From many lines of evidence, it appears probable that GABA is a major inhibitory transmitter in the invertebrate and vertebrate CNS (8).

An outline of the chief known reactions of GABA is shown in Fig. 1. GABA is formed in the CNS of vertebrate organisms to a large extent, if not entirely, from L-glutamic acid. The reaction is catalyzed by an L-glutamic acid decarboxylase (GAD I), an enzyme found in mammalian organisms only in the CNS, largely in gray matter. For a number of years it was assumed that there was only one GAD in the vertebrate organism and that it was located entirely in neurons in the CNS. With more sensitive methods, it was found that GAD activity can be detected in glial cells, kidney, adrenal and pituitary glands, and blood vessels. The GAD in the latter tissues (GAD II) shows different properties from the neuronal enzyme (11).

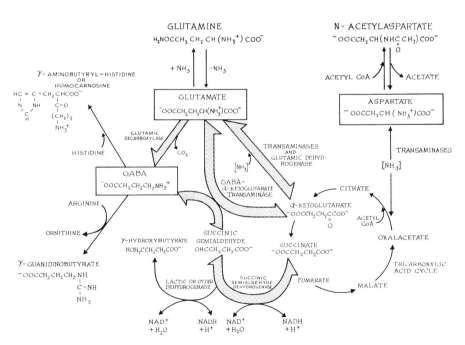

FIG. 1. Outline of main known reactions of GABA.

We now have succeeded in purifying GAD I to homogeneity (12). It has a molecular weight of 85,000, a sharp pH optimum at 7.0, and catalyzes the rapid α-decarboxylation only of L-glutamic acid of the naturally occurring amino acids, and to a very slight extent that of L-aspartic acid. Further studies of the properties of this enzyme are in progress. Henceforth, when mention is made of GAD in this chapter, it will be assumed that reference is being made to GAD I. Further work is also in progress in our laboratories on the purification and properties of GAD II.

The reversible transamination of GABA with α-ketoglutarate is catalyzed by an aminotransferase, GABA-T, which in the CNS is found chiefly in the gray matter, but also is found in other tissues. The products of the transaminase reaction are succinic semialdehyde and glutamic acid. A dehydrogenase is present which catalyzes the oxidation of succinic semialdehyde to succinic acid, which in turn can be oxidized via the reactions of the tricarboxylic acid cycle. Only recently have we succeeded in purifying GABA-T to homogeneity, and its properties are being studied in detail (13). In lobsters and in other invertebrates, similar enzymes are present in *both* peripheral and central nervous systems (14).

The steady-state concentrations of GABA in various brain areas probably are normally governed by the GAD activity and not by the GABA-T. In many inhibitory nerves, both GAD and GABA are present and are distributed throughout the neuron, the GAD being somewhat more highly concentrated in the presynaptic endings than elsewhere. The GABA-T is contained in mitochondria of all neuronal regions, but it seems to be richer in the mitochondria of those neuronal sites onto which GABA might be liberated. Such regions would be expected to exist in perikarya and dendrites that receive inhibitory inputs and possibly in the glial and endothelial cells that are in the vicinity of inhibitory synapses (8, 9).

There is evidence for presynaptic release of GABA. Stimulation of axons of several nerves inhibiting different lobster muscles was shown to result in the release of GABA in amounts related to the extent of stimulation, while stimulation of the excitatory nerve did not produce GABA release (14). Data showing the liberation of GABA on stimulation of specific inhibitory neurons in the vertebrate nervous system are extremely difficult to obtain, but there are many experiments that indicate that this does take place (15–19).

The ionic basis of the inhibitory effect of GABA on the postsynaptic regions of vertebrate and invertebrate neurons is known (see 8 for review). Applied GABA alters the membrane conductance to chloride ions, with the membrane potential staying near the resting level. GABA also has a presynaptic inhibitory action at the crayfish neuromuscular junction, imitating the action of the natural inhibitory transmitter by increasing permeability to chloride, thus decreasing the probability of release of quanta of excitatory transmitter (20). There is as yet no hint about the manner in which chemical or physical interaction of GABA with membranes produces increases in the chloride ion conductance of the membranes, and to date all of our attempts to isolate the GABA receptor have failed. Recent evidence suggests that GABA may be the transmitter mediating presynaptic inhibition in a number of regions in the vertebrate CNS (21–23), and that it may act by producing depolarization of primary afferent terminals. Although it was suggested that sodium may be the chief ion involved in the mechanism (23), recent unpublished data in several laboratories suggest the participation of the chloride ion.

The cessation of action of a synaptically active substance could be brought about by the removal of the substance from the sensitive sites by destruction, by transport, or by diffusion. In the case of GABA, it is likely that active transport out of the synaptic gap is the major inactivating mechanism (8).

WHERE GABA FUNCTIONS

Biochemical analytical data have shown the presence of GAD and GABA in many regions of the vertebrate CNS. However, in no instance have the functional relationships been worked out to the same extent as they have in the cerebellum (8). GABA probably mediates the inhibitory actions of stellate and basket cells upon the Purkinje cells and of the Golgi type 2 cells at the mossy fiber endings. It also transmits the inhibitory messages that go from the Purkinje cells to each other and to the cells in the intracerebellar nuclei. GABA also takes part in information processing beyond the Purkinje cell synapses. For example, rabbit oculomotor neurons may be inhibited by GABA neurons found in the vestibular nuclear complex (24).

In the retina, the cellular layers all contained GABA and GAD activity, higher contents of GABA being accompanied by higher levels of GAD activity (25). The highest values for GABA and GAD were found in the third layer, the ganglion cell layer, and the next highest in the receptor-containing layer. The region of the optic fibers showed no GABA and only traces of GAD. Therefore, the GABA neurons probably are not the retinal ganglion cells, whose axons furnish the bulk of the fibers of the optic nerve. The GABA neurons of the retina, therefore, are probably indigenous to the retina. Although it appears likely that at least some of the amacrine cells are GABA neurons, much further work is required to determine which of them are the GABA neurons.

The hippocampal formation is another structure suitable for laminar analysis. Recent data suggest strongly that GABA plays an important regulatory role in the activity of the hippocampus, possibly mediating the inhibition of the pyramidal cells by the basket cells (26, 27).

There is relatively convincing physiological evidence that inhibition in the mammalian cortex may be mediated by GABA neurons (28). In the spinal cord, the chief enzymes of GABA metabolism, GAD and GABA-T, are higher in the dorsal than in the ventral gray matter (29, 30), and recent data suggest that there may be an extensive system of indigenous GABA neurons in the dorsal part of the cord (31) and that these may be involved in the phenomenon of presynaptic inhibition (32).

We have succeeded in obtaining antibodies to homogeneous preparations of GAD (33) and currently are trying to develop methods for the direct visualization of GABA neurons at the histological and ultrastructural levels in the regions of the nervous system. The achievement of this goal would greatly facilitate understanding of the function of the GABA system and the experimental determination by physiologists as to whether or not GABA neurons may be inhibiting in a tonic fashion pacesetter neurons at key sites in the nervous system.

THE RELATIONS OF THE GABA SYSTEM TO OTHER TRANSMITTER SYSTEMS

Throughout this discussion it will be assumed that inhibitory neurons can interact with other inhibitory neurons regardless of the transmitter which they employ. This is based on the knowledge that the Purkinje cells, which probably are GABA-releasing neurons (34), are inhibited by basket and stellate cells, which also probably are GABA-releasing neurons (35, 36); and, likewise, that Purkinje cells are inhibited through noradrenergic endings of nerve fibers (37), which have their origin in the locus coeruleus (38). Thus, inhibitory neurons utilizing GABA as a transmitter can be inhibited by other GABA neurons and by noradrenergic neurons. Serotonin-releasing neurons from the raphe nuclei inhibit noradrenergic neurons in the brainstem, an inhibition that may play a key role in slow-wave sleep mechanisms (39). It is likely that in the complex arrangements of various regions of the CNS a variety of combinations of inhibitory neurons can act on each other. In most instances in which they have been studied by iontophoretic application, the biogenic amines have been found to exert an inhibitory action on neurons (40, 41).

Excitatory information coming in from receptors can go to neurons in the spinal cord or in the brainstem, increasing their probability of firing. Sensory input comes in via excitatory endings that may impinge directly on pacesetter neurons and also on inhibitory neurons (GABA-releasing, catecholaminergic, serotoninergic) lying entirely in the immediate neighborhood, which would disinhibit pacesetter neurons by liberating them from the tonic inhibition of GABA neurons. The identity of the excitatory transmitter (or transmitters) is not known with certainty, but it may be a polypeptide (42), or possibly glutamic acid (43). In addition, some of the GABA neurons could inhibit adjacent sensory endings by presynaptic inhibition via axo-axonic connections. If a stimulus is sufficiently great, it may affect cholinergic spinal motor neurons so that their discharge would elicit a spinal reflex prior to detailed processing of the incoming signals in CNS regions beyond the spinal cord segment involved. The latter situation must be clearly distinguished from that in which motor units would be used as part of a coordinated behavioral sequence resulting from a processing of the incoming stimulus pattern in the higher centers of the CNS. Contrary to much previous belief, it is obvious that the simple spinal reflex cannot be used as a model for CNS function.

Analytical data for GABA itself (31) and for the enzyme GAD (44), which makes GABA from glutamic acid, indicate that indigenous GABA neurons probably are richest in the substantia gelatinosa and the upper laminae of the dorsal horn (see Table 1). Inhibitory interneurons employing glycine as transmitter seem to be richer in the ventral portions of the spinal cord (45). Neurons in the substantia gelatinosa appear to modulate the input from primary cutaneous afferents in the spinal cord. Fluorescent microscopic studies in mice and rats have shown there to be a system of fine, longitudinally oriented fibers in the substantia gelatinosa which appear to be noradrenergic, whereas morphologically similar terminals in the cat probably contain serotonin (46). The noradrenergic fibers appear to be in synaptic contact with each other as well as with dendrites of other neurons in the substantia gelatinosa. The latter probably are descending fibers from the pons. The results in Table 1 indicate that the GAD activity in the

TABLE 1. *Glutamic decarboxylase activity in monkey cortex and spinal cord*

Structure	Activity (mmoles/kg dry wt/hr)
Occipital cortex	
Layers 1–2	25.0
Layers 3–4a	57.7
Layers 4b–5	19.4
Layer 6	13.3
White	0
Spinal cord	
Dorsal ganglion	1.6
Dorsal root	1.6
Lumbar gray matter	
Substantia gelatinosa	19.9
Dorsal horn-dorsal region	25.6
(probably laminae 1–3)	
-medial region	16.9
(probably laminae 4–6)	
Ventral horn-medial region	11.5
-ventral region	6.8
Ventral root	2.5
Lateral pyramidal tract	0

From (44).

monkey spinal cord also shows a marked dorsal-ventral gradient and that the substantia gelatinosa and the dorsal regions involving laminae 1–3 of the spinal cord contain by far the highest amount of the enzyme that makes GABA. It is, therefore, not at all unreasonable to conjecture that there are synapses between the noradrenergic or serotoninergic fibers with the GABA neurons in the substantia gelatinosa.

Directly, and/or after processing in the spinal cord, the sensory input can enter the brainstem, where it may act on monoaminergic interneurons lying entirely within the brainstem that can inhibit the tonically active GABA neurons that are holding in check intersystem monoaminergic neurons. This action could result in the disinhibition, and therefore activation, of the input of the brainstem neurons to the higher brain centers. It is well known that ascending pathways from the reticular formation of the brainstem are very important in increasing the background activity of neurons in higher brain centers. When the connections between the brainstem region and the cortex are cut, the activity of cortical neurons either stops completely or the frequency of discharge becomes much lower than in the brain of an intact animal, while stimulation of this region in an intact animal increases the activity of cortical neurons. In a study of neuronal units in rabbit visual cortex, it was shown that destruction of the mesencephalic reticular formation or its blockade by drugs reduced the frequency of appearance of groups of spikes from a given cortical neuron but did not change the number of spikes appearing in a group when a neuron did fire (47). This decrement in discharge frequency was not observed when the lateral geniculate body or the superior colliculi, specific relay stations of the visual system, were destroyed. The above data are consistent with the idea that the impulses from the brainstem serve to release cortical units for firing in their own characteristic fashion, and that the pathways from the brainstem are much more important for maintaining cortical activity than those from the specific sensory nuclei. There is abundant evidence that the excitatory information of the brainstem to the cortex is largely mediated by a neuronal system employing norepinephrine (NE) as transmitter (46). The NE innervation comes along a dorsal NE bundle that originates from NE neurons in the locus coeruleus area of the pons, and recent data suggest that a single NE neuron from this area can innervate both cerebral and cerebellar cortices and also in its course can give off collaterals to the colliculi, the geniculate bodies, and part of the thalamus (38). It is this system of neurons that may be importantly involved in EEG arousal. Since most of the direct cellular experiments with NE have shown that this substance exerts an inhibitory effect on the neurons being studied (40, 41), the only logical way in which it can be envisioned that a neuronal system employing NE as a transmitter may be an excitatory one is if it were to be acting through inhibition of inhibitory interneurons, or by disinhibition. If we postulate that the primary inhibition within the cortex is exerted by a system of tonically active inhibitory GABA interneurons, a proposition not without considerable electrophysiological support (28), then the well-known system of NE endings in the cortex could be envisioned to be acting in such a way as to inhibit the GABA neurons, which are themselves holding cortical activity in check. Although there exists a diffuse network of very fine, varicose NE nerve terminals in practically all parts of the cerebral cortex, the highest density of terminals appeared in the four outer cortical layers (48). It is instructive in this regard to look at the distribution in the cerebral cortex of GAD, the enzyme that synthesizes GABA. The data in Table 1 show the GABA-forming neurons probably have by far the highest density in the four outer cortical layers of the occipital or visual cortex in the monkey, the highest being in layers 3–4A. Since this is also a region of high density of NE nerve endings, it is not unreasonable to presume that the NE neurons, activated by incoming sensory input, send signals from the brainstem region to the cortex, releasing the activity of cortical pyramidal neurons from inhibition by GABA neurons. The input of brainstem NE neurons occurs both to the inhibitory neurons which are restraining the activity of cortical pacesetter neurons and to centers involved in perceptual integration, such as the hippocampus, cerebellum, thalamus, basal ganglia, and so on. The input from brainstem neurons is not sufficient in itself to release a preprogrammed effector circuit. Instead, it is suggested that perceptual integration must take place within the various analyzing regions of the nervous system (see ref. 49 for pertinent discussion) and that from the central visceromotor system [hypothalamus, septum, and paramedian region of the mesencephalon (50)] there must come either a GO or NO GO signal. Within the structures of this system, the emotionally significant aspects of the total stimulus pattern, external and internal, are summated, and a signal is generated which causes the organism to act by releasing or withholding behavior options already available to it. If a decision is reached that a particular behavioral option is *not* to be employed, then an inhibitory signal may go out to the cortical pacesetter neurons related to the control of that behavioral option, so that they will be sure not to discharge at all or, at least, not to increase their basal rate of discharge. On the other hand, if a decision is reached that a particular behavioral option should be employed, then there might be inhibition of the same tonically active inhibitory GABA neurons that were acted on by the inhibitory brainstem (NE) neurons, so that the additive effect would result in the disinhibition of pacesetter neurons. From the above, it is suggested that the disinhibitory signal from brainstem neurons alone is a necessary but not sufficient condition for the release of the activity of pacesetter cortical neurons in an intact conscious organism. As a result of the disinhibition of pacesetter neurons in a higher brain center, excitatory signals to monoaminergic interneurons located in the brainstem disinhibit descending intersystem monoaminergic neurons which, together with other disinhibitory and excitatory influences communicated by the same pacesetter neurons through the pyramidal tract, release neurons in the spinal cord from inhibition by tonically active GABA neurons. This finally allows motor neurons to fire and cause those effectors to respond which are involved in the particular behavioral option that has been selected. Thus, spinal circuits would be released for action at least in part by the disinhibitory action of descending NE fibers.

Recently, striking experimental support has appeared for some aspects of the above scheme (51). Acute spinal cats ordinarily show neither postural nor locomotor activity. However, after intravenous administration of Clonidine® [2-(2,6-dichlorophenylamine)-2-imidazoline hydrochloride], a specific stimulator of noradrenergic receptors that passes the blood–brain barrier, it was possible to elicit walking behavior on a moving treadmill with a speed that can be adjusted by the speed of the treadmill, and in the best preparations, "this locomotion looks normal to the eye with smooth alternating movements in all joints" (51). Thus, stimulation of noradrenergic receptors in the cord, combined with stimulation by a treadmill, can release the expression of neural programs for coordinated postular control and locomotion that are located entirely in the cord! What other programs remain to be discovered, and how may this knowledge be applied to problems of paraplegia, and so on?

The type of interaction discussed above illustrates the general principle by which I believe the nervous system as a whole, as well as many neuronal subsystems, might operate, so that if one were to go into detailed consideration of the relations of the neuronal subsystems involved in mechanisms of perceptual integration, in hypothalamic relations, and so on, one would come out with the same general type of scheme, varying, of course, in detail and complexity from region to region.

THE GABA SYSTEM IN THE BASAL GANGLIA

Although the nature of all of the connections among the basal ganglia and between them and other brain structures is not known and all of their functions have not been delineated, it appears that they are largely concerned with processing information related to proprioceptive, vestibular, and visual stimuli in the service of coordinating postural mechanisms. As far as it is possible for a biochemist to gather the sense of present neuro anatomical opinion, it seems that the caudate nucleus, putamen, and substantia nigra all exchange fibers with each other and that efferent outputs from the caudate and putamen go to the globus pallidus, which also may receive some fibers from the substantia nigra. The globus pallidus has two-way communication with the subthalamic nucleus. There are thalamic and cortical inputs to the caudate and putamen. The final results of the computations in the basal ganglia are sent out via a fiber system from the globus pallidus to the ventral lateral nuclei of the thalamus.

The globus pallidus and substantia nigra have the highest contents of GABA and highest activities of GAD in the brain (52–55). A recent detailed regional analysis for GABA in human substantia nigra showed there to be an uneven distribution, the content being higher in the pars reticulata than in the pars compacta and highest in the middle portion at the border between the two regions (56). Stimulation of the head of the caudate produced inhibition in nigral neurons, and it was concluded that caudato-nigral fibers inhibit nigral cells monosynaptically (57). This inhibition was blocked by picrotoxin (58). A microiontophoretic study of nigral neurons that were inhibited by caudate stimulation showed them also to be strongly inhibited by GABA, but not by glycine, acetylcholine, or dopamine (59). GABA levels in the substantia nigra were considerably reduced after destruction of the striatum by suction (60). The above results all are in keeping with the interpretation that there are GABA-inhibitory synapses on dendrites of nigral neurons in the pars reticulata formed by axons that are striatal in origin. Since there is monosynaptic inhibition in pallidal neurons mediated by axon collaterals of the caudato-nigral fibers, it would appear possible that GABA also plays an inhibitory role here. On the other hand, destruction of the substantia nigra did not show significant reduction of GAD activity in the caudate nucleus, even when dopamine was reduced to undetectable levels (61). The latter shows that there probably are no nigro-caudatal GABA fibers. Pallidal lesions were shown to reduce nigral GAD activity, but not that of the caudate (62). The latter results suggest that the globus pallidus also may exert inhibitory effects in the substantia nigra via a GABA input and that the known pallidal inhibitory effects in the ventral lateral thalamic nuclei also might be mediated by fibers from pallidal GABA neurons. The inhibitory dopamine tracts from the nigral neurons to the striatum are, of course, well known.

Normal relations in the basal ganglia must involve *minimally* a coordinated functioning of different groups of inter- and intrasystem neurons whose transmitters are GABA, dopamine, acetylcholine (63), and an excitatory transmitter which is glutamic acid, or whose action externally applied glutamic acid can mimic (64).

Let us suppose that the basal ganglia [by analogy with the spinal cord (51), the abdominal ganglia of the crayfish (1, 2), and the stomatogastric ganglion of the spiny lobster (7)] contain preprogrammed neural circuits for patterned postural control that are held in tonic inhibition by indigenous, closely lying GABA neurons. The chief switching mechanisms for turning on the patterned activities within the non-nigral regions may be the dopamine fibers emanating from the substantia nigra. Afferent inputs to the nigral neurons may release patterns of firing. In analogy to the activating effects of noradrenergic input to the cortex, the nigro-fugal fibers release dopamine in the caudate and putamen, inhibiting indigenous tonically inhibitory GABA neurons and, acting together with excitatory and/or disinhibitory inputs from the thalamus and cortex, release specific coded neural patterns in a sequential manner. The results of this activity are communicated to the pallidum and thence to regions in the thalamus where integration with other incoming information takes place. The final postural instructions are then sent to the appropriate regions of the motor cortex, where after further refinement the activity of appropriate pyramidal neurons is released to signal the effectors. The circuits that are fired in the basal ganglia inform the other units about their activity via intersystem-inhibitory GABA fibers, particularly to the appropriate nigral neurons, thus preventing their own further activation until the need arises again.

How does the above model correlate with what is known about the basal ganglia? If postural-regulating circuits can be released for firing only when there is sufficient inhibitory action of dopaminergic neurons on GABA neurons, a relative deficiency or excess in monoamine input should result in the failure of coordination of postural behavior. Hypofunction or non-function of the nigral neurons does lead to the failure to release appropriate circuits necessary for maintenance of postural control. Indeed, a "striatal dopamine deficiency" produced by naturally induced or experimental destruction of the nigral neurons or by blocking of their function by decreasing the content of dopamine (α-methyl tyrosine or reserpine) or by blocking the action of dopamine on its postsynaptic sites (chlorpromazine or haloperidol) leads to akinesia and rigidity, the classic symptoms of Parkinson's disease (65)—the programs for postural controls cannot be released. The ameliorative effects of treatment with high doses of L-DOPA in parkinsonism probably can be largely attributed to an increased transmission by the remaining striatal dopaminergic neurons (65). Relative hyperactivity of the nigral dopamine neurons should lead to inappropriate release of action patterns; the reversible, amphetamine-induced stereotyped behavioral patterns in animals and humans may be attributable to the extra release of monoamines that this drug produced in the basal ganglia (4). If the nigral dopamine neurons act directly on the GABA neurons, their destruction typically should lead to atrophic changes in the GABA neurons; in untreated Parkinson's disease, the GAD activity in the caudate was found to be reduced to less than half the normal value (65). Does treatment with L-DOPA bring striatal GAD levels back to normal?

In contrast to what one sees with dopamine deficiency, specific degeneration or functional blockade of GABA neurons in the basal ganglia should lead to the expression of inappropriate and dissociated movement patterns. Because of its ubiquitous occurrence and function throughout the CNS, it has not been possible to observe effects of pharmacological blockade of GABA that are specific to the basal ganglia; usually, running fits followed by tonic-clonic convulsions are induced. Recently, however, relatively specific and remarkable decreases in GABA levels have been found in the substantia nigra, putamen-globus pallidus, and caudate nucleus of patients with Huntington's chorea (66), a hereditary disease in which slight, inconstant, irregular choreiform movements eventually progress into constant twitching, stretching, gesturing, facial grimaces, and so on. Since orally or parenterally administered GABA usually does not pass the blood-brain barrier and often causes undesirable peripheral effects, the search is on for a suitable GABA-mimetic substance as a possible treatment in Huntington's chorea. The occasionally helpful effects of haloperidol, a blocker of dopamine receptors, in patients with Huntington's chorea might be attributable to a decreased extent of inhibition of GABA neurons, allowing the less-than-normally effective GABA neurons to maintain their tenuous hold on the neurons requiring their restraints.

A NOTE ON CEREBRAL MICROCIRCULATION

The lesion that leads to the degeneration of nigral neurons in parkinsonism may be secondary to the loss of close contacts between capillaries and nigral neurons in the zona compacta because of infiltration of proliferated glia between cell surface and capillary wall (67). Thus, the statement that "striatal dopamine deficiency has been found to be characteristic for the parkinsonian symptoms of any etiology" (65) may be understood in terms of a characteristic response of the nigral region to almost any kind of injury. The neuropathological specificity may reside in the characteristic series of events that occur when the relation of the nigral neurons to their blood supply is disturbed. An analysis similar to the above would be interesting in Huntington's chorea. This brings up the very important role that the microcirculation must play in every brain region and the importance of studying the effects of local disturbances in neuronal-vascular relationships on pathological manifestations of morphological, neurochemical, neurophysiological, and behavioral parameters.

LOCALIZING GABA NEURONS—A BASIS FOR FURTHER PROGRESS

It is not enough to determine GABA levels and GAD activities in different neural regions. In the last analysis we must be able to visualize directly GABA neurons and to determine their numbers and the details of their connections in specific sites of the nervous system in order to be able to elucidate their relationships to the neurons upon which they impinge and those which act on them. We have made many attempts to develop such procedures in recent years, but they all have failed because of the difficulties in localizing histochemically the products of the enzymatic reaction of GAD, GABA, and CO_2. We were left with the difficult alternative approach of locating GABA neurons by immunohistochemical procedures. The ideal specific marker for GABA neurons is GAD, the enzyme that produces GABA. This required the preparation of pure GAD, developing antibodies to the enzyme, and visualizing the antibodies by a suitable labeling technique specifically at those cellular and subcellular sites where GAD, the antigen, is located.

Currently available to us is pure GAD from mouse brain, and we have prepared antibody to this enzyme in rabbits. The antibodies to mouse brain GAD formed in rabbits have been found to cross-react with the GAD of several other mammalian species. Many experiments now are in progress relevant to this field of activity. We are hopeful, but not certain, that procedures currently being developed in our laboratory eventually will make it possible to determine whether or not variant types of GAD occur in different brain areas under normal and disease conditions, whether deficiencies might exist in the relative numbers of GABA neurons or defects may occur in their relationships to other neurons in pathological states in animals or in humans. An example of an experiment that might give interesting results would be to follow the sequence of changes in GABA neurons and their cellular relationships during the course of events following the destruction of the nigro-striatal tract. The latter kind of study could be correlated closely with electrographic, behavioral, and histological studies. It should be possible to determine whether or not relatively selective degenerative processes take place in GABA neurons.

ACKNOWLEDGMENTS

This investigation was supported in part by grant NB-01615 from the National Institute of Neurological Diseases and Stroke, and grant MH–22438–01 from the National Institute of Mental Health.

REFERENCES

1. Ikeda, K., and Wiersma, C. A. G., *Comp. Biochem. Physiol.* 12, 107 (1964).
2. Wiersma, C. A. G., and Ikeda, K., *Comp. Biochem. Physiol.* 12, 509 (1964).
3. Roeder, K. D., Tozian, L., and Weiant, E. A., *J. Insect Physiol.* 4, 45 (1960).
4. Randrup, A., and Munkvad, I., in: *International Symposium on Amphetamines and Related Compounds,* p. 695, Raven Press, New York (1970).
5. Roberts, E., *Neurosci. Res. Program Bull.* 10, 468 (1972).
6. Maynard, D. M., *Proceedings of the 6th Winter Conference on Brain Research,* p. 63 (1973). (Held Jan. 13–19, 1973, Vail, Colorado.)
7. Maynard, D. M., *Ann. N.Y. Acad. Sci.* 193, 59 (1972).
8. Roberts, E., and Kuriyama, K., *Brain Res.* 8, 1 (1968).
9. Roberts, E., and Hammerschlag, R., in: *Basic Neurochemistry,* p. 131, Little, Brown and Co., Boston (1972).
10. Roberts, E., and Frankel, S., *Fed. Proc.* 9, 219 (1950).
11. Wu, J.-Y., and Roberts, E., *Trans. Am. Soc. Neurochem.* 4, 70 (1973).
12. Wu, J.-Y., Matsuda, T., and Roberts, E., *J. Biol. Chem.* 248, 3029 (1973).
13. Schousboe, A., Wu, J.-Y., and Roberts, E., *Biochemistry* 12, 2868 (1973).
14. Otsuka, M., Iversen, L. L., Hall, Z. W., and Kravitz, E. A., *Proc. Nat. Acad. Sci.* 56, 1110 (1966).
15. Jasper, H. H., Khan, R. T., and Elliott, K. A. C., *Science* 147, 1448 (1965).

16. Mitchell, J. F., and Srinivasan, V., *Nature* 224, 663 (1969).
17. Obata, K., and Takeda, K., *J. Neurochem.* 16, 1043 (1969).
18. Srinivasan, V., Neal, M. J., and Mitchell, J. F., *J. Neurochem.* 16, 1235 (1969).
19. Bradford, H. F., *Brain Res.* 19, 239 (1970).
20. Takeuchi, A., and Takeuchi, N., *J. Physiol. (London)* 183, 433 (1966).
21. Davidson, N., and Southwick, C. A. P., *J. Physiol.* 219, 689 (1971).
22. Nicoll, R. A., *Brain Res.* 35, 137 (1971).
23. Barker, J. L., and Nicoll, R. A., *Science* 176, 1043 (1972).
24. Obata, K., and Highstein, S. M., *Brain Res.* 18, 538 (1970).
25. Kuriyama, K., Sisken, B., Haber, B., and Roberts, E., *Brain Res.* 9, 165 (1968).
26. Fonnum, F., and Storm-Mathisen, J., *Acta Physiol. Scand.* 76, 35A (1969).
27. Curtis, D. R., Felix, D., and McLennan, H., *Brit. J. Pharmacol.* 40, 881 (1970).
28. Dreifuss, J. J., Kelly, J. S., and Krnjević, K., *Exp. Brain Res.* 9, 137 (1969).
29. Albers, R. W., and Brady, R. O., *J. Biol. Chem.* 234, 926 (1959).
30. Salvador, R. A., and Albers, R. W., *J. Biol. Chem.* 234, 922 (1959).
31. Qtsuka, M., and Miyata, Y., in: *Advances in Biochemical Psychopharmacology*, Vol. 6, Costa, E., Iversen, L. L., and Paoletti, R., p. 61, Raven Press, New York (1972).
32. Davidoff, R. A., *Brain Res.* 36, 218 (1972).
33. Saito, K., Wu, J.-Y., Matsuda, T., and Roberts, E., *Trans. Am. Soc. Neurochem.* 4, 70 (1973).
34. Obata, K., Ito, M., Ochi, R., and Sato, N., *Exp. Brain Res.* 4, 43 (1967).
35. Curtis, D. R., Duggan, A. W., Felix, D., and Johnston, G. A. R., *Nature* 226, 1222 (1970).
36. Woodward, D. J., Rushmer, D., Hoffer, B. J., Siggins, G. R., Oliver, A. P., and Armstrong, C., *Fed. Proc.* 30, 318 (1971).
37. Bloom, F. E., Hoffer, B. J., and Siggins, G. R., *Brain Res.* 25, 523 (1971).
38. Olson, L., and Fuxe, K., *Brain Res.* 28, 165 (1971).
39. Jouvet, M., *Science* 163, 32 (1969).
40. Bradley, P. B., *Internat. Rev. Neurobiol.* 11, 1 (1968).
41. Curtis, D. R., and Crawford, J. M., *Ann. Rev. Pharmacol.* 9, 209 (1969).
42. Otsuka, M., *Proceedings of the Fifth International Congress on Pharmacology, Abstracts of Invited Presentations*, p. 16 (1972).
43. Graham, L. T., Jr., Shank, R. P., Werman, R., and Aprison, M. H., *J. Neurochem.* 14, 465 (1967).
44. Albers, R. W., and Brady, R. O., *J. Biol. Chem.* 234, 926 (1959).
45. Aprison, M. H., Davidoff, R. A., and Werman, R., *Handbook of Neurochem.* 3, 381 (1970).
46. Fuxe, K., Hökfelt, T., and Ungerstedt, U., *Intern. Rev. Neurobiol.* 13, 93 (1970).
47. Velikaya, R. R., and Sycheva, T. M., *Neurosci. Translations* 15, 11 (1970–71); original, *Neirofiziologiya* 2, 43 (1970).
48. Fuxe, K., Hamberger, B., and Hökfelt, T., *Brain Res.* 8, 125 (1968).
49. Roberts, E., and Matthysse, S., *Ann. Rev. Biochem.* 39, 777 (1970).
50. Nauta, W. J. H., in: *Limbic System Mechanisms and Autonomic Function*, p. 21, Charles C Thomas, Springfield, Ill. (1972).
51. Forssberg, H., and Grillner, S., *Brain Res.* 50, 184 (1973).
52. Fahn, S., and Coté, L. J., *J. Neurochem.* 15, 209 (1969).
53. Perry, T. L., Berry, K., Hansen, S., Diamond, S., and Mok, C., *J. Neurochem.* 18, 513 (1971).
54. Perry, T. L., Hansen, S., Berry, K., Mok, C., and Lesk, D., *J. Neurochem.* 18, 521 (1971).
55. Okada, Y., Nitsch-Hassler, C., Kim, J. S., Bak, I. J., and Hassler, R., *Exp. Brain Res.* 13, 514 (1971).
56. Kanazawa, I., Miyata, Y., Toyokura, Y., and Otsuka, M., *Brain Res.* 51, 363 (1973).
57. Yoshida, M., and Precht, W., *Brain Res.* 32, 225 (1971).
58. Precht, W., and Yoshida, M., *Brain Res.* 32, 229 (1971).
59. Feltz, P., *Can. J. Physiol. Pharmacol.* 49, 1113 (1971).
60. Kim, J. S., Bak, I. J., Hassler, R., and Okada, Y., *Exp. Brain Res.* 14, 95 (1971).
61. Hockman, C. H., Lloyd, K. G., Farley, I. J., and Hornykiewicz, O., *Brain Res.* 35, 613 (1971).
62. McGeer, P. L., McGeer, E. G., Wada, J. A., and Jung, E., *Brain Res.* 32, 425 (1971).

63. McGeer, P. L., and McGeer, E. G., *Fed. Proc.* 30, 1085 (1971).
64. Krnjević, K., in: L-*DOPA and Parkinsonism*, p. 189, F. A. Davis Co., Philadelphia (1970).
65. Hornykiewicz, O., *Fed. Proc.* 32, 183 (1973).
66. Perry, T. L., Hansen, S., and Kloster, M., *New Engl. J. Med.* 288, 337 (1973).
67. Issidorides, M. R., *Brain Res.* 25, 289 (1971).

Advances in Neurology, Vol. 5
Raven Press, New York © 1974

Some Neuroactive Compounds in the Substantia Nigra

K. Krnjević

Department of Research in Anaesthesia, McGill University, Montreal 101, Quebec, Canada

Not the least interesting feature of the substantia nigra is its remarkably high content of at least three agents which have been proposed as central neurotransmitters: dopamine (DA), gamma-aminobutyric acid (GABA), and Substance P.

DA is well known in this context, and much of this volume is devoted to various aspects of its biochemistry, physiology, and pharmacology. The exceptionally high levels of GABA and Substance P are less widely known.

DOPAMINE

The wealth of evidence concerning DA and a postulated dopaminergic pathway projecting from the substantia nigra to the striatum is extensively reviewed elsewhere in this volume, especially by Fuxe and by Ungerstedt. There is little to be added in the way of neurochemical information, but it seems pertinent to review the situation from an electrophysiological point of view. However overwhelming the evidence obtained by purely neuro-chemical, histochemical, and pharmacological techniques, the problem of the nature and function of nigrostriatal pathways will be solved only when there is adequate support from corroborative electrical studies. Un-fortunately, this is far from being the case: in some respects the situation is even less satisfactory than a few years ago (1, 2).

The general postulate is that DA is released in the striatum as a "classi-cal" neurotransmitter, which either excites or inhibits striatal neurons. If we consider the first alternative — DA as an excitatory transmitter — what picture do we get?

Dopaminergic Excitation

There is good agreement between the results of recent morphological and electrophysiological studies of the caudate nucleus, both of which indicate a purely excitatory input to the caudate. According to Kemp and Powell (3), "afferent fibres to the caudate nucleus all terminate with asymmetrical membrane thickening associated with round vesicles." This kind of synaptic morphology is widely accepted as characteristic of excitatory synapses (4–6). The systematic survey of neuronal responses in the caudate to various types of inputs by Hull and his colleagues (7) showed excitatory post-synaptic potentials to be always the earliest recordable events; from this evidence they conclude that all inputs into the caudate are indeed excitatory. It is particularly relevant in this context that the only direct *(monosynaptic)* nigrostriatal connection demonstrated so far (8–10) is clearly excitatory. This pathway conducts impulses slowly but can do so at a high frequency, and it excites a characteristic population of cells, distributed throughout all regions of the caudate. Unfortunately, there is no ground at all for thinking that this pathway could be dopaminergic: (a) the caudate cells in question have consistently failed to show *any* excitatory effects of DA (11–13); (b) although excitation by this pathway is depressed by haloperidol, this is

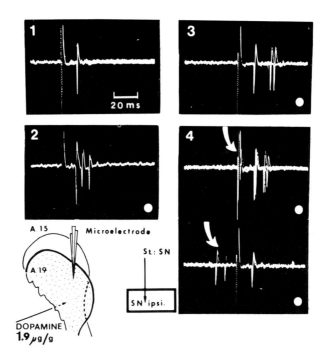

FIG. 1. Orthodromic response of a caudate neuron to ipsilateral substantia nigra (SN) stimulation in a cat showing 84% DA depletion in the left caudate nucleus 15 days after 6-hydroxydopamine treatment. (DA concentration in caudate: 1.9 μg/g.) *1:* Superimposed sweeps showing constant response latency. *2–4:* Microiontophoresis of < 10 nA glu-tamate (traces with dot), single trace in *2* showing multiple spike discharge, and super-imposed tracings in *3* and *4* showing absence of collision extinction after glutamate-induced spikes (arrows). *Left diagram:* Sites of stimulation (st: SN) and recording (A19); frontal stereotaxic plane A15 in caudate was also stimulated to identify cells activated antidromically by nigral stimulation (from ref. 15, by permission of Elsevier Publishing Co.).

probably a nonspecific action, unrelated to a block of "DA receptors" (14); and (c) very substantial chronic destruction of nigrostriatal fibers rich in DA by 6-hydroxydopamine (Figs. 1 and 3) or their inactivation by a combination of reserpine and alpha-methyl-paratyrosine both fail to abolish the activity of this pathway (15).

Only in the putamen have excitatory effects of DA been reported to be predominant (16). However, their significance remains to be determined, especially as they have not yet been confirmed, and other evidence suggests that interruption of nigro-putamen connections leads to an *increase* in firing of putamen neurons (17).

A different kind of facilitatory action of DA, a very prolonged potentiation of muscarinic excitation by acetylcholine, has been observed in sympathetic ganglia by Libet and Tosaka (18). The possibility of such an effect in the striatum should be kept in mind, even though there is no evidence that it occurs in the central nervous system: several tests performed in the cerebral cortex, where ACh has a comparable excitatory action, have failed to reveal any comparable effect of DA (Fig. 2).

Dopaminergic Inhibition

It is usually believed that a nigrostriatal dopaminergic pathway has a moderating action on the striatal cells, and thus on extrapyramidal motor control (19). Can DA therefore be an inhibitory transmitter?

Judging by its widespread—although hardly dramatic—depressant action on neuronal firing in the caudate (11, 12, 20, 21), DA, if released by nerve fibers, would tend to reduce the activity of caudate neurons. According to Feltz and de Champlain (12), DA appears to be unusually effective after treatment with 6-hydroxydopamine. This change was attributed mainly to a loss of DA-containing terminals, which would presumably slow down the removal of the applied DA. It is well known, of course, that nigral stimulation causes an inhibition of unit firing in the caudate (10, 21) as well as a release of metabolites of DA (22).

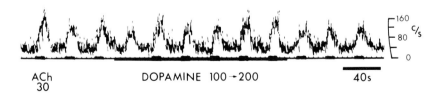

ACh
30   DOPAMINE 100→200   40s

FIG. 2. Firing frequency of a cortical neuron in the motor cortex of a cat (lightly anesthetized with nitrous oxide and methoxyflurane) excited at regular intervals by microiontophoretic applications of acetylcholine (upward signals). DA was applied in addition for a period of 3 min (downward signal), but it did not potentiate significantly the responses evoked by acetylcholine. Iontophoretic currents are indicated in nanoamperes (P. Feltz, K. Krnjević, and A. Mauro, *unpublished observations*).

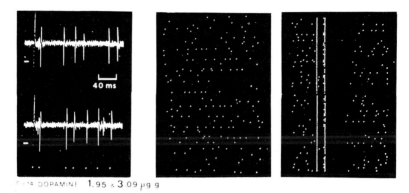

' ‍'4 DOPAMINE   1.95 л 3 09 µg g

FIG. 3. Extracellular recording, with multibarrelled pipette, of a caudate unit excited orthodromically and inhibited by stimulation of the substantia nigra. The firing is maintained by release of glutamate. The examined caudate nucleus of cat Cd 14 had its dopamine content lowered by 84% (concentrations in left and right caudate nuclei indicated below). *Left:* Two oscilloscope traces showing response to a single shock (0.2 msec) just above threshold. Note fixed latency of first spike, better seen in right-hand dot displays showing the discharge. Each dot represents a spike and each horizontal row a sequence (see also bottom at extreme left). The sequences are repeated from above down at intervals of 1 sec. *Middle:* Ongoing firing, without stimulus. *Right:* Stimulus (first alignment of dots) followed by response (second alignment) and pause in firing, usually also seen without preceding excitation (from ref. 12, by permission of Elsevier Publishing Co.).

However, the simple hypothesis of a tonic moderating influence by a direct inhibitory dopaminergic pathway is hard to reconcile with some other evidence: (a) the inhibitory effect of nigral stimulation is not obviously diminished after treatment with 6-hydroxydopamine (Fig. 3) (12); and (b) the mean frequency of spontaneous unit firing recorded in monkeys with chronically implanted electrodes is not significantly altered by lesions which cut the nigrostriatal connection so as to lower the caudate DA content by more than 90% (23).

Thus, although DA could have an inhibitory function, there is a blatant discrepancy between, on the one hand, the morphological and electrophysiological evidence that all demonstrable inputs into the caudate (including that from the substantia nigra) are probably excitatory, and, on the other hand, the histochemical evidence of a direct DA-containing nigrostriatal projection—especially since destruction of this projection does not abolish nigrostriatal inhibition and produces little change in the activity of caudate neurons. There seem to be only two possible explanations for these contradictory results: one is that inhibitory dopaminergic terminals have an unconventional morphology and that their function can be effectively maintained by relatively few surviving fibers, perhaps because the removal of DA is much slower after denervation (see ref. 12). The other possibility is that the role of DA is of only marginal importance and that the function of the nigrostriatal system normally depends primarily on the activity of other kinds of fibers.

GABA

The very high concentration of GABA and glutamic decarboxylase in the substantia nigra is well established (24–26). It is associated with an unusually high capacity for GABA uptake (27, 28) and is likely to be due to the presence of a powerful *descending* striatonigral inhibitory pathway whose action appears to be mediated by GABA (29, 30) (see Fig. 4). Since section of this pathway causes a loss of GABA from the substantia nigra (31), it is likely — although not certain — that the inhibitory fibers have their cells of origin in the striatum rather than within the substantia nigra.

Caudate neurons are also very sensitive to GABA (11); it is not improbable that the inhibitory effects of nigro-caudate stimulation which persist after destruction of the DA-containing terminals are mediated by the release of GABA (15) from the numerous caudate inhibitory interneurons (3). Although one cannot make any more precise statements about the function of GABA — and very possibly of L-glutamic acid acting as an excitatory transmitter (32, 33) — it would be very surprising if these amino acids did not have a major role to play in the organization of activity in the nigrostriatal complex. It is very relevant that as a result of lesions in animals and in parkinsonian patients there is a significant disturbance in the nigral metabolism of GABA (26).

SUBSTANCE P

This 11-amino acid polypeptide was originally discovered in the gut (34). It has a powerful excitatory action on smooth muscle and it is a potent sialogogue. Although it has been studied over a number of years, in particular as perhaps the transmitter released by afferent nerve fibers (35, 36) and various central pathways (37), more precise studies have become possible only recently, since the isolation of pure Substance P and its synthesis by Leeman and her colleagues (38, 39). Their recent experiments *(personal communication)* have confirmed the previous finding of an outstandingly high concentration of Substance P in the substantia nigra, much higher than in any other part of the brain.

The function of this polypeptide is very much a matter of conjecture. So far there has been no serious evidence in support of the suggestion that it might be the transmitter at primary afferent synapses. According to some experiments of Otsuka et al. (40), Substance P causes a depolarization of amphibian spinal motoneurons. Recent tests on dorsal column nuclei of cats by Krnjević and Morris (41), however, have not shown any quick exci-

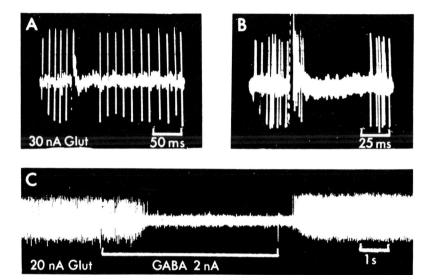

FIG. 4. Extracellular recording with multibarrelled pipette of a nigral unit discharge inhibited by caudate stimulation and depressed by GABA. The firing is maintained by release of glutamate (Glut). *A:* Single shock (0.2 msec) stimulation (1.5 × threshold) inducing a pure inhibition. *B:* 2.0 × threshold: superimposed tracings (four or five sweeps at 3/sec) show an early excitation but only slightly longer inhibition. *C:* Firing of the same unit (note reduced voltage scale) depressed by a 6-sec injection of 2 nA of GABA (white bar) (from ref. 30, by permission of *Canadian Journal of Physiology and Pharmacology*).

tatory action compatible with the requirements of an excitatory transmitter at these particularly rapidly acting synapses. On the other hand, there was evidence in some cases of a slow and prolonged (but ultimately reversible) excitatory action, whereas some other cells showed a marked inactivation of evoked unitary responses. These effects are consistent with the possibility that Substance P may in some way change the level of excitability of at least some central neurons. Although we have no evidence about the sensitivity of nigral or striatal cells to Substance P or related polypeptides, its presence in exceptionally high concentration in this region may be a significant element in the operation of nigrostriatal mechanisms and their disturbance in diseased states.

CONCLUSIONS

The marked beneficial action of L-DOPA in the treatment of parkinsonism has necessarily — and rightly — caused most investigators to focus on the function of a possible dopaminergic pathway. But it seems advisable to widen this narrow perspective now to include other neuro-agents that are concentrated in the substantia nigra, particularly in view of some striking discrepancies between present neurochemical and electrophysiological findings. One should perhaps remember that neurons and other cells of the nervous system are remarkably easily loaded with various exogenous compounds, and that these can be released during activity — perhaps instead of the normal transmitters. It would not be very surprising if parkinsonism were the manifestation of a more general disorder of metabolism (42). The therapeutic effects of L-DOPA may well be due to its unusual ability to penetrate the blood-brain barrier — in contrast to many other amino acids — and in this way to restore a generally flagging supply of neuroactive substances.

ACKNOWLEDGMENTS

I am grateful to the Canadian Medical Research Council for its financial support of some of the research reported here.

REFERENCES

1. Krnjević, K., in: *L-Dopa and Parkinsonism*, edited by A. Barbeau and F. H. McDowell, p. 189. F. A. Davis Co., Philadelphia (1970).
2. Krnjević, K., in: *The Neuroleptics. Modern Problems in Pharmacopsychiatry*, Vol. 5, p. 12. S. Karger, Basel (1970).
3. Kemp, J. M., and Powell, T. P. S., *Phil. Trans. R. Soc. Ser. B*, 262, 403 (1971).
4. Gray, E. G., *J. Anat.*, 93, 420 (1959).
5. Colonnier, M., *Brain Res.*, 9, 268 (1968).
6. Peters, A., Palay, S. L., and Webster, H. de F., *The Fine Structure of the Nervous System: The Cells and their Processes*. Harper & Row, New York (1970).
7. Hull, C. D., Levine, M. S., and Buchwald, N. A., Abstracts, *2nd Ann. Meet. Soc. Neuroscience*, Houston, p. 180, (1972).
8. Frigyesi, T. L., and Purpura, D. P., *Brain Res.*, 6, 440 (1967).
9. Feltz, P., and MacKenzie, J. S., *Brain Res.*, 13, 612 (1969).
10. Feltz, P., and Albe-Fessard, D., *Electroenceph. Clin. Neurophysiol.*, 33, 179 (1972).
11. Feltz, P., *J. Physiol.*, 205, 8P (1969).
12. Feltz, P., and de Champlain, J., *Brain Res.*, 43, 601 (1972).
13. Feltz, P., and de Champlain, J., *Proc. Catecholamines* Symposium, Strasbourg, May 1973 *(in press)*.
14. Feltz, P., *Eur. J. Pharmacol.*, 14, 360 (1971).
15. Feltz, P., and de Champlain, J., *Brain Res.*, 43, 595 (1972).
16. York, D. H., *Brain Res.*, 20, 233 (1970).
17. Ohye, C., Bouchard, R., Boucher, R., and Poirier, L. J., *J. Pharmac. Exp. Ther.*, 175, 700 (1970).
18. Libet, B., and Tosaka, T., *Proc. Nat. Acad. Sci.*, 67, 667 (1970).
19. Hornykiewicz, O., in: *Handbook of Neurochemistry*, Vol. 7, p. 465. Plenum Press, New York (1972).
20. McLennan, H., and York, D. H., *J. Physiol.*, 189, 393 (1967).
21. Connor, J. D., *J. Physiol.*, 208, 691 (1970).
22. Portig, P. J., and Vogt, M., *J. Physiol.*, 204, 687, (1969).
23. Buchwald, N. A., Levine, M. S., Hull, C. D., and Heller, A., Abstracts, *2nd Ann. Meet. Soc. Neuroscience*, Houston, p. 136 (1972).
24. Fahn, S., and Côté, L. J., *J. Neurochem.*, 15, 209 (1968).
25. Okada, Y., Nitsch-Hassler, C., Kim, J. S., Bak, I. J., and Hassler, R., *Exp. Brain Res.*, 13, 514 (1971).
26. McGeer, P. L., McGeer, E. G., Wada, J. A., and Jung, E., *Brain Res.*, 32, 425 (1971).
27. Hökfelt, T., Jonsson, G., and Ljungdahl, A., *Life Sci.*, 9, 203 (1970).

28. Okada, Y., and Hassler, R., *Brain Res.*, 49, 214 (1973).
29. Precht, W., and Yoshida, M., *Brain Res.*, 32, 229 (1971).
30. Feltz, P., *Can. J. Physiol. Pharmacol.*, 49, 1113 (1971).
31. Kim, J. S., Bak, I. J., Hassler, R., and Okada, Y., *Exp. Brain Res.*, 14, 95 (1971).
32. Krnjević, K., *Int. Rev. Neurobiol.*, 7, 41 (1964).
33. Krnjević, K., *Nature*, 228, 119 (1970).
34. von Euler, U. S., and Gaddum, J. H., *J. Physiol.*, 72, 74 (1931).
35. Lembeck, F., *Arch. Exp. Path. Pharmakol.*, 219, 197, (1953).
36. Stern, P., *Ann. N.Y. Acad. Sci.*, 104, 403 (1963).
37. Zetler, G., in: *Handbook of Neurochemistry*, Vol. 4, p. 135. Plenum Press, New York (1970).
38. Chang, M., Leeman, S. E., and Niall, H. D., *Nature New Biol.*, 232, 86 (1971).
39. Tregear, G. W., Niall, H. D., Potts Jun., J. T., Leeman, S. E., and Chang, M. M., *Nature New Biol.*, 232, 87 (1971).
40. Otsuka, M., Konishi, S., and Takanashi, T., *Proc. Jap. Acad.*, 48, 342 (1972).
41. Krnjević, K., and Morris, M. E., Abstracts, *3rd Ann. Meet. Society Neuroscience*, San Diego, p. 349 (1973).
42. McGeer, P. L., in: *L-Dopa and Parkinsonism*, edited by A. Barbeau and F. H. McDowell, p. 61. F. A. Davis Co., Philadelphia (1970).

Advances in Neurology, Vol. 5
Raven Press, New York © 1974

Evidence for Descending Pallido-Nigral GABA-Containing Neurons

P. L. McGeer, H. C. Fibiger, L. Maler, T. Hattori, and
E. G. McGeer

*Division of Neurological Sciences, Department of Psychiatry, University of British
Columbia, Vancouver 8, B. C., Canada*

There is increasing evidence that γ-aminobutyric acid (GABA) acts as a neurotransmitter. It has a typical unequal distribution in brain, and so does its synthetic enzyme glutamic acid decarboxylase (GAD) (1–6). Both these materials are highly concentrated in the synaptosomal fraction of sub-cellular homogenates (6–9). GABA is preferentially taken up by nerve endings (10–13) and, when applied iontophoretically, inhibits the firing of single neurons (14). Since high levels of GABA and GAD are found in the basal ganglia, particularly the globus pallidus and substantia nigra (1–6), it might be expected that GABA-containing neuronal pathways are as-sociated with extrapyramidal function.

If the cell body of a GABA-containing neuron is destroyed, or its axon is cut, there should be anterograde degeneration with a loss of GABA and GAD in the distal segment. Depending on whether or not there is significant branching proximal to the cut, there may be retrograde degeneration as well. The fact that destruction of Purkinje cell axons leads to losses of GAD in Deiters' and the interpositus nuclei has led to the hypothesis that Purkinje cells use GABA as their transmitter agent (15).

It has been reported that electrolytic lesions of the globus pallidus (16), hemitransections at the levels of the subthalamus (17) or ventro-medial hypothalamus (18), or destruction of the striatum by suction (17) produce significant decreases in GABA and GAD in the substantia nigra. This can be taken as initial evidence in favor of long, GABA-containing axons origi-nating in rostrally located structures in the basal ganglia and descending to terminations in the substantia nigra. The experiments reported here suggest that the principal origin may be the globus pallidus.

MATERIALS AND METHODS

Under pentobarbital sodium (Nembutal®) anesthesia (50 mg/kg i.p.), hemitransections were carried out on rats weighing 355 to 475 g using the stereotaxic atlas of König and Klippel (20). Coordinates were chosen to produce hemitransections at the level of the anterior commissure just rostral to the globus pallidus (anterior hemitransection) or at the level of the ventro-medial hypothalamus (posterior hemitransection) by the method of McGeer et al. (18). Two weeks after the lesions, the animals were killed by cervical fracture, the brains quickly removed, placed on a freezing microtome, and sectioned. The caudate-putamen, globus pallidus, and substantia nigra were dissected out. The GAD activity was measured by the method of Chalmers et al. (2), and tyrosine hydroxylase by the method of McGeer et al. (21) using exogenous co-factor on each area.

In some rats 1 μl of solution containing 10 μC of ^{3}H-leucine (specific activity 38.6 C/mmole) was injected stereotaxically into the globus pallidus by the method of Fibiger et al. (19). After 24 hr the animals were sacrificed by perfusion with a solution containing 4% paraformaldehyde and 0.5% glutaraldehyde. The brains were examined by light and electron microscopic autoradiography (11).

RESULTS

The posterior hemitransections brought about sharp reductions in GAD activity in the substantia nigra without changing GAD values in the caudate-putamen and globus pallidus (Table 1). The anterior hemitransections produced a slight reduction in GAD activity in the caudate-putamen and globus pallidus but had no effect on the substantia nigra GAD in 11 of the 14 rats studied (Table 1). In the three rats that did show a decrease in substantia nigra GAD, the globus pallidus was noted on gross inspection to have been damaged in its more rostral region by the hemitransection. In these three animals a significant reduction (to 69% of controls) of nigral GAD activity was found ($p < 0.01$). Tyrosine hydroxylase activity was significantly reduced in all brain regions measured in both the anterior and posterior hemitransected groups.

A light microscopic radioautograph of one of the rats injected with

TABLE 1. *Effect of hemitransections of rat brain on GAD and tyrosine hydroxylase activities in various brain regions (expressed as % of control values)*

Area	Posterior hemitransections		Anterior hemitransections	
	GAD	Tyrosine hyd.	GAD	Tyrosine hyd.
Substantia nigra	17.8 ± 3.5	55.8 ± 8.7	100.1 ± 9.2	65.9 ± 9.6
Globus pallidus	98.5 ± 16.6	18.8 ± 12.4	76.8 ± 9.1	53.8 ± 10.1
Caudate-putamen	107.6 ± 6.9	15.5 ± 8.2	86.0 ± 7.7	19.7 ± 4.9

V_{max} of GAD (in μmoles/g/hr) in the control samples was: caudate-putamen 15.8; globus pallidus 24.9; substantia nigra 29.0. V_{max} of tyrosine hydroxylase (in nmoles/g/hr) was: caudate-putamen 102.7; globus pallidus 53.2; substantia nigra 64.1. N = 10 to 11 animals for each group.

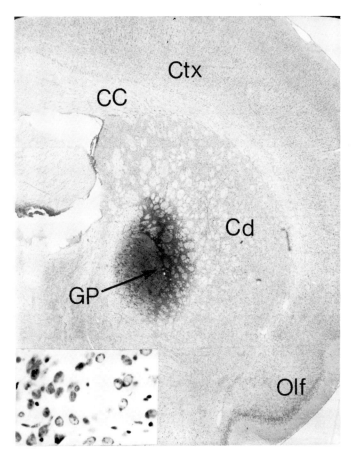

FIG. 1. Injection site of ³H-leucine in the globus pallidus, 16.5 ×. Insert shows that the caudate is free of grains, 325 ×. Abbreviations: CC, corpus callosum; Cd, caudate; Ctx, cortex; GP, globus pallidus; Olf, olfactory cortex. The stereotaxic plane of this injection is A6360µ in the König and Klippel atlas (20).

³H-leucine in the globus pallidus is shown in Fig. 1. In this animal the injection was reasonably well confined to the globus pallidus proper. It is significant that no grains could be detected in the caudate putamen. There was heavy labeling in the subthalamic nucleus adjacent to the globus pallidus which is the principal known efferent pathway of the external globus pallidus (Fig. 2). There was also significant labeling in the rostral substantia nigra, particularly the pars compacta (Fig. 3). There was no labeling of the thalamus as would be expected had there been diffusion from the globus pallidus to the entopeduncular nucleus. Thus, the labeling in the substantia nigra in this case is unlikely to have arisen from diffusion of the leucine into cell bodies in the entopeduncular nucleus. However, injections into both the

FIG. 2. Autoradiograph of subthalamic nucleus of Luys following injection of ^{3}H-leucine in the globus pallidus. 325 ×.

globus pallidus and entopeduncular nucleus produced far more extensive labeling throughout the rostro-caudal extent of the substantia nigra. The localization of grains in the substantia nigra in nerve endings is shown in Fig. 4, which is an electron microscopic radioautogram of a labeled type 1 synapse, typical of that described by Rinvik and Grofova (22).

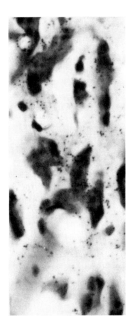

FIG. 3. Autoradiograph of the substantia nigra pars compacta following injection of ^{3}H-leucine in the globus pallidus. 650 ×.

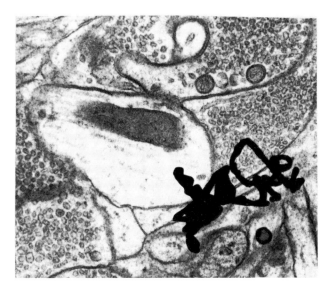

FIG. 4. Electron microscopic autoradiograph of the substantia nigra pars compacta following injection of ³H-leucine in the globus pallidus. 35,280 ×.

DISCUSSION

The posterior hemitransection experiments indicate quite clearly that procedures which destroy the connections between the globus pallidus and the substantia nigra result in significant losses in nigral GAD activity. On the other hand, anterior hemitransections which destroy most of the caudato-nigral projection have no influence on nigral GAD activity. This strongly suggests that the source of most of the GABA terminals in the substantia nigra is the globus pallidus and/or some closely related structure such as the entopeduncular nucleus.

Although a caudato-nigral projection is well established, a projection from the external division of the globus pallidus to the substantia nigra has so far not been established by classical neuroanatomical techniques in the rat or other species. The axoplasmic flow of labeled protein, synthesized from ³H-leucine in the globus pallidus (Fig. 1), to terminals in the rostral substantia nigra provides evidence of such a tract. The principal known output of the external globus pallidus is to the subthalamic nucleus (23), and this was by far the most heavily labeled area from the globus pallidus injection (Fig. 2). The projection to the substantia nigra is much less heavily labeled, indicating that the substantia nigra receives only a minor proportion of the output of the globus pallidus. Had the grains in the substantia nigra been derived from protein transport originating in entopeduncular nucleus cell bodies, then heavy labeling would have been expected in the thalamus since this is the principal efferent projection of that nucleus. Since no such labeling was observed, the entopeduncular nucleus could not have been the principal source of the radioactive protein in the rostral substantia nigra pars compacta. Furthermore, had the protein been only in fibers of passage going through the substantia nigra, then the electron microscopic radio-autograms would not have revealed grains principally over nerve endings as in Fig. 4. Injections of leucine into both the globus pallidus and the ento-peduncular nucleus produced far more extensive labeling of the substantia nigra throughout its extent. This indicates that, in accord with suggestions from classical results (22), there is an extensive projection from the ento-peduncular nucleus to the substantia nigra.

The posterior hemitransections failed to reduce GAD activity in the caudate-putamen or globus pallidus. This observation agrees with previous results (17) which indicated that striatal GABA levels were not reduced by hemitransection at the level of the subthalamus (17). The apparent lack of a retrograde effect may indicate the existence of other GABA systems which terminate or originate in the striatum, or it may indicate a lack of retrograde degeneration because of axon collaterals from the GABA-containing neurons.

The anterior hemitransections may have reduced slightly GAD levels in both the caudate-putamen and the globus pallidus without any effect on nigral GAD activity. This may indicate that GABA neurons project from the striatum to the pallidum, but further research on this point is required.

Yoshida and Precht (24) have demonstrated that the substantia nigra is inhibited monosynaptically by stimulation of the head of the caudate nucleus and that the effect is blocked by picrotoxin. Kim et al. (17) found a decrease in nigral GAD following extirpation of the striatum. These data have been interpreted as indicating that the well-established caudato-nigral projection is GABA-containing. However, the decrease in nigral GAD noted by Kim et al. (17) was small, comparable to those in the anterior hemitransections reported here where a slight amount of damage was done to the globus pallidus. It thus seems unlikely that the major caudato-nigral tract could be due to GABA-containing neurons. This does not explain why the caudato-nigral inhibitory effect should be blocked by picrotoxin unless picrotoxin is a somewhat nonspecific agent.

Although the source of GAD in the substantia nigra cannot yet be con-sidered proven, the evidence to date supports a descending GABA-con-taining pathway in the rat with its origin in the globus pallidus and ento-peduncular nucleus and its terminations in the substantia nigra. The high level of activity in the caudate and the small decreases seen after anterior hemitransection suggest the possibility of internally organized GABA-containing neurons in the neostriatum with the possibility of some projec-tions to the globus pallidus.

The physiological role of GABA in the basal ganglia remains unproved although it is quite possible that one of its functions is to inhibit dopaminergic neurons of the substantia nigra.

The possible importance of GABA and GAD to Parkinson's disease is also unknown. However, pathological changes in the substantia nigra and globus pallidus have long been reported as features of this disease. We have measured the GAD distribution in normal and neurologically diseased brains including Parkinson's disease cases (25). The substantia nigra and globus pallidus GAD was found to be selectively decreased in Parkinson's disease as compared with the GAD levels in other areas of brain. The substantia nigra in the cases of Parkinson's disease had a ratio of 0.53 relative to cortical areas, whereas accident cases had a ratio of 2.05 ($p < 0.001$). The significance of these decreases is not yet known.

SUMMARY

Posterior hemitransections of rat brain at the level of the ventromedial hypothalamus reduced GAD levels in the substantia nigra to 17.8% of control values. GAD values in the caudate-putamen and globus pallidus were unchanged. Anterior hemitransections at the level of the anterior commissure brought about no change in the substantia nigra GAD in those cases where the globus pallidus was clearly undamaged. The GAD of the caudate-putamen was reduced to 86% of the control value and that in the globus pallidus to 76.8%. In three animals where anterior hemitransections did visible damage to the globus pallidus, the GAD levels in the substantia nigra were mildly reduced to 70% of control values.

^{3}H-Leucine injected stereotaxically into the globus pallidus resulted in protein being transported by axoplasmic flow into the subthalamic nucleus and the substantia nigra. The transported protein in the substantia nigra was highly localized to nerve endings and the related postsynaptic elements. The evidence developed to date, although not yet complete, supports the concept of a descending GABA-containing pathway with terminations in the substantia nigra and a probable origin in the globus pallidus and entopeduncular nucleus.

ACKNOWLEDGMENTS

This research project was supported by MRC Grant 68–4013, MRC Grant 68–3633, MRC Grant 68–4674, MRC Scholarship 68–8202, Muscular Dystrophy Association Grant 65–6042, Alfred P. Sloan Foundation Grant 65–7245, and Province of B.C. Grant 65–6875.

REFERENCES

1. Albers, R. W., and Brady, R. O., *J. Biol. Chem.* 234, 926 (1959).
2. Chalmers, A., McGeer, E. G., Wickson, V., and McGeer, P. L., *Comp. Gen. Pharmacol.* 1, 385 (1970).
3. Fahn, S., and Côté, L. J., *J. Neurochem.* 15, 209 (1968).
4. Muller, P. B., and Langemann, H., *J. Neurochem.* 9, 399 (1962).

5. Lowe, I. P., Robins, E., and Eyerman, G. S., *J. Neurochem.* 3, 8 (1958).
6. Okada, Y., Nitsch-Hassler, C., Kim, J. S., Bak, I. J., and Hassler, R., *Exp. Brain Res.* 13, 514 (1971).
7. Kuriyama, K., Roberts, E., and Kakefuda, T., *Brain Res.* 8, 132 (1968).
8. Neal, M. J., and Iversen, L. L., *J. Neurochem.* 16, 1245 (1969).
9. Salganicoff, L., and DeRobertis, E., *J. Neurochem.* 12, 287 (1965).
10. Kuhar, M. J., Green, A. I., Snyder, S. H., and Gfeller, E., *Brain Res.* 21, 405 (1970).
11. Hattori, T., McGeer, P. L., Fibiger, H. C., and McGeer, E. G., *Brain Res.* 54, 103 (1973).
12. Iversen, L. L., and Bloom, F. E., *Brain Res.* 41, 131 (1972).
13. Hökfelt, T., and Ljungdahl, A., *Brain Res.* 22, 391 (1970).
14. Krnjevic, K., and Schwartz, S., *Exp. Brain Res.* 3, 320 (1967).
15. Fonnum, F., Storm-Matheson, J., and Walberg, F., *Brain Res.* 20, 259 (1970).
16. McGeer, P. L., McGeer, E. G., Wada, J. A., and Jung, E., *Brain Res.* 32, 425 (1971).
17. Kim, J. S., Bak, I. J., Hassler, R., and Okada, Y., *Exp. Brain Res.* 14, 95 (1971).
18. McGeer, E. G., Fibiger, H. C., McGeer, P. L., and Brooke, S., *Brain Res.* 52, 289 (1973).
19. Fibiger, H. C., Pudritz, R. E., McGeer, P. L., and McGeer, E. G., *J. Neurochem.* 19, 1697 (1972).
20. König, J. F. R., and Klippel, R. A., *The Rat Brain.* Williams and Wilkins, Baltimore (1963).
21. McGeer, E. G., McGeer, P. L., and Wada, J. A., *J. Neurochem.* 18, 1647 (1971).
22. Rinvik, E., and Grofova, I. *Exp. Brain Res.* 11, 229 (1970).
23. Nauta, W. J. H., and Mahler, W. R., *Brain Res.* 1, 3 (1966).
24. Yoshida, M., and Precht, W., *Brain Res.* 32, 225 (1971).
25. McGeer, P. L., McGeer, E. G., and Wada, J. A., *Neurology* 21, 1000 (1971).

DISCUSSION

Dr. Calne: I have two questions in relation to Baclofen or Lioresal, which is reputed to be a GABA analogue: what is the reaction of Baclofen on GABA systems and dopamine systems, and is there any experience with this drug which has been used in man for spasticity?

Dr. McDowell: Dr. Roberts, do you have an answer for that?

Dr. Roberts: What is the chemical name of the compound you are talking about?

Dr. Calne: I do not know its chemical structure.

Dr. Roberts: I guess it may be *para*-chlorophenyl-GABA. As far as I know, there is no evidence that it is GABA-mimetic. Do you know of any?

Dr. Calne: I think that there may be some experience on this point with its use in parkinsonism.

Dr. Roberts: The only data that I would consider would be empirical observation showing a system that is sensitive to GABA and that would respond when this material was put onto it. Our experience has been that very small alterations in the molecule of GABA destroy its properties and change membrane conductance to chloride.

My guess is that adding the *para*-chlorophenyl group completely changes its properties. Maybe Dr. Krnjevic knows something about this point.

Dr. Krnjevic: I have never seen any data on this particular compound, but I think any substitution like this would probably knock out the action.

Dr. Roberts: It would have some pharmacological activity, but I do not think it would be related to GABA at all.

Dr. Fuxe: I would like to ask Dr. Krnjevic why he doesn't think that the inhibitory effects obtained in the striatum by stimulation of the substantia nigra could be mediated by the dopamine. There is the concept of super-sensitivity and we know that there is always a sparse plexus of dopamine terminals remaining from which dopamine can be released and reach the supersensitive receptors. What do you think about the possibility that it is still, in spite of the effect on dopamine of the 6-hydroxydopamine treatment, related to the concept of supersensitivity?

Dr. Krnjevic: I do not think the data are sufficiently quantitative to exclude the possibility, as you suggest. There is a great deal of inhibition left there, and I think one really has to assume that there is another inhibitory effect present. One simple way of looking at this is to think of the GABA neurons as being strictly within the caudate, and they themselves may be acted upon (as Dr. Roberts suggested) by a dopaminergic pathway.

There is one possibility that perhaps should be kept in mind: some inhibitory neurons at any rate do not necessarily generate spikes and they may not necessarily be evident in electrophysiological recording, especially with extracellular recording. Electrophysiologists are biased in favor of the larger spikes, and one of the problems in recording the monosynaptic pathway (I mentioned that Paul Feltz has worked it out so beautifully) is that those spikes are smaller than the most obvious ones. This may be partly why that pathway had not really been analyzed very much before.

It is conceivable that there may be interneurons which, because they are Golgi type II cells with only local branches, do not have spikes. This assumption that cells have to generate spikes is, of course, unfounded, and cells of that type could be acted upon by a dopaminergic pathway. If this were an inhibitory pathway, one would not necessarily see very much electrical activity recording extracellularly.

Dr. McDowell: Dr. Ungerstedt, do you have a comment?

Dr. Ungerstedt: May I just relate a few experiments we have done on extracellular activity in the caudate? We first degenerated cells with 6-hydroxydopamine and then tested for the efficacy of this degeneration by the rotational response to apomorphine. We then selected animals that actually were denervated or had many supersensitive receptors and recorded extracellular activity in the denervated caudate. We find first of all that there is a higher incidence of firing cells and secondly that the cells that are not firing can very easily be excited by applying DLH iontophoretically. In our experiments there was really a great difference between the denervated and the innervated caudate.

Dr. Krnjevic: I would like to answer that because Buchwald's experiments were done not by using 6-hydroxydopamine but by actually making a lesion. He made the point that if they made the lesion close to the substantia nigra then there was a definite, although not very large, increase in firing in the caudate. However, if they made the lesion much closer to the caudate, which was at least as effective in reducing the dopamine content, then there was no significant change in firing. Buchwald recently concluded that you cannot correlate the changes in firing with the dopamine content.

Dr. Ungerstedt: If you make this lesion closest to the nigra, you also abolish the behavioral response to a dopamine receptor-stimulating drug.

Dr. Krnjevic: Yet you reduce the dopamine.

Dr. Ungerstedt: Yes, but my belief is that you are actually manipulating another pathway, possibly the efferent pathway from the caudate and this adds another factor.

Dr. Forno: Is the large amount of GABA in the compact zone or in the reticular zone; or is the distribution known?

Dr. Roberts: A paper has just been published on this point; the content is higher in the pars reticulata than in the pars compacta, and it is highest in the middle portion between the two.

Dr. Poirier: I think the observation that you just made concerning this gradient concentration within the middle portion of the substantia nigra is interesting because most of the nigral cells are in the medial part in the cat and the monkey.

Dr. Sibley: I would like to ask if Dr. Roberts knows if the total concentration of GABA in the substantia nigra or caudate is reduced in animals who are treated with excessive amounts of levodopa or in DOPA-induced chorea.

Dr. Roberts: I do not know that because I have not done experiments in that area.

Dr. Tyce: We have a colony of rats that were fed 1% DOPA for several months. In this group of animals we measured the concentration of GABA in the whole brain and found no change. However, we have found changes in the rate of formation of GABA from ^{14}C-glucose in the rats that have been fed DOPA for several months. Not after a single injection of DOPA but after DOPA feeding for several months the incorporation of ^{14}C and ^{14}C-glucose is reduced.

Advances in Neurology, Vol. 5
Raven Press, New York © 1974

Continuing Studies of the Peripheral Vascular Actions of Dopamine

Leon I. Goldberg, T. Budya Tjandramaga, Aaron H. Anton, and
Noboru Toda

Clinical Pharmacology Program, Emory University School of Medicine, Atlanta, Georgia
30322; Department of Anesthesiology, Case Western Reserve University School of Medicine, Cleveland, Ohio 44106, and Department of Pharmacology, Faculty of Medicine,
Kyoto University, Kyoto, Japan

At the last meeting of this group (1), unusual vasodilating actions of dopamine on renal and mesenteric arteries were described. Those results suggested the existence of a peripheral dopamine vascular receptor. New information is presented here concerning two separate problems relating to the peripheral action of dopamine. The first deals with the action of dopamine on isolated arteries, and the second concerns the apparent lack of correlation between dopamine plasma levels and the cardiovascular and renal actions of the amine in animals and man.

I. AN ISOLATED VASCULAR SYSTEM TO STUDY DOPAMINE-INDUCED VASODILATION

The cardiovascular and renal actions of dopamine have recently been reviewed (2). Dopamine has three qualitatively different actions on the cardiovascular system: (a) Dopamine stimulates the heart, both by a direct action on *beta*-adrenergic receptors and indirectly through the release of norepinephrine. These effects can be completely blocked by *beta*-adrenergic blocking agents such as propranolol. (b) Vasoconstriction is caused by action on *alpha*-adrenergic receptors. This effect predominates with large doses and results in elevation of arterial pressure. The vasoconstriction can be completely blocked by *alpha*-adrenergic blocking agents, such as phentolamine and phenoxybenzamine. After *alpha*-adrenergic blockade, dopamine lowers blood pressure in all species studied. (c) Dopamine causes vasodilation in renal and mesenteric vascular beds by action on the proposed dopamine receptor. The amine also appears to dilate selectively coronary blood vessels, but this effect is more difficult to observe because of the complications involved in studying the beating heart. More recently, von Essen (3) provided evidence that similar vasodilation occurs in intracerebral arteries.

The following evidence supports a specific vascular dopamine receptor: (a) Dopamine-induced vasodilation is selective. (b) It is not blocked by *beta*-adrenergic blocking agents or the classic antagonists. (c) Structure-activity studies have shown that only the N-methyl analogue epinine causes similar vasodilation. Apomorphine also produces selective renal vasodilation, but the effect is less than that produced by dopamine or epinine. (d) Vasodilation is selectively attenuated by haloperidol, phenothiazines, bulbocapnine, and apomorphine. As stated above, apomorphine also has a vasodilating action, so it possibly acts as both a partial agonist and antagonist. More recently, Goldberg and Musgrave *(unpublished data)* have found that 3-methoxy-4-hydroxy-phenylethylamine also exerts a weak antagonistic action. Similar effects were not exhibited by 4-methoxy-3-hydroxy-phenylethylamine or 3,4-methoxy-phenylethylamine.

Most of the above studies were carried out in intact animals, primarily the dog. Studies in intact animals, however, do not prove the existence of a specific receptor for two important reasons: (a) The effect may be due to a metabolite of dopamine. Typical vasodilation is not produced by 3-methoxy-4-hydroxy-phenylethylamine, dopacetic acid, homovanillic acid, or tetrahydropapaveroline. But an unknown metabolite could still be responsible. (b) The effect may be due to the release of an endogenous vasodilating material such as a kinin or a prostaglandin. There is no evidence for or against such an argument.

Thus, it is important to develop an isolated arterial preparation which relaxes in the presence of dopamine.

Attempts have been made to find such a preparation, but most investigations have demonstrated only *alpha*-adrenergic contractions. For example, Strandhoy, Cronnely, Long, and Williamson (4) reported that superfusion of isolated renal canine arteries resulted in vasoconstriction. Similarly, Kelly (5) found that isolated dog renal and mesenteric arterial strips contracted when dopamine was added to the bathing medium. Only two reports have described relaxation of isolated blood vessels. In 1958 Burn and Rand (6) reported that dopamine caused contraction of the untreated rabbit aortic strip. However, when the strip was maximally contracted by norepinephrine, a large dose of dopamine caused relaxation. Antagonists were not studied. These investigators concluded that the effect was due to the weaker agonist, dopamine, replacing norepinephrine at receptor sites. Kohli (7) found that dopamine caused relaxation of the rabbit aortic strip contracted with carbachol and treated with phenoxybenzamine. This relaxation, however, was completely reversed by the *beta*-adrenergic blocking agent propranolol.

For the past several months, we (Toda and Goldberg) have utilized a different approach in the Department of Pharmacology of Kyoto University Faculty of Medicine. Helical strips of canine renal, mesenteric, basilar, coronary, and femoral arteries ranging in size from 0.3 to 3 mm (outside diameter) were placed in isolated organ baths containing nutrients maintained at 37°C and bubbled with 95% oxygen and 5% CO_2. The method has previously been described (8). As observed by previous investigators, most preparations exhibited dose-related contractions when dopamine was added to the bath. However, relaxation was also found to occur in some strips. These different responses could have been due to variations in initial contractile state and *alpha*-adrenergic sensitivity. Accordingly, all preparations were treated with a contracting agent. In most of the preliminary work potassium was used in concentrations ranging from 10 to 30 mM. As described by Furchgott and Bhadrakom (9), potassium markedly potentiates the contracting actions of sympathomimetic amines. Accordingly, in order to demonstrate dopamine-induced relaxation, the preparations were pretreated with phenoxybenzamine, 10^{-5} M, which was applied for 60 min, and then removed. After these modifications, relaxation to dopamine (10^{-6} to 5×10^{-4} M) was consistently demonstrated in renal, mesenteric, coronary, and basilar arterial strips. This relaxing effect of dopamine could not be prevented by prior administration of the *beta*-adrenergic blocking agents sotalol (10^{-4} M) or propranolol (10^{-6} M) at doses which markedly antagonized the relaxing action of isoproterenol. The relaxation produced by dopamine also appeared to be different from that produced by papaverine, since the latter drug almost uniformly caused further relaxation after the maximum response to dopamine. As in the intact animal, similar dopamine-induced relaxation was not observed in femoral arteries (10). In addition to the above studies, relaxation was observed when the vessels were contracted with barium, vasopressin, or prostaglandin $F\alpha_2$. Typical dopamine-induced relaxation occurring in a phenoxybenzamine-treated, barium-contracted mesenteric arterial strip is shown in Fig. 1. Note that both isoproterenol and papaverine caused further relaxation after the maximum effect of dopamine.

Initial structure-activity studies have indicated that epinine (N-methyl-dopamine) appears to exert similar relaxing actions as dopamine. On the other hand, 3-methoxy-4-hydroxy-phenylethylamine was inactive until very large doses were given. Possible antagonistic effects of haloperidol, bulbo-capnine, and chlorpromazine are currently being explored.

In summary, we have demonstrated for the first time a consistent dopamine-induced relaxation of isolated dog renal, mesenteric, basilar, and coronary arteries *in vitro*. Preliminary data suggest that this effect is due to an action on specific dopamine vascular receptors.

II. CORRELATION OF CARDIOVASCULAR EFFECTS AND PLASMA LEVELS OF DOPAMINE

Because L-DOPA is decarboxylated to dopamine, the administration of sufficient doses of the amino acid causes cardiovascular and renal actions

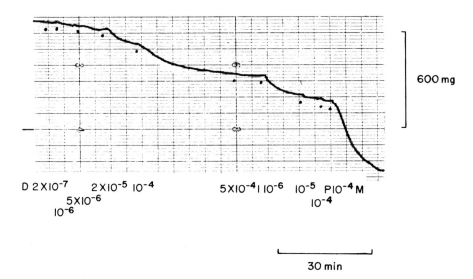

FIG. 1. Relaxation produced by dopamine (D), isoproterenol (I), and papaverine (Pa) in an isolated canine mesenteric arterial strip contracted with barium, 1 mM. The strip had previously been exposed to phenoxybenzamine, 10^{-5} M, for 60 min. The horizontal line at the left denotes tension of the strip before application of barium. The vertical scale signifies tension in milligrams; horizontal scale, time in minutes.

identical to those produced by dopamine. Thus, it should be possible to correlate plasma levels of dopamine with pharmacological action observed after administration of the amino acid and the amine. Whitsett and Goldberg (11) demonstrated that measurements of the externally recorded pre-ejection period was a sensitive indicator of the positive inotropic effects of L-DOPA. The positive inotropic effect of 1.5 g of L-DOPA was completely eliminated by prior administration of 10 mg of the *beta*-adrenergic blocking agent propranolol. Interestingly, shortening of the pre-ejection period was no longer observed after 3 months of L-DOPA therapy. In order to investigate the mechanism responsible for the tolerance, we (Tjandramaga, Goldberg, and Anton, 12) measured DOPA and dopamine levels in patients who did and did not have shortening of the pre-ejection period. Our results indicated that there was no correlation between the plasma levels of dopamine and cardiac activity. Furthermore, dopamine plasma levels were extremely high in some patients, but there was no sign of excessive cardiovascular activity such as cardiac arrhythmias or hypertension.

In order to make more direct correlations between the cardiac and renal actions and plasma levels of DOPA and dopamine, this subject was investigated in the anesthetized dog (13). Cardiac contractility was measured by a Walton-Brodie strain gauge arch sutured to the right ventricle, and renal blood flow was measured with an electromagnetic flowmeter. A marked discrepancy was observed in the plasma levels produced by dopamine and L-DOPA and the cardiac and renal actions. This discrepancy was not the result of the action of L-DOPA or its metabolites to block receptors or to cause nonspecific depression, since a superimposed dopamine infusion produced marked increments in cardiac contractile force, with only slight elevations in dopamine plasma levels after the peak effects of L-DOPA were recorded.

We are currently exploring the possibility that removal of the blood from the animal or patient and the analytical procedures somehow cause an overestimation of free dopamine level in the plasma.

Imai, Sugiura, and Tamura (14) demonstrated that the dopamine present in the normal human plasma is mostly in a conjugated form. These investigators (15) reported that acid hydrolysis liberates extremely high levels of dopamine from the plasma of patients receiving L-DOPA. We also have found that acid hydrolysis as well as enzymatic hydrolysis with β-glucuronidase (Ketodase, Endo) and sulfatase (Sulfatase type II, Sigma) cause a pronounced increase in measured plasma dopamine in patients treated with L-DOPA. There are a number of steps in the Anton and Sayre (16) method which could conceivably cause release of free dopamine from an acid labile conjugate. First, the protein is precipitated with 0.4 normal $HClO_4$. Secondly, dopamine is eluted from the aluminum oxide with 0.05 normal HCl, and thirdly, the hydrolysis might occur during the formation of the fluorophor with sodium periodate. The first two have been ruled out by the use of an organic solvent extraction procedure that eliminates these acid treatments. Other possibilities include the release of bound dopamine from albumin, platelets, or red cells. The known metabolites of dopamine have been tested in the analytical procedure and ruled out as a possible artifact.

In summary, there is a marked discrepancy between the measured concentrations of dopamine in the plasma and its cardiovascular actions in patients and experimental animals receiving L-DOPA. The basis for this discrepancy is still under investigation.

ACKNOWLEDGMENT

This work was supported in part by U.S Public Health Service grant GM-14270.

REFERENCES

1. Goldberg, L. I., in: *L-DOPA in Parkinsonism,* p. 305, A. Davis Company, Philadelphia (1970).
2. Goldberg, L. I., *Pharmacol. Rev.,* 24, 1 (1972).
3. Essen, von C., *J. Pharm. Pharmacol.,* 24, 668 (1972).
4. Strandhoy, J. W., Cronnely, R., Long, J. P., and Williamson, H. E., *Proc. Soc. Exp. Biol. Med.,* 141, 336 (1972).

5. Kelly, M. J., *Brit. J. Pharmacol.*, 46, 575 (1972).
6. Burn, J. H., and Rand, M. J., *Brit. J. Pharmacol.*, 13, 471 (1958).
7. Kohli, J. D., *Can. J. Physiol. Pharmacol.*, 47, 171 (1969).
8. Toda, N., Usui, H., Nishino, N., and Fujiwara, M., *J. Pharmacol. Exp. Ther.*, 181, 512 (1972).
9. Furchgott, R. F., and Bhadrakom, S., *J. Pharmacol. Exp. Ther.*, 108, 129 (1953).
10. Toda, N., Goldberg, L. I., and Fujiwara, M., *Jap. J. Pharmacol.*, 23 (Suppl.), 45 (1973).
11. Whitsett, T. L., and Goldberg, L. I., *Circulation*, 35, 97 (1972).
12. Tjandramaga, T. B., Goldberg, L. I., and Anton, A. H., *Fed. Proc.*, 32, 798 (1973).
13. Tjandramaga, T. B., Goldberg, L. I., and Anton, A. H., *Proc. Soc. Exp. Biol. Med.*, 142, 424 (1973).
14. Imai, K., Sugiura, M., and Tamura, Z., *Chem. Pharm. Bull.*, 18, 2134 (1970).
15. Imai, K., Sugiura, M., Tamura, Z., Hirayama, K., and Narabayashi, H., *Chem. Pharm. Bull.*, 19, 439 (1971).
16. Anton, A. H., and Sayre, D. F., *J. Pharmacol. Exp. Ther.*, 145, 326, (1964).

DISCUSSION

Dr. McDowell: Dr. Anton, have you any comments about the methodology?

Dr. Anton: I have one comment. One of the things that we have done recently to rule out acid hydrolysis is to devise a technique for carrying out dopamine analysis without using acid at all. We run the analysis at just about neutral pH. We find exactly the same results doing a simultaneous assay in a sample using the acid precipitate method with aluminum hydroxide and absorption. It does not seem that acid hydrolysis is necessary.

Dr. Carlsson: I wonder if Dr. Goldberg has considered the possibility or probability that the distribution of dopamine after DOPA administration in the body is entirely different from that of administered dopamine.

The dopamine formed after giving DOPA is formed intracellularly, and then it probably leaks out. Outside these cells you probably have a rather high concentration of dopamine. Moreover, are not some of the cardiovascular actions of DOPA central in origin?

Dr. Goldberg: Yes, that would be fine if it were going the other way, that is, if we had low dopamine levels with changes in cardiac activity, but we found high dopamine levels and no changes in cardiac activity.

Dr. Carlsson: Yes, but you have so many different actions and you have pointed out that they go in different directions.

Dr. Goldberg: If you give a dose of DOPA achieving plasma levels of 25 and produce a 50% increase in cardiac contractility, this is blocked by propanolol. If we take the same animal and give him 1 microgram per kilogram per minute of dopamine, we can produce the same effect at plasma levels of 1 microgram. These are exactly the same effects: I do not see how there can be something different at the receptor.

Dr. Carlsson: You may also have to consider the possibility of a presynaptic effect. You could have a presynaptic adrenergic blocking action, perhaps by dopamine inside the adrenergic neurons.

Dr. Goldberg: I cannot think that fast, but I do not see it; I think we are dealing with the receptor for now.

Dr. Goldstein: Dr. Goldberg, how do you exclude the possibility that some of the effects are not due to the formation of norepinephrine from dopamine?

Dr. Goldberg: We cannot exclude that as far as the heart is concerned, but we can certainly exclude it with regard to the kidney since norepinephrine constricts vessels in the kidney. The cardiac effect is due to two things: release of norepinephrine and direct action of dopamine on the receptor. I do not know whether dopamine is converted to norepinephrine or not. That is a possibility. You suggest the possibility that the reason we are not having more cardiac effect with high DOPA levels is that we may be releasing more norepinephrine with the infusion than we do with the DOPA.

Dr. Goldstein: With regard to the methodology, I wonder whether it would be possible for you to hydrolyze those conjugates enzymatically and measure before and after enzymatic hydrolysis. This will give you a clear-cut answer about how much conjugation is present.

Dr. Goldberg: I may not have made that clear, but Dr. Anton is doing that; he is using ketolase and sulfatase.

Dr. Tyce: Dr. Manfred Muenter and I have been doing some studies on the concentrations of conjugated and free dopamine in plasma, and we have results that are very similar to those of Dr. Goldberg and Dr. Anton. The procedure used is a perchloric acid precipitation of proteins and then alumina separation, which would not hydrolyze the conjugates. In the isolated perfused rat liver we have these conjugates and they are not hydrolyzed by this mild treatment.

We have found that quite high or very low concentrations of free dopamine in various patients seem to bear no relation to any cardiovascular side effects.

Since the conjugate is hydrolyzed by glucolase but not by glucuronidase, we believe it to be a sulfur.

Dr. Reis: Dr. Goldberg, under normal circumstances what is the source of dopamine which is reaching these receptors? Do you believe it is from a neural source? Is the receptor a nonspecific reader of levels of dopamine within the circulation?

Dr. Goldberg: I think it just reads dopamine in the circulation. If you administer L-DOPA to a dog, the response is just like that following a slow infusion of dopamine. We are quite certain that this is caused by dopamine, because if you give a decarboxylase inhibitor the response is completely blocked. We do not think it has much to do with interneural release. In the heart there is some release of norepinephrine.

Dr. Reis: I don't mean pharmacologically. In the natural life of the animal, is the circulating dopamine serving a function? What is the source of the dopamine which would be acting on the receptor under normal circumstances?

Dr. Goldberg: Where is the dopamine coming from? There is some from the brain, some from the diet, and some from the gut.

Dr. Sandler: A methodological point, Dr. Anton. My colleague Kim Ping Wong has recently developed a gas chromatographic method for detection of catecholamines in urine. In the course of this, she has detected an unknown oxidation metabolite of dopamine with fluorescence characteristics identical to those of dopamine. So far we have been quite unable to pinpoint what it is, but if this compound were to form *in vivo,* it might shed some light on the sort of problems that Dr. Goldberg has been mentioning.

Dr. Krnjević: I wondered whether you have completely excluded the possibility that DOPA itself is changing the sensitivity of the dopamine receptors.

Dr. Goldberg: As far as we can tell, DOPA itself is totally inactive. That is, if one gives DOPA and then a decarboxylase inhibitor, nothing happens to any of the "receptors" that we have studied. Also, D-DOPA is inactive. You know we can give alpha-methyldopa or any of the decarboxylase inhibitors, and none of these effects takes place.

Dr. Krnjević: No, but if you give the DOPA and the decarboxylase inhibitor and dopamine, is the effect of dopamine more or equal to the normal effect?

Dr. Goldberg: The dopamine effect will be seen whatever else we have done; this does not block the receptor.

Dr. Anton: I have two comments to both points. As far as Dr. Sandler's point is concerned, we have also taken samples from patients who have rather high dopamine levels and have done paper chromatography on them. The only compounds we find on paper chromatograms are those we find by the other techniques. The values are in agreement within 50%.

I would also like to point out, in response to the last question, that if dogs have these high levels (detectable chemical levels at least) of DOPA and if dopamine is infused even though these high levels are still present, you get the cardiovascular effects at these low levels of dopamine, which is a weird puzzle we cannot explain.

Dr. Goldberg: We give L-DOPA and we get a 40% increase in cardiac contractility and a level of dopamine of, say, 50 nanograms. Then we give dopamine (6 micrograms per kilogram per minute) intravenously and increase the dopamine level from 50 to 51, and the cardiac contractility goes up three times. That is, for less than a 1% increase in the plasma level, we get that much more cardiac response.

Dr. Brossi: Dr. Goldberg, when you give large amounts of L-DOPA, what do you measure afterward: L-DOPA or just DOPA or D-DOPA?

Dr. Goldberg: Dr. Anton measures DOPA and dopamine.

Dr. Anton: The method does not distinguish between L- and D-DOPA.

Dr. Brossi: Do you mean that D-DOPA is not active? Is it not feasible that the L-DOPA is being converted by some mechanism into D-DOPA?

Dr. Anton: I do not know of any evidence for that. Can someone else answer that? We do infuse L-DOPA, and these are the responses we get; and we assume we are measuring L-DOPA. I do not know if there is a conversion to D-DOPA.

Dr. Carlsson: Let me suggest this explanation. When you give DOPA through a central action you get a reduction in sympathetic tone to the heart and this is compensated for by the dopamine level that you have at the receptors in the heart to some extent.

Dr. Goldberg: If this were true, should we not also block the dopamine we give intravenously?

Dr. Carlsson: No, I don't think so. If the sympathetic tone goes down, the heart still is capable of responding to the circulating dopamine.

Advances in Neurology, Vol. 5
Raven Press, New York © 1974

The Pathology of Parkinsonism: A Comparison of Degenerations in Cerebral Cortex and Brainstem

Ellsworth C. Alvord, Jr., Lysia S. Forno, John A. Kusske,
R. Jerry Kauffman, J. Scott Rhodes, and Charles R. Goetowski

Department of Pathology, University of Washington School of Medicine, Seattle, Washington 98195, Laboratory of Neuropathology, Palo Alto Veterans Administration Hospital and Department of Pathology, Stanford University School of Medicine, Palo Alto, California 94304, and Pathology Laboratory, Swedish Hospital and Medical Center, Seattle, Washington 98104

In our previous analysis of the pathology of parkinsonism (1, 2) we concluded that the substantia nigra and locus ceruleus bore the brunt of the diseases which produced the parkinsonian state. These diseases were of at least two (possibly three) types: 1. the Lewy body type of unknown etiology and 2. the Alzheimer's neurofibrillary tangle type usually following epidemic encephalitis lethargica but possibly including a third type of unknown etiology. Since many parkinsonian patients appear to be demented, and since a fourth type of parkinsonism has been recognized in the Chamorros on Guam and associated specifically with dementia and amyotrophic lateral sclerosis, it became of interest to see if any of the types of parkinsonism commonly found in the United States was associated with any of the lesions commonly found in dementia (Alzheimer's neurofibrillary tangles and senile plaques in the neocortex and limbic lobe and Simchowicz's granulo-vacuolar inclusion bodies in the hippocampus). Thus began the present study to reexamine all of the cases of parkinsonism coming to autopsy in Seattle and Palo Alto, in which we looked for various degrees of each change in specific anatomic sites and compared the various types and severities of parkinsonism with each other and with age- and type-matched nonparkinsonian controls.

CASE MATERIAL

The 532 cases in this study consisted of 129 definite parkinsonians (90 from the Neuropathology Laboratory of the Palo Alto Veterans Administration Hospital and 39 from the Neuropathology Laboratory of the University of Washington), 25 questionable parkinsonians (from Palo Alto), 322 consecutive autopsies in 1969 and 1970 (from Palo Alto, containing

289 nonparkinsonians), and 56 miscellaneous cases (13 from Seattle and 43 from Palo Alto).

All of the histologic observations on the 532 cases were made by Dr. Lysia Forno, who graded the changes for each of 13 site-lesion combinations, as follows: nerve cells with Lewy bodies or Alzheimer's neurofibrillary tangles were counted in the substantia nigra on one side and in the locus ceruleus bilaterally. For purposes of coding, one to two nerve cells with one or more Lewy bodies or Alzheimer's tangles were graded as +, three to five cells as ++, six to 10 cells as +++, and more than 10 as ++++. Nerve cell loss in the substantia nigra, locus ceruleus, and cerebral cortex was graded on an arbitrary scale from 0 to ++++ (cf. Figs. 1 and 2). Alzheimer's neurofibrillary tangles, senile plaques, and Simchowicz's granulovacuolar degeneration in the cerebral cortex were graded semiquantitatively, taking into account the number of lesions in the entire slide or slides examined, but roughly corresponding to the following distribution of the changes: one to two abnormal cells per medium power field +, three to 10 cells ++, and more than 10 per medium power field +++ (cf. Figs. 2, 3, and 4). The sections from the cerebral cortex were examined in the hippocampal formation and in the neocortex (usually superior frontal cortex, often from additional cortical areas, but occasionally restricted to the fusiform gyrus). Intermediate degrees of each semiquantitative change were recognized.

Relatively few cases had insufficient material for some of these observations; in such situations the blanks were arbitrarily coded as zero. All blocks were stained by H & E and many by periodic acid-Schiff (usually combined with luxol fast blue and hematoxylin) and various silver stains for axons. The parkinsonian cases had more blocks and more stains per block than the nonparkinsonian cases, but an attempt was made to keep these variables relatively fixed and to examine the slides in the absence of knowledge of the clinical observations, but the slides were not reassigned random numbers, and the only serious attempt to control the histologic observations was by the inclusion of 13 nonparkinsonian cases in the 52 cases sent from Seattle to Dr. Forno with no clinical records. Her clinicopathologic correlations in these cases were practically perfect, so that the senior author was convinced that all of the observations were reasonably accurate.

All of the clinical observations relating to parkinsonism and dementia were obtained from the medical records at the appropriate hospitals. Dr. Forno graded the severity of the parkinsonism from the charts in the Palo Alto Veterans Administration Hospital in the following manner: cases with some components of parkinsonism (resting tremor, rigidity, and akinesia) described but without a diagnosis actually made were called ?; those with all of the components described or the diagnosis of mild parkinsonism actually recorded by the attending physicians were called ±; cases with definite but not severe parkinsonism were rated +; cases with moderately severe parkinsonism necessitating treatment and cases with very severe

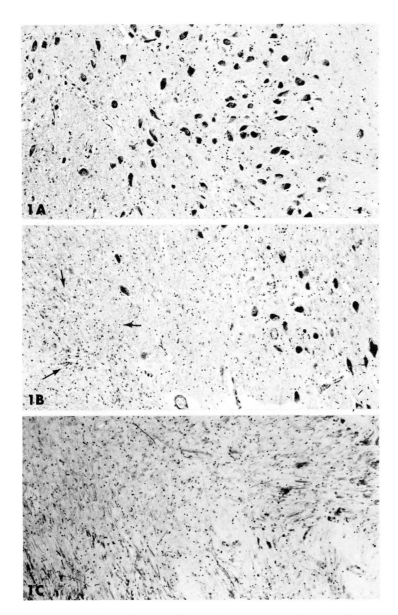

FIG. 1. *A*. Substantia nigra with no cell loss. Normal control (49-year-old man without parkinsonism). Hematoxylin-Eosin stain, × 72 (72 A 155). *B*. Substantia nigra with slight to moderate nerve cell loss (+ to ++). Idiopathic parkinsonism with Lewy bodies (not seen at this magnification). Glial scar with focal nerve cell loss indicated by arrows. Hematoxylin-Eosin stain, × 72 (72 A 138). *C*. Substantia nigra with severe nerve cell loss (+++). Postencephalitic parkinsonism. Luxol fast blue — cresyl violet stain, × 72 (64 A 158).

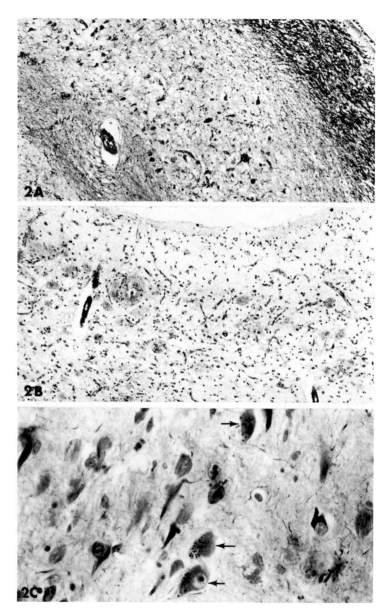

FIG. 2. *A.* Pyramidal cell layer of hippocampus with slight to moderate (+ to ++) nerve cell loss. Luxol fast blue – Bielschowsky stain, × 72 (68 A 169). *B.* Frontal cortex with moderate to severe (++ to +++) nerve cell loss. Luxol fast blue, periodic acid-Schiff, hematoxylin stain, × 72 (68 A 169). *C.* Pyramidal cell layer of hippocampus with moderate (++) granulovacuolar degeneration *(arrows)* and Alzheimer's neurofibrillary tangles. Luxol fast blue – Bielschowsky stain, × 360 (72 A 58).

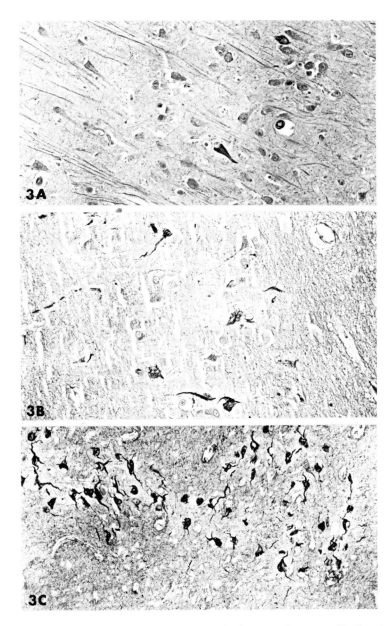

FIG. 3. Alzheimer's neurofibrillary tangles in cerebral cortex: *A.* + neurofibrillary tangles in pyramidal cell layer. Palmgren silver impregnation, × 144 (67 A 156). *B.* ++ neurofibrillary tangles in pyramidal cell layer. Holmes silver impregnation, × 144 (Np 1283). *C.* +++ neurofibrillary tangles in subiculum. Holmes silver impregnation, × 144 (Np 3025).

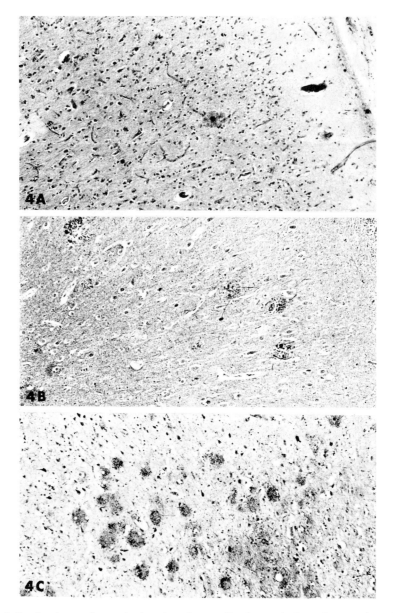

FIG. 4. Senile plaques in cerebral cortex: A. + senile plaques in frontal cortex. Luxol fast blue, periodic acid-Schiff, hematoxylin stain, × 72 (70 A 81). B. ++senile plaques in hippocampal gyrus. Bielschowsky silver impregnation, × 72 (70 A 81). C. +++senile plaques in hippocampal gyrus. Luxol fast blue−Bielschowsky silver impregnation, × 72 (69 A 169).

disease with total disability were rated ++. Dementia, admittedly more difficult to estimate retrospectively, was graded similarly, an attempt being made to differentiate "organic dementia" from "functional psychiatric" (usually schizophrenic) disorders. Dr. John Kusske graded similar observations on the Seattle cases from 0 to ++++; but in order to make the scales comparable, the following simplification was used: 0, ?, definite (±, +), and severe (++ to ++++).

The notations of Drs. Forno and Kusske were transcribed to numbers $(0 = 0, \pm = 1, + = 3, ++ = 5, +++ = 7, ++++ = 9)$ for computer analysis, the print-out of which provided the number of cases for each decade of age at the time of death and the mean degree of lesion (± 1 standard error of the mean) for each of the 13 site-lesion combinations. Nine major categories were considered and designated as follows:

1. all cases: 154 parkinsonians, 377 nonparkinsonians.
2. those without Lewy bodies in either the substantia nigra or the locus ceruleus (L+): 80 parkinsonians, 84 nonparkinsonians.
3. those with Lewy bodies in either the substantia nigra or the locus ceruleus (L+); 80 parkinsonians, 84 nonparkinsonians.
4. those without Alzheimer's tangles in either the substantia nigra or the locus ceruleus (A0): 74 parkinsonians, 237 nonparkinsonians.
5. those with Alzheimer's tangles in either the substantia nigra or the locus ceruleus (A+): 80 parkinsonians, 140 nonparkinsonians.
6. those without either Lewy bodies or Alzheimer's tangles in either the substantia nigra or the locus ceruleus (L0 A0): 25 parkinsonians, 187 nonparkinsonians.
7. those without Lewy bodies but with Alzheimer's tangles in either the substantia nigra or the locus ceruleus (L0 A+): 49 parkinsonians, 106 nonparkinsonians.
8. those with Lewy bodies but without Alzheimer's tangles in either the substantia nigra or the locus ceruleus (L+ A0): 49 parkinsonians, 50 nonparkinsonians.
9. those with both Lewy bodies and Alzheimer's tangles in either the substantia nigra or the locus ceruleus (L+ A+): 31 parkinsonians, 34 nonparkinsonians.

Each category was subdivided into eight groups with four degrees of parkinsonism (P0, P?, P+, or P++) and history of encephalitis (E0, E+); but since only some of the severe cases of parkinsonism had such a history, there were effectively only five groups, which could be designated as P0 E0 (377 cases), P? E0 (25 cases), P+ E0 (66 cases), P++ E0 (51 cases), and P++ E+ (12 cases). One case was coded P0 E+. In addition, all of the parkinsonians (including ? = 1) were combined into one group regardless of the degree of parkinsonism or past history of encephalitis. In this manner, the mean degree of each variable (± 1 SEM) was calculated for each decade in each clinical group of each histologic category for various populations of patients (19 operatively and 20 nonoperatively treated parkinsonians in Seattle and all the parkinsonians in Palo Alto plus the 1969 and 1970 consecutive series of autopsies of nonparkinsonians).

The age-matched comparisons could, therefore, be readily obtained and plotted graphically. Figure 5 indicates the numbers of patients per decade in each group. Note that the distribution and number of controls is similar to the total number of cases, especially above age 60.

Specific subpopulations were compared with each other before pooling the cases. In view of the different rates of accumulation of various lesions, it was necessary to restrict these initial comparisons to those age groups with an adequate number of cases. Among the Seattle cases those aged 60 to 69 years and either operated or not operated on could be compared as total cases or as restricted to those with Lewy bodies. Fifty to 69% of the comparisons were identical, and the discrepancies were symmetrically distributed on either side; but it appeared that the cases which had been operated on had more severe parkinsonism and more cell loss in the substantia nigra, more Lewy bodies in the locus ceruleus, and less Alzheimer's tangles in the locus ceruleus than those which had not been operated on. The differences seemed relatively slight, so that the Seattle cases were pooled and compared with the Palo Alto cases. Age groups up to 79 years contained an

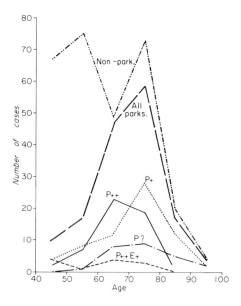

FIG. 5. Number of cases per decade of age at death in 289 nonparkinsonian controls (1969 and 1970) and in patients with varying degrees of parkinsonism (25 P?, 66 P+, 51 P++ without a past history of encephalitis, and 12 P++ E+ with a past history of encephalitis).

adequate number of cases for the total population of parkinsonians and ages 60 to 79 for Lewy body cases. Sixty-one to 71% of all these comparisons were identical, and again the discrepancies were symmetrically distributed on either side: the Palo Alto cases had more senile plaques in the neocortex and less Alzheimer's tangles in the locus ceruleus. The original gradings of the degree of parkinsonism and dementia were known to have been different and were rescaled, as described above, so that they became more comparable.

Since Dr. Forno (3) has been oversampling her autopsy material for many years for cases with Lewy bodies, the total population of nonparkinsonian cases would not necessarily be the proper source of normal controls, but the consecutive series of 322 cases examined in 1969 and 1970 and containing 289 nonparkinsonians served admirably for these base lines of "normal" aging. Indeed, when the various nonparkinsonian cases were compared, it was obvious that there were relatively fewer cases with Lewy bodies in either the substantia nigra or the locus ceruleus and with associated neuronal loss in the same situation in the 1969 and 1970 consecutive series than in the total population, as would be expected from her oversampling for Lewy body cases. Only one other change (neuronal loss in the hippocampus) showed a comparable difference, for reasons which are not yet apparent.

From these preliminary analyses it seemed that the comparisons which would be most meaningful would be as follows:

1. Normal (nonparkinsonian) controls (289 cases from the 1969 and 1970 Palo Alto consecutive series of 322 cases), as well as all 377 nonparkinsonians included in the whole series.

2. Patients with parkinsonism of three degrees of severity (25 questionable, 66 definite, and 63 severe) from the combined 39 cases from Seattle and the 115 cases from Palo Alto.

3. Patients with or without either Lewy bodies or Alzheimer's tangles in the substantia nigra or locus ceruleus in each of the above groups.

RESULTS

To begin with the 289 nonparkinsonians in the 1969 and 1970 consecutive series of autopsies, Fig. 6 illustrates the development of each of the 13 changes studied as a function of age at the time of death. Since most of the curves were relatively straight lines, their equations could be easily determined (Figs. 7 and 8) and a weighted average of all the cerebral cortical degenerations developed (Fig. 9). This weighted average cortical degeneration included seven alterations: Alzheimer's tangles, senile plaques, and neuronal loss in both hippocampus and neocortex and Simchowicz's granulovacuolar change in the hippocampus.

Figures 10 and 11 illustrate the mean degree of this weighted average

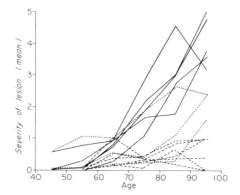

FIG. 6. Mean severity of each lesion in 289 nonparkinsonian controls (1969 and 1970) as a function of decade of age at death. Identification and equations of each curve are provided in Figs. 7 and 8.

cortical degeneration in each clinical group for the whole population (Fig. 10) and for various subpopulations (Fig. 11). It should be noted that each point represents the mean of at least three patients in the particular decade. For the two largest groups (all nonparkinsonians and all parkinsonians), the standard error of the mean is indicated by the shading, but, for simplicity, the overlapping standard errors of each of the groups representing different degrees of parkinsonism are not included. Note that all of the groups of parkinsonians have greater degrees of cortical degeneration than the nonparkinsonian controls, but that there is no consistent pattern with respect to the severity of parkinsonism (Fig. 10). That each group from Seattle is similar to the comparable one in Palo Alto (Fig. 11) justifies the

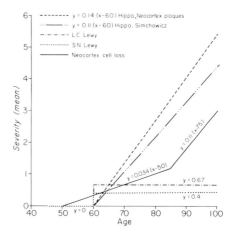

FIG. 7. Equations expressing the approximate age-severity of lesions illustrated in Fig. 6.

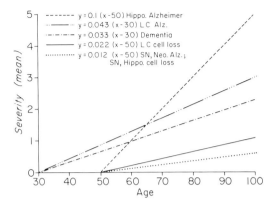

FIG. 8. Equations expressing the approximate age-severity of lesions illustrated in Fig. 6.

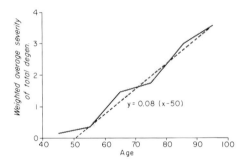

FIG. 9. Equation *(dashed line)* approximately expressing the age-severity of the weighted average severity of seven cerebral cortical degenerations in 289 nonparkinsonian controls (1969 and 1970). The shaded area includes ± 1 standard error of the actual mean.

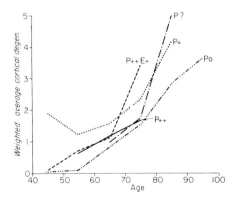

FIG. 10. Weighted average cortical degeneration as a function of age at death in patients with varying degrees of parkinsonism (PU = 1969 and 1970 nonparkinsonian controls).

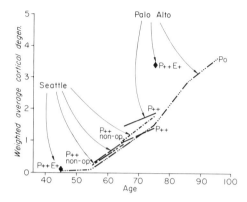

FIG. 11. As in Fig. 10, but limited to those cases in Seattle who could be compared with cases of the same severity of parkinsonism in Palo Alto.

pooling of all the cases to achieve a greater number of cases and smoother curves. Only the ages at death of the severe postencephalitic cases (P++ E+) are different in Seattle as compared to Palo Alto, for reasons not yet apparent.

Figures 12 and 13 similarly illustrate the mean degrees of dementia in each group for the whole population (Fig. 12) or for various subpopulations (Fig. 13). Again, each group of parkinsonians is more demented, on the average, than the age-matched nonparkinsonian controls (Fig. 12), and the cases in Seattle are reasonably comparable to those in Palo Alto (Fig. 13).

Figure 14 compares the mean degrees of dementia and weighted average cortical degeneration in each clinical group for the whole population. Note that all but the oldest cases have relatively more dementia than cortical degeneration.

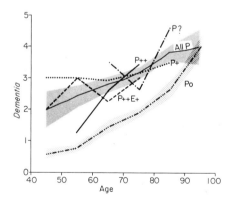

FIG. 12. Mean degree of dementia in nonparkinsonian controls (P0 = 1969 and 1970 nonparkinsonian controls) and in patients with varying degrees of parkinsonism. The shaded areas include ± 1 SEM for all the parkinsonians (all P) and for the nonparkinsonians (P0).

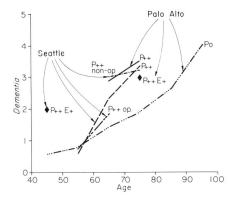

FIG. 13. As in Fig. 12, but limited to those cases in Seattle who could be compared with cases of the same severity of parkinsonism in Palo Alto.

Similar graphic illustrations of the degree of neuronal loss occurring in the substantia nigra as functions of age and severity of parkinsonism are given in Figs. 15–17, for each clinical group in the whole population (Fig. 15), in those with Lewy bodies in either the substantia nigra or locus ceruleus (Fig. 16), and in those without Lewy bodies (Fig. 17). It is obvious that the Lewy body cases (Fig. 16) show an orderly quantitative pattern of increasing neuronal loss with increasing degrees of parkinsonism, relatively independent of age (except that the more severe cases tend to die earlier), whereas the cases without Lewy bodies (Fig. 17) are a mixture of severe cases (with appropriately severe neuronal loss in the substantia nigra) and mild-to-moderate cases (without sufficient neuronal loss in the substantia nigra).

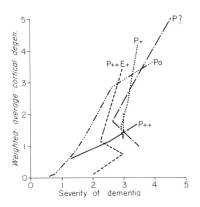

FIG. 14. Weighted average cortical degeneration and severity of dementia in nonparkinsonian controls and in patients with varying degrees of parkinsonism. (Each line includes increasing ages of patients, the oldest cases occurring at the labeled end of each line; cf. Figs. 10 and 12.)

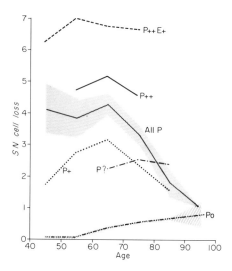

FIG. 15. Mean degree of neuronal loss in the substantia nigra as a function of age at death in patients with varying degrees of parkinsonism (P0 = all 377 nonparkinsonian controls). The shaded areas include ± 1 SEM for all the parkinsonians (all P) and for the nonparkinsonians (P0).

Another view of these relationships is given in Fig. 18, which attempts to define "thresholds" of neuronal loss in the substantia nigra associated with increasing degrees of parkinsonism. The relatively straightforward pattern for the Lewy body cases contrasts with that for the cases without

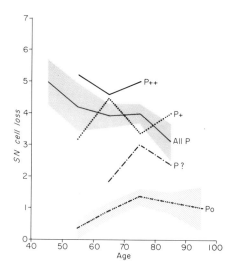

FIG. 16. As in Fig. 15, but limited to those cases with Lewy bodies in either the substantia nigra or locus ceruleus (80 parkinsonians and 84 nonparkinsonians).

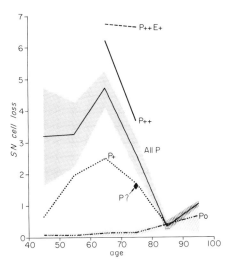

FIG. 17. As in Figs. 15 and 16, but limited to those cases without Lewy bodies in either the substantia nigra or locus ceruleus (74 parkinsonians and 293 nonparkinsonians).

Lewy bodies, in whom only the most severe cases (generally postencephalitic) have lost cells in the substantia nigra to the same (or greater) degree as the Lewy body cases.

In an attempt to find an "extranigral cause" (4) for the parkinsonism in

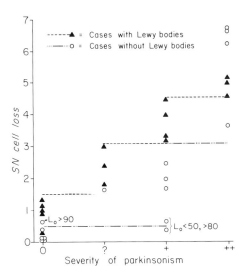

FIG. 18. "Thresholds" for developing increasing degrees of parkinsonism. Each point represents one decade (*cf.* Figs. 16 and 17). The exceptional groups of cases without Lewy bodies are those dying over age 90 without parkinsonism and those definite (+) parkinsonians dying below age 50 or above age 80 (*cf.* Fig. 17).

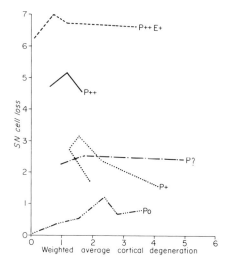

FIG. 19. Neuronal loss in the substantia nigra and weighted average cortical degeneration in patients with varying degrees of parkinsonism. (Each line includes increasing ages of patients, the oldest cases occurring at the labeled end of each line; *cf.* Figs. 10 and 15.)

those cases without Lewy bodies, Figs. 19–21 were constructed, comparing the degrees of substantia nigra neuronal loss and weighted average cerebral cortical degeneration in the various clinical groups in the whole population (Fig. 19), in various subpopulations (Fig. 20), and in the cases without Lewy bodies (Fig. 21). The Lewy body cases (not illustrated) were straightforward (as in Figs. 16 and 18), but the cases without Lewy bodies (Fig. 21) are

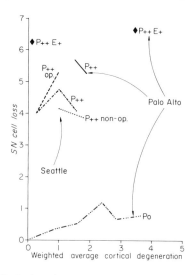

FIG. 20. As in Fig. 19, but limited to those cases in Seattle who could be compared with cases of the same severity of parkinsonism in Palo Alto.

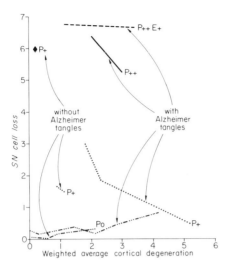

FIG. 21. As in Fig. 19, but limited to those cases without Lewy bodies in either substantia nigra or locus ceruleus, subdivided according to presence or absence of Alzheimer's tangles in either substantia nigra or locus ceruleus.

obviously heterogeneous, divisible into those with and those without Alzheimer's tangles in either the substantia nigra or locus ceruleus. In those moderate (+) parkinsonians without Lewy bodies but with Alzheimer's tangles, there is a tendency for the older cases (indicated by the label P+ at the end of the line in Fig. 21) to have disproportionately greater cortical degeneration, suggestive of a variant of senile dementia (2) with more diffuse changes not yet defined.

DISCUSSION

The pathoanatomic analysis of degenerative diseases occurring in the older ages is complicated by the necessity for making comparisons not only between the normal controls and the cases with the disease but also between at least two types of each of these groups: (1) within the normal controls there are the "optimal normals," i.e., those in their 20's, whose brains on the average are fully developed and relatively free of any degenerative changes and, therefore, relatively easily distinguished from the cases; but there are also "age-matched controls," whose brains on the average contain increasing degrees of degenerative changes which are still more or less subclinical, which may also be expected to occur within the cases but which may play little or no role in the production of the particular disease under consideration. (2) Within the cases of the particular disease there are those who are only slightly, moderately, or severely affected at the time the patient dies (with, but not necessarily of, the disease), whose brains should show qualitative or quantitative changes proportionate to the severity of the clinical disease.

Of course, with a disease as pleomorphic clinically as parkinsonism is, one may expect to find a pleomorphism histologically, with different lesions correlating with tremor, rigidity, bradykinesia, etc. Our current lumping together of all of these into one summary diagnosis of mild, moderate, or severe parkinsonism may obscure important relationships. All the more so is this true when one considers what is lumped together in the diagnosis "dementia." But in spite of these limitations, most of the important comparisons have been accomplished in this study of parkinsonism. The analysis is not yet complete, but the current tentative conclusions can be summarized briefly, as follows:

1. All of the 13 site-type age changes considered in this study begin at approximately 50 to 60 years of age and increase approximately linearly, except for the following: (a) the number of neurons in the substantia nigra containing Lewy bodies (which appear at about age 60 and remain rather constant), (b) the number of neurons in the locus ceruleus containing either Lewy bodies or Alzheimer's tangles (which do not appear in increasing numbers of affected cells per case but rather as increasing percentages of cases affected), and (c) the number of neurons in the locus ceruleus containing Alzheimer's tangles and dementia (which begin at about 30 years of age).

2. The severity of parkinsonism generally correlates with the degree of neuronal loss in the substantia nigra. Those patients with Lewy bodies in either the substantia nigra or locus ceruleus have relatively clear thresholds for the development of progressively severe parkinsonism. However, those patients without Lewy bodies have lower and less well-defined thresholds for less severe parkinsonism and appear to be a heterogeneous mixture of diseases not yet satisfactorily defined as (a) those without Alzheimer's neurofibrillary tangles (and, therefore, especially poorly defined merely in negative terms) and (b) those with Alzheimer's tangles and either definitely postencephalitic (and "well understood") or not known to be postencephalitic. In this last group those cases over 80 years of age possibly are a variant of senile dementia with disproportionately more cortical degeneration and less degeneration of the substantia nigra.

3. All parkinsonians have more cortical degeneration and disproportionately more dementia than age-matched nonparkinsonian controls, but these differences are not proportionate to the degree or type of parkinsonism.

4. It would appear, therefore, that parkinsonism occurs in people with diffuse degenerative changes in the brain and that at least two major types can be distinguished: (a) "Lewy body disease," which is relatively stereotyped, in which the degree of parkinsonism is correlated with the degree of neuronal loss in the substantia nigra and the degree of dementia with the

degree of all cerebral cortical degenerations; and *(b)* "Alzheimer's tangle disease(s)," which include(s) postencephalitic cases and others, possibly a variant of senile dementia, in which the degree of cortical degeneration correlates with the dementia but the degree of neuronal loss in the substantia nigra correlates only with the more severe degrees of parkinsonism.

ACKNOWLEDGMENTS

The research reported in this chapter was supported in part by a training grant in neuropathology (5 T01 NS05231–15) from the National Institute of Neurological Diseases and Stroke, U.S. Public Health Service, and by the Veterans Administration Medical Research Program.

We are greatly indebted to Dr. William B. Hamlin, Director of Laboratories, Swedish Hospital and Medical Center, for providing facilities for the computer analysis of these cases.

REFERENCES

1. Forno, L. S., and Alvord, E. C., Jr., in: *Recent Advances in Parkinson's Disease*, p. 120. F. A. Davis Co., Philadelphia (1971).
2. Alvord, E. C., Jr., in: *Recent Advances in Parkinson's Disease*, p. 131. F. A. Davis Co., Philadelphia (1971).
3. Forno, L. S., *J. Amer. Geriat. Soc.* 17, 557 (1969).
4. Alvord, E. C., Jr., in: *Pathogenesis and Treatment of Parkinsonism*, p. 161. Charles C Thomas, Springfield, Ill. (1958).

Advances in Neurology, Vol. 5
Raven Press, New York © 1974

Depigmentation in the Nerve Cells of the Substantia Nigra and Locus Ceruleus in Parkinsonism

Lysia S. Forno and Ellsworth C. Alvord, Jr.

Laboratory Service, Palo Alto Veterans Administration Hospital and Department of Pathology (Neuropathology), Stanford University School of Medicine, Stanford, California 94304, and Department of Pathology (Neuropathology), University of Washington, Seattle, Washington 98104

Decrease of the normal dark pigmentation in the substantia nigra and locus ceruleus is a well-documented feature of parkinsonism. We have, until recently, regarded this as well explained by the loss of nerve cells in these nuclei. When the nerve cells die, the neuromelanin is set free and is phagocytized by microglial or histiocytic cells, and a certain amount of pigment is removed through the blood stream in the course of time. In cases of postencephalitic parkinsonism of long duration, very few nerve cells remain in the substantia nigra, and scanty fine pigment granules are left in the tissue.

Duffy and Tennyson's electron microscopic observations on neuro-melanin and Lewy bodies in idiopathic parkinsonism (1) first brought the possibility to our attention that changes in the neuromelanin pigment granule might take place within the nerve cell as part of the degenerative process. They described a decrease in the very dense particulate material in the pigment granule in many nerve cells in substantia nigra and locus ceruleus in brains from patients with parkinsonism.

Neuromelanin is probably related to the catecholamine formation in pigmented nerve cells, and it is therefore possible that an abnormality of catecholamine metabolism could manifest itself in the neuromelanin. It has also been suggested (1) that neuromelanin may participate in the formation of the Lewy inclusion. For these reasons we decided to have a closer look at the pigmentation of the nerve cells in the parkinsonism material from the Palo Alto Veterans Hospital and the University of Washington (2, 3). This is not a quantitative study; biochemical abnormalities not visible with the methods used cannot be ruled out; and the electron microscopic findings are preliminary.

We have separated our material into cases with Lewy bodies and cases with Alzheimer's neurofibrillary tangles in the substantia nigra and have included only cases with well-pronounced changes in the form of nerve cell loss, Lewy inclusions, and tangles. Electron microscopic examination was carried out on autopsy material, fixed in glutaraldehyde and prepared according to routine electron microscopic methods. The locus ceruleus was examined in this way in 24 cases. Five were parkinsonism cases of Lewy body type, two were of Alzheimer tangle type, and four had clinical symptomatology vaguely suggestive of parkinsonism but did not belong in the Lewy body or tangle category on pathological examination. The remaining 13 did not have parkinsonism, but some of them showed incidental neurofibrillary tangles in the locus ceruleus in paraffin sections.

RESULTS: PARAFFIN SECTIONS

In the cases of idiopathic parkinsonism with Lewy bodies, all cases showed similar findings. In contrast to the normally pigmented substantia nigra in nonparkinsonians (Fig. 1A), the nerve cells displayed unpigmented areas either in the form of pale, often rounded areas devoid of organelles or in the form of characteristic Lewy bodies (4) (Fig. 1B–E). Many nerve cells appeared swollen, especially the normally more rounded nerve cells in the locus ceruleus. Neuromelanin in the abnormal cells was often displaced to the periphery and appeared more scanty than usual. Where Lewy bodies were present, abundant neuromelanin at the periphery of the inclusion was the rule, but occasionally this pigment was sparse or absent (Fig. 1C). Unpigmented cells, not thought to belong to adjacent nonpigmented structures, were extremely rare in Lewy body parkinsonism. The small, unpigmented nerve cells which form a normal part of the locus ceruleus were easily distinguished from the larger cells.

The overall impression of these cases was that of normal pigmentation of the cells except for the focal areas. The depigmentation here appeared to be due to displacement of melanin, rather than depigmentation, although some reduction in pigment in certain cells could not be ruled out.

The cases with neurofibrillary tangles (with and without a history of encephalitis lethargica) showed much more convincing depigmentation of nerve cells, but only in cases with severe substantia nigra nerve cell loss (Fig. 2A), and not to any marked degree in the locus ceruleus, where nerve cell loss was less pronounced. Focal areas of depigmentation were rare, and when present were often associated with neurofibrillary tangle formation. The depigmentation noted was a diffuse scarcity of pigment as well as nerve cells without visible melanin pigment (Fig. 2C–F). Cells with neurofibrillary tangles had all gradations from relatively abundant melanin pigment over a reduced amount to complete absence of pigment (Fig. 2B–E). Extraneuronal melanin was more finely granular and of a lighter yellow color. With less nerve cell loss, the depigmentation became less convincing.

By comparison, our normal control material showed very rare focal unpigmented areas within nerve cells and equally rare unpigmented nerve cells.

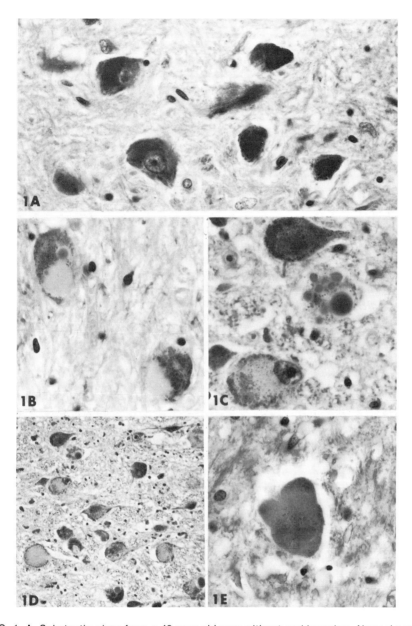

FIG. 1. A. Substantia nigra from a 49-year-old man without parkinsonism. Normal nerve cells. Hematoxylin-Eosin, ×550. B–E. Examples of nerve cell changes in substantia nigra and locus ceruleus in idiopathic parkinsonism with Lewy bodies. B. Lewy bodies and focal pale areas in nerve cells in the substantia nigra. Hematoxylin-Eosin, ×640. C. Nerve cell with numerous Lewy bodies and scant neuromelanin pigment. Locus ceruleus. Hematoxylin-Eosin, ×640. D. Locus ceruleus. Same case as Fig. 1C. Several Lewy bodies and varying amounts of neuromelanin pigment are present. Hematoxylin-Eosin, ×250. E. Locus ceruleus. Swollen nerve cell with faintly visible Lewy bodies surrounded by sparse neuromelanin granules. Hematoxylin-Eosin, ×640.

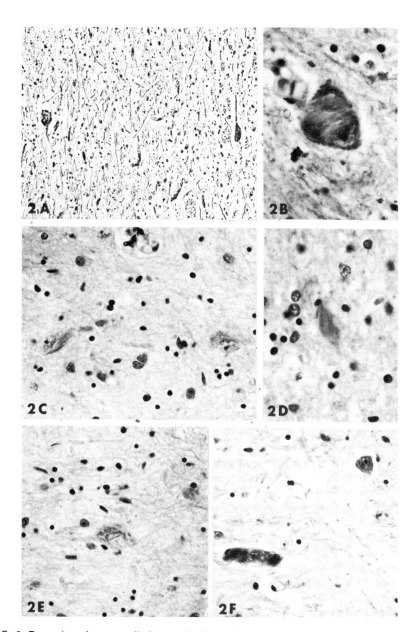

FIG. 2. Examples of nerve cell changes in the substantia nigra in cases of parkinsonism with neurofibrillary tangles. A. Substantia nigra. Few nerve cells remain. Silver, ×400. Seventy-year-old man with postencephalitic parkinsonism for 33 years. B. Neurofibrillary tangle and neuromelanin in nerve cell in the substantia nigra from 63-year-old man with parkinsonism for 9 years. No history of encephalitis. Hematoxylin-Eosin, ×640. C. Substantia nigra from 69-year-old man with postencephalitic parkinsonism. Two unpigmented nerve cells, one with a neurofibrillary tangle. Hematoxylin-Eosin, ×400. D. Substantia nigra from the same case as C. Neurofibrillary tangle. No melanin seen. Hematoxylin-Eosin, ×640. E. Substantia nigra from same case as C and D. Nerve cell with minute neuromelanin pigment. Hematoxylin-Eosin, ×640. F. Substantia nigra from same case as Fig. 2B. One unpigmented and one normally pigmented nerve cell. Hematoxylin-Eosin, ×400.

ELECTRON MICROSCOPIC OBSERVATIONS

Neuromelanin was easily demonstrated as lobulated, membrane-bound structures with lipid globules, a medium-dense granular matrix, and coarse patches of extremely dense material. The dense material represents the melanin portion of the complex, while the other two components resemble lipofuscin (1, 5, 6) (Figs. 3 and 4). The majority of melanin granules in the locus ceruleus, from parkinsonism material as well as from controls, had a large dense component, but in all cases some neurons had lesser amounts of the dense material, and this variation could also be found within the cytoplasm of individual nerve cells. Figures 3 and 4 show such variations at lower and higher magnifications, in association with Lewy bodies or twisted neurotubules and in normal controls. In Fig. 4E, a macrophage with ingested neuromelanin is seen.

COMMENT

We have reached no definite conclusion, and it is still possible that the nerve cell loss is the only cause of depigmentation in the substantia nigra and locus ceruleus in parkinsonism. Loss of pigment in individual nerve cells is most convincing in parkinsonism of long duration with neurofibrillary tangles in the substantia nigra. But there is the possibility that unpigmented nerve cells from neighboring structures, especially from the reticular zone of the substantia nigra, could be mistaken for compact zone nerve cells in the shrunken, gliotic tissue. Electron microscopy was of no help here, since it was done on the less involved locus ceruleus and in only two cases of the neurofibrillary tangle type. In the Lewy body cases, we could not confirm Duffy and Tennyson's findings of a decrease in the dense component of the melanin granule. We attribute any apparent decrease to normal variations in the dense particulate material. The wide normal variation is also suggested by our own observations in the sympathetic ganglia, where the dense patches tend to be quite small and discrete.

A crucial question is whether neuromelanin is capable of degradation *in vivo* once it is formed. Melanins in general are well known for their insolubility and resistance to enzymes. But there are reports (7, 8) that melanosomes may be broken down by lysosomes within melanocytes. In Chediak-Higashi syndrome (7), the abnormal giant melanosomes degenerate at a certain stage of development, beginning in the protein matrix. Numerous vacuolated areas are formed, and much of the osmiophilia disappears. In nerve cells, the neuromelanin may form a part of a residual lysosomal body (9). More complex vacuolated pigment bodies have been described with age (5), but we know of no other details concerning neuromelanin degradation. An abnormal neuromelanin formation in parkinsonism rather than an alteration in previously normal melanin should also be considered, and might be associated with the formation of the Lewy inclusion.

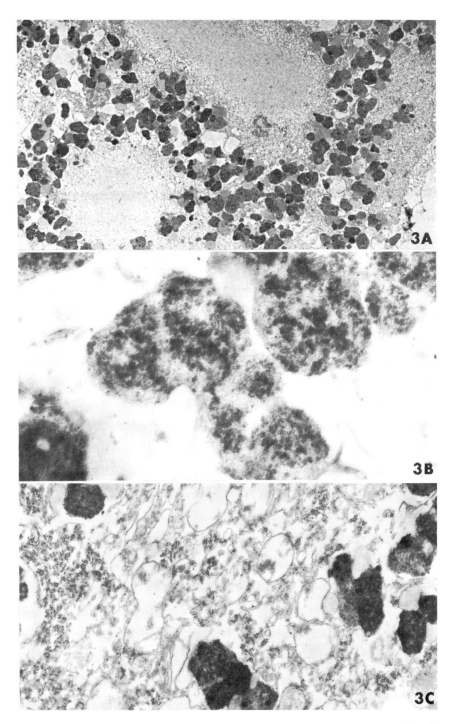

FIG. 3. A. Locus ceruleus from 82-year-old man with idiopathic parkinsonism. Two fila-
mentous Lewy bodies with amorphous to faintly granular core are seen surrounded by
neuromelanin granules. No membrane separates the Lewy inclusion from the neuromelanin. Electron micrograph ×2400. B. Neuromelanin granules in the locus ceruleus from a
61-year-old man with slight parkinsonism of less than 1 year duration. Lewy bodies were
present only in the sympathetic ganglia. Electron micrograph ×22,500. C. Neuromelanin
in nerve cell in the locus ceruleus from a 54-year-old man with diabetes and myocardial
infarction. No clinical parkinsonism. Electron micrograph ×10,500.

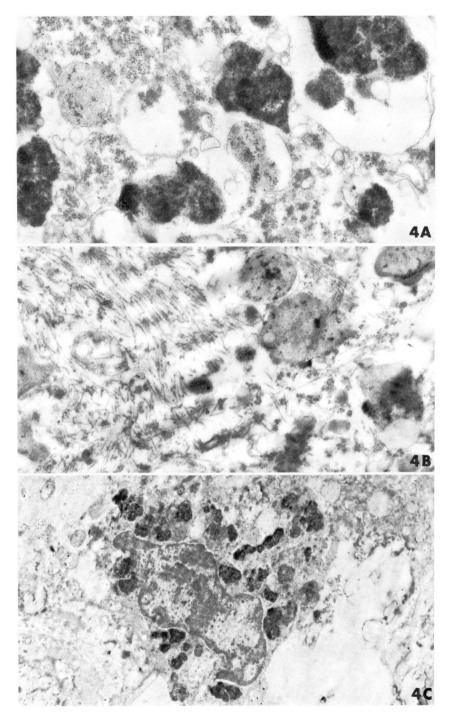

FIG. 4. A. Neuromelanin in nerve cell in the locus ceruleus from a 63-year-old man with Alzheimer tangles type parkinsonism (same case as Fig. 2B and F). Electron micrograph ×10,500. B. Twisted neurotubules and neuromelanin granules in the cytoplasm of a nerve cell in the locus ceruleus. Sixty-four-year old nonparkinsonian with incidental neuro-fibrillary tangles. Electron micrograph ×3690. C. Macrophage with ingested neuromelanin in the locus ceruleus from a 102-year-old black male with vascular disease. No definite parkinsonism. Electron micrograph ×3300.

Further studies of neuromelanin and of Lewy body formation in both pigmented and unpigmented nerve cells, for example in the sympathetic ganglia (10) and in the innominate substance and dorsal motor vagus nucleus, may give us clues to the part played by the neuromelanin in the nerve cell degeneration in parkinsonism.

ACKNOWLEDGMENTS

This work was supported by the Veterans Administration Medical Research Program.

REFERENCES

1. Duffy, P. E., and Tennyson, V. M., *J. Neuropathol. Exp. Neurol.* 24, 398 (1965).
2. Forno, L. S., and Alvord, E. C., in: *Recent Advances in Parkinsonism,* F. A. Davis, Philadelphia, 1971, p. 120.
3. Alvord, E. C. et al., in: *This Volume.*
4. Greenfield, J. G., and Bosanquet, F. D., *J. Neurol. Neurosurg. Psychiat.* 16, 213 (1953).
5. Moses, H. L., Ganote, C. E., Beaver, D. L., and Schuffman, S. S., *Anat. Rec.* 155, 167 (1966).
6. Hirosawa, K., *Zeitschr. f. Zellforschung* 88, 187 (1968).
7. Zelickson, A. S., Windhorst, D. B., White, J. G., and Good, R. A., *J. Invest. Dermatol.* 49, 575 (1967).
8. Zelickson, A. S., Mottaz, J., and Hunter, J. A., in: *Pigmentation: Its Genesis and Biologic Control,* Appleton-Century-Crofts, New York, 1972, p. 445.
9. Barden, H., *J. Neuropathol. Exp. Neurol.* 28, 419 (1969).
10. Forno, L. S., *J. Neuropathol. Exp. Neurol.* 32, 159 (1973) (abstract).

Advances in Neurology, Vol. 5
Raven Press, New York © 1974

Corpus Striatum in Paralysis Agitans and in Perphenazine-Injected Rats

H. Pakkenberg and J. Bøttcher

Department of Neurology, Kommunehospitalet, DK 1399 Copenhagen K, Denmark

It is generally agreed that there is a loss of nerve cells in the substantia nigra in parkinsonism (1, 2, 3). Denny-Brown (4) studied the globus pallidus, in particular, and found demyelinization and abnormal vessels. Pakkenberg (5) found a normal cell count in this nucleus, although there were changes in the RNA content in the cells. On the other hand, descriptions of the neostriatum are scanty, and contain only vague general information with no attempts at quantification (6, 7, 8). Using pneumoencephalography, Selby (9) found cortical atrophy in 57% and dilatation of the ventricles in 30% of 250 brains from parkinsonian patients.

Harman and Carpenter (10) made direct determinations of the volume of the basal ganglia in one normal human brain, and found a volume of 13.93 cm³. Von Bonin and Shariff (11) found a volume of 11.89 cm³ in one normal human brain.

DETERMINATION OF THE VOLUME OF STRIATUM

The volume determinations described here were made by Dr. J. Bøttcher. The volume of globus pallidus, putamen, and nucleus caudatus was determined in eight brains from human subjects aged from 53 to 79 years (mean 68.5 years) dying suddenly from coronary thrombosis or as a result of accident without head trauma and in nine brains from patients with paralysis agitans, aged 67 to 85 years (mean 74.8 years). The latter brains constitute those parkinsonian brains submitted consecutively to the laboratory of neuropathology of the Kommunehospital during a period of approximately 2 years. The control brains, which were obtained from the Institute of Forensic Medicine of the University of Copenhagen, were only selected with regard to cause of death and age.

Following fixation in formalin, each brain was cut into slices 5 mm thick in a specially constructed cutting apparatus, and each section was then photographed. The thickness of the brain slice was determined. The blocks were embedded in paraffin, cut into sections 12 to 15 μ in thickness, and the area of the basal ganglia mentioned above determined by projection and

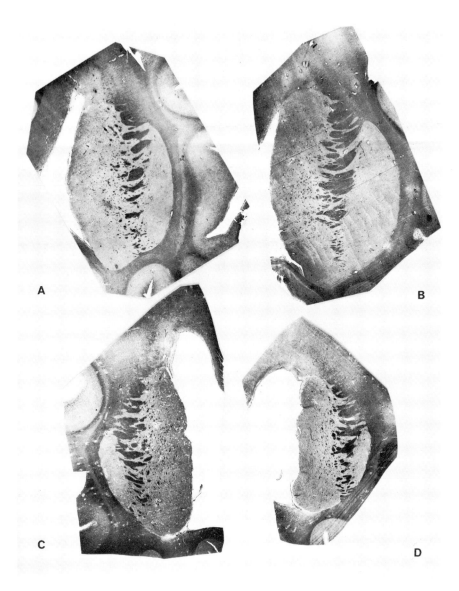

FIG. 1. Selected examples of slides from two control brains *(top)* and two parkinsonian brains *(bottom)*.

planimetry. A correction was made for shrinkage by correlating fixed lines in the photograph and the histological preparation. The volume was calculated for each slice using the formula for a truncated cone, and the results added. Thus, it is the volume of the fixed brain which is determined, but as the difference in weight between the unfixed and the formalin-fixed brain is only 40 g on the average, the volume obtained will be very close to the value for the unfixed brain. The shrinkage was equal in the control and the parkinsonian group.

Figure 1 shows that the ventricles are enlarged in the parkinsonian brains represented. This accords with the experience gained by neurosurgeons in stereotaxic intervention. It is of course not possible to know whether this enlargement of the ventricular system is due to atrophy of striatum or of other parts of the hemisphere. Table 1 shows that there is no reduction in the three regions of the striatum in the parkinsonian brains.

In order to obtain more precise information on the nervous elements of the striatum, a count of the nerve cells has been instituted (by Dr. Bøttcher). Unfortunately, it is not possible to differentiate biochemically between the various types of nerve cell before the count, but only to group the cell population according to size.

STRIATUM IN RAT BRAINS

It is well known that it is possible to cause selective destruction of adrenergic nerve endings in rat brain by means of 6-hydroxy-dopamine (12).

TABLE 1. *Volume of the three parts of striatum (in arbitrary units) in nine paralysis agitans brains and eight control brains*

Parkinsonian patients								
	Right				Left			
Age	Caud.	Putam.	Pall.	Total	Caud.	Putam.	Pall.	Total
72	5.71	6.65	1.67	14.03	4.46	6.09	1.55	12.10
67	5.32	5.63	1.33	12.28	4.91	6.30	1.53	12.74
83	3.62	4.50	1.23	9.35	3.89	4.99	1.61	10.49
77	4.14	5.09	1.50	10.73	4.34	5.68	1.72	11.74
78	4.24	5.97	1.23	11.44	3.00	3.78	0.92	7.70
71	2.38	3.54	1.11	7.03	2.91	3.68	1.26	7.85
70	3.97	5.50	1.77	11.24	3.55	5.25	1.58	10.38
85	3.54	5.75	1.24	10.53	3.04	5.20	1.39	9.63
71	5.56	6.25	1.51	13.32	3.91	5.48	1.42	10.81
Mean: 74.9 years				11.10				10.38
Control patients								
	Right				Left			
Age	Caud.	Putam.	Pall.	Total	Caud.	Putam.	Pall.	Total
70	3.81	5.43	1.43	10.69	3.86	5.95	1.52	11.35
64	3.28	4.53	0.95	8.77	2.51	4.48	0.86	7.86
69	3.61	6.52	1.57	11.70	3.12	6.77	1.69	11.59
53	3.85	4.86	1.25	9.97	4.91	7.06	1.77	11.98
78	3.57	4.49	1.28	9.35	3.30	4.62	1.19	9.13
65	4.78	6.73	1.43	12.96	4.99	6.05	1.43	12.49
79	3.80	5.93	1.48	11.21	4.02	4.52	1.33	9.88
70	4.18	5.15	1.61	10.95	4.18	4.84	1.53	10.56
Mean: 68.5 years				10.70				10.60

However, it is also possible to produce a loss of nerve cells in the striatum in rats by means of other drugs (13). We injected perphenazine enanthate every second week for a year into rats in a dose of the same order of magnitude as that administered to human subjects (3.4 mg/kg rat/injection). The nerve cells were then counted both in the cortex and in the basal ganglia. The basal ganglia count was 20% lower in the perphenazine-injected animals than in the controls ($p < 0.005$). The cortex counts were the same in both groups. We are unable to decide whether there is a particular type of nerve cell which is particularly sensitive to perphenazine. A number of the animals were given injections of ^{3}H-uridine or ^{3}H-lysine and sacrificed after 1 hr. Microautoradiography demonstrated that labeling of the cortical cells in the treated animals was slightly greater than in the controls. In the basal ganglia, the results were the reverse in the case of uridine. None of these differences was significant.

In a further series of experiments we examined how amphetamine-induced stereotyped behavior is influenced by quaternary chlorpromazine injected into the corpus striatum (14). The stereotypies are inhibited. The same is the case if quaternary neuroleptic drugs of the butyrophenone type are injected intrastriatally (15). Injection of p-hydroxy-amphetamine or dopamine into the corpus striatum gave rise to a stereotyped hyperactive behavior, similar to that seen after subcutaneous injection of amphetamine (16). Bilateral lesions (30 to 90%) of corpus striatum inhibited the stereotyped behavior in rats injected subcutaneously with amphetamine (17). We conclude from these and other observations that the action of amphetamine in the brain is mediated through dopaminergic mechanisms in corpus striatum.

REFERENCES

1. Greenfield, G., and Bosanquet, F., J. Neurol. Neurosurg. Psychiat. 16, 213 (1953).
2. Hassler, R., J. Psychol. Neurol. 48, 387 (1938).
3. Klaue, R., Arch. Psychiat. Nervenkrankh. 111, 251 (1940).
4. Denny-Brown, D., in: The Basal Ganglia and Their Relation to Disorders of Movement. Oxford Univ. Press, London (1962).
5. Pakkenberg, H., Acta Neurol. Scand. Suppl. 4, 39, 139 (1963).
6. Lewy, F., Dtsch. Z. Nervenheilk. 50, 50 (1914).
7. Keschner, M., and Sloane, P., Arch. Neurol. Psychiat. 25, 1011 (1931).
8. Bielschowsky, M., J. Psychol. Neurol. 25, 1 (1920).
9. Selby, G., J. Neur. Sci. 6, 517 (1968).
10. Harman, R., and Carpenter, M., J. Comp. Neurol. 93, 125 (1950).
11. von Bonin, G., and Shariff, G., J. Comp. Neurol. 94, 427 (1951).
12. Hedreen, J., and Chalmers, J., Brain Res. 47, 1 (1972).
13. Pakkenberg, H., Fog, R., and Nilakantan, B., Psychopharmacologia 29, 329 (1973).
14. Fog, R., Randrup, A., and Pakkenberg, H., Psychopharmacologia 12, 428 (1968).
15. Fog, R., Randrup, A., and Pakkenberg, H., Psychopharmacologia 19, 224 (1971).
16. Fog, R., and Pakkenberg, H., Exper. Neur. 31, 75 (1971).
17. Fog, R., Randrup, A., and Pakkenberg, H., Psychopharmacologia 18, 346 (1970).

DISCUSSION

Dr. Barbeau: I would like to ask if anyone could give us some data on pathologic changes in the other pigmented areas of the brain. The dorsal nucleus of the vagus is well known, but we also need to know about the other areas of the brain in Parkinson's disease that have dopamine normally. I am thinking of the median eminence and the hippocampus. These areas should be carefully looked at for cell changes. Dr. Forno, do you have any data on these parts of the brain?

Dr. Forno: As part of our study, the changes that were described there were mainly the senile plaques and granulovacuolar degeneration. We had a few cases that had Lewy bodies in these areas when there were Lewy bodies elsewhere. We have not studied the median eminence that systematically, but we have sometimes looked at the hippocampal and septal areas. These areas also have Lewy bodies when they are extensive in the other cases.

Dr. Barbeau: Dr. Forno, did you also look at the sympathetic ganglia?

Dr. Forno: I have not looked at them in all cases, but I have looked at a number of sympathetic ganglia. Seventy percent of the sympathetic ganglia that I have examined when there were Lewy bodies elsewhere would have Lewy bodies of a peculiar sausage shape in the sympathetic ganglia. The electron microscopic features of these are somewhat different. We observed a granular vesicular body that looks as if it could be composed of degenerating and dense core vesicles. This is a very intriguing finding for me. I have not yet been able to find out quite how this kind of Lewy body relates to the other Lewy bodies.

Dr. Barbeau: I think it is very important to decide whether this is a generalized or a specific nigral disease we're talking about.

Are there other questions?

Dr. Roberts: About a year or so ago I saw a very interesting paper by Isidoriedes Redes from Athens, in which he did a series of studies of people who had parkinsonian symptoms of different severity and duration. He looked at the brains both with the light and the electron microscope. He inferred that there were normally very close contacts between the capillaries in the substantia nigra and the nigral cells. Even before there was degeneration of the cells, there was the beginning of the separation of this close contact with glial end feet coming in there, and the thought was that maybe all the degeneration was secondary to a disruption of the normal contacts or of the normal relations between the vasculature and the particular susceptible cells in that region.

Secondly, Frank Dixon and Mike Oldstone of La Jolla have recently been finding deposition of viral antigen-antibody complexes in blood vessels, particularly in the choroid plexus. In one case in the mouse hippocampus these were similar to the degenerations seen with glomerulonephritis. One of the possibilities suggested from this is that the lesion in the blood vessels might be related to these antigen-antibody complexes which settle on the endothelial cells and affect them primarily. I wonder if this kind of change I have mentioned has any relationship to the consequent pathology that you might be seeing.

Dr. Forno: I'd like to comment on the paper by Redes. If it is the one that I recall, it was not an electron microscopic study but a histochemical one. I felt that it was very difficult from that kind of material with so much shrinkage to be really sure that there were valid observations. But electron microscopy in autopsy material would have the same difficulties.

Dr. Fahn: I wonder if any of the three speakers can tell us if there are regional differences within the substantia nigra in the pathologic changes seen in Parkinson's disease and in the perphenazine-treated rat. In other words, is there a regional difference in the zona compacta or recticulata?

Dr. Pakkenberg: We counted the cells in the substantia nigra years ago, but since we counted the two parts of the substantia nigra together, I cannot give you an exact answer.

Dr. Van Woert: Are there any changes in the drug-induced Parkinson's disease? I know there are two papers now describing a degeneration of nigral cells in drug-induced parkinsonism.

Dr. Forno: I've not been impressed by these reports; in fact, when I examined a case with parkinsonian symptoms and there was no change in the substantia nigra or locus ceruleus, then I was more willing to accept it as a true drug-induced parkinsonism.

Dr. Boshes: Dr. Alvord and Dr. Forno have presented a large number of data, which gives you an idea of the enormity of the problem. However, I have some difficulty understanding some of the collation of the data. If they held rigidly to neuropathological correlations, I would have no problem, but the moment one begins to correlate this with a term such as dementia, then we have real problems. If the term *dementia* is used to indicate senile or presenile dementia as neuropathological entities, I see no problem. The moment you began to correlate that with the term clinical dementia, then we're in trouble. Clinical dementia is too broad a term, and is too uncritically used. We cannot correlate exquisite staining of neurofibrillary tangles, Lewy bodies, the various types of macrophages, degeneration of the neuronal elements with a word dementia. In the group of patients who died demented, we have seen many types of memory changes. Memory changes may be, for example, problems of short-term memory storage, memory retrieval, long-term memory, ancient memory, recent memory, and so on. These are different processes. Some memory changes occur with hippocampal lesions, some with mamillotemporal lesions, and some are combination lesions of the cortex. The brain of an old person is certainly different from the brain of a young person in terms of memory implantation and memory processing. As we have watched the large series of patients on L-DOPA and compared them to those not on L-DOPA, we find two types of memory changes. In some the L-DOPA seems to decompensate the brain, and we see a severe, dementing, organic decompensation. Others are not affected. In others, the process seems to stimulate the brain to higher functions, at least as seen by measurable tests. Intellectual functions are better, but they are not better uniformly; they are better in a cognitive sphere. Some patients, however, at the end of 3 years, begin to slip in the affective sphere; they become disinterested and depressed. We then see some changes which make the patient appear demented. Actually if you were to test him for cognitive function you might find him nearly normal, although affectively he may be functioning poorly. I would caution using correlations between neuroanatomical substrates and clinical phenomena such as dementia.

Dr. Barbeau: I think your point is well taken, Dr. Boshes. Dr. Cotzias, do you have a question?

Dr. Cotzias: Just a very quick technical point. Melanins are dense to visible light because they are black, but they are dense to electrons because they have a lot of metal in them. One is never going to see a resolution in melanin granules unless the metal is removed with chelating agents.

Advances in Neurology, Vol. 5
Raven Press, New York © 1974

Neuromelanin

Aaron B. Lerner

Department of Dermatology, Yale University School of Medicine, New Haven, Connecticut 06510

Melanin in skin, hair, and eyes is derived from the oxidation of DOPA, an *ortho*-dihydroxyphenyl compound. But the term melanin should have a more general meaning. Most aromatic organic compounds with hydroxyl and/or amino groups *ortho* or *para* to each other can be oxidized and polymerized to colored substances (Figs. 1 and 2). The structures of melanin pigments are difficult to determine because the molecules are usually insoluble as well as complicated. Examples of melanins other than those from DOPA are the black hair dye obtained from the oxidation of *para*-phenylenediamine, and the pigment in the large bowel in melanosis coli resulting from the oxidation of emodin present in cascara used as a laxative by the patient. The color of red hair in man and animals is a melanin that results from DOPA first combining with cysteine to form 5-S-cysteine-DOPA, and then the oxidation and polymerization of this substance to the red pigment (Fig. 3). In describing a melanin, one should specify the tissue that is under consideration as well as the name of the initial compound from which the pigment was derived. Thus, we could speak of skin melanin obtained from 5-S-cysteine-DOPA, melanin dye from *para*-phenylenediamine, and so on. The term neuromelanin was introduced by Lillie (1, 2) to identify brown-to-black, intracytoplasmic granules found in parts of the nervous system. The term is a useful one. It is generally assumed that this melanin is derived from dopamine, adrenaline, and/or noradrenaline. There may be more than one neuromelanin in various parts of the nervous system, and some day it may be possible to specify the compound from which it comes.

Using their own modification of the silver reaction of Lillie (1, 2), Cole-

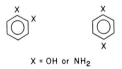

X = OH or NH₂

FIG. 1. The oxidation and polymerization of mono or polycyclic carbon or heterocyclic aromatic compounds with hydroxyl and/or amino groups ortho or para to each other give rise to melanins. The melanin of skin, hair, and eyes is derived from DOPA after it is converted to DOPA quinone. Neuromelanin may come from DOPA after it forms dopamine.

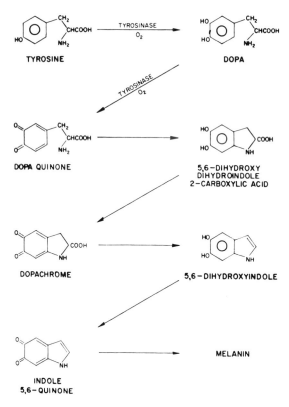

FIG. 2. Steps in the oxidation of tyrosine to melanin by oxygen and tyrosinase in melanocytes. One of the final products (Fig. 3) is an irregular polymer made up to a large extent
of groups of six units of the three quinones, viz., DOPA quinone, three molecules; indole-
5,6-quinone, two molecules; and dopachrome, one molecule.

man and Fenichel (3, 4) studied the location of melanin in the brainstem of
children and adults. They not only pinpointed tracts of melanin granules in
parts of the nervous system, but they also determined the age at which the
pigment appears. In all instances, pigmentation increased with age. This
characteristic also occurs where other kinds of melanin are produced; for
example, eye color, as well as skin and hair color, slowly but definitely
darkens with age, and the darkening continues throughout life. Hair becomes
white not only because there is less tyrosinase, but also because melanocytes
disappear from hair bulbs.

Melanin in the central nervous system does not come from DOPA in
melanocytes. If melanocytes were present, there would be examples of
melanomas originating from the nervous system. The only place melanomas
appear in the nervous system is in the leptomeninges.

The chemical structure is not known in detail of any melanin. Biological

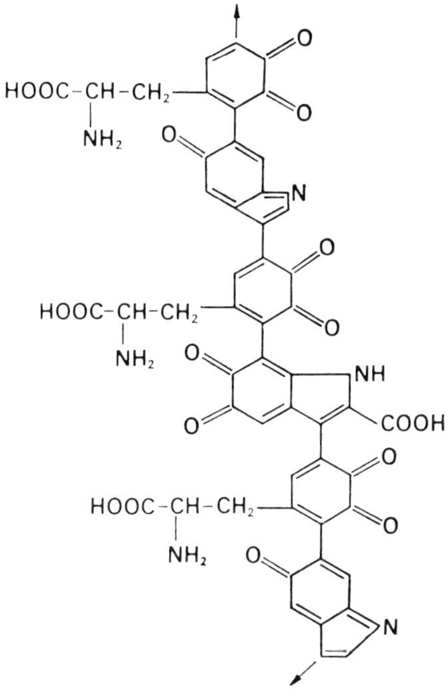

FIG. 3. Melanoma melanin according to Hempel.

polymers are usually considered as being made up of subunits in a definite sequence; for example, proteins, peptides, glycogen, DNA, and RNA all have definite sequences. Melanin polymers, however, are irregular, and the final product need not be the same as that produced in an adjacent position (5–7). The careful and detailed analytical approach by Nicolaus and his co-workers (8) on a study of degradative products from melanin, the labeling experiments by Swan (9) and his associates, and the labeling experiments of Hempel (10) have shown that melanin is not a regular polymer (Fig. 4). The techniques used by these investigators should be applied to a study of neuro-melanins to determine the compounds of origin. The melanins are probably

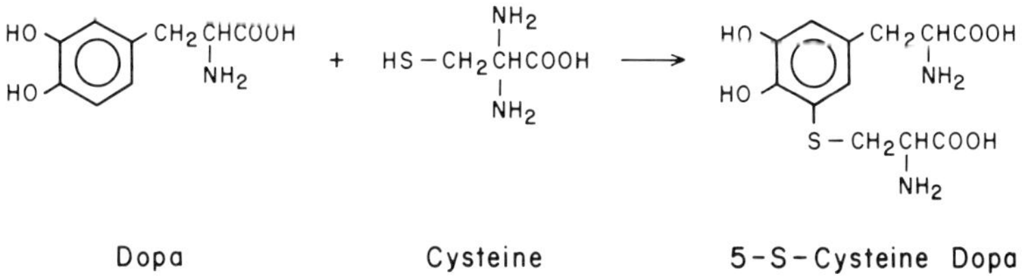

Dopa Cysteine 5-S-Cysteine Dopa

FIG. 4. The pigment of red hair is probably a melanin obtained from the oxidation and polymerization of 5-S-cysteine-DOPA that forms from DOPA reacting with cysteine in melanocytes.

amenable to analysis with a mass spectrograph after the pigment has been degraded by physical means.

The importance of melanin as a marker for the presence of the metabolism of DOPA and dopamine derivatives must be studied further.

REFERENCES

1. Lillie, R. D., *J. Histochem. Cytochem.* 3, 453 (1955).
2. Lillie, R. D., *J. Histochem. Cytochem.* 5, 325 (1957).
3. Coleman (Bazelon), M., and Fenichel, G. M., *Neurology* 17, 512 (1967).
4. Fenichel, G. M., and Coleman (Bazelon), M., *Neurology* 18, 817 (1968).
5. Mason, H. S., in: *Advances in Biology of Skin, Vol. VIII: The Pigmentary System,* edited by W. Montagna and F. Hu, Pergamon Press, New York, 1967, p. 293.
6. Nicolaus, R. A., Hempel, K., and Mason, H. S. Comments on Howard S. Mason's Paper, p. 313 (ref. 5).
7. Blois, M. S., A Note on the Problem of Melanin Structure, p. 319 (ref. 5).
8. Nicolaus, R. A., *Melanins,* Hermann, Paris, 1968.
9. Swan, G. A., *Ann. N.Y. Acad. Sci.* 100, 1005 (1963).
10. Hempel, K., in: *The Biologic Effects of Ultraviolet Radiation,* edited by Frederick Urbach, Pergamon Press, New York, 1969, p. 305.

Advances in Neurology, Vol. 5
Raven Press, New York © 1974

Biochemistry of Neuromelanin

Melvin H. Van Woert and Lalit M. Ambani

*Departments of Internal Medicine and Pharmacology, Yale University School of Medicine,
New Haven, Connecticut 06510*

Much less is known about the structure, synthesis, and function of the melanin present in the neurons of the central nervous system than the melanin found in the skin. However, the differences as well as similarities between neuromelanin and skin melanin may be relevant to the function of the extrapyramidal system. In this chapter we have summarized the present state of our knowledge of the biochemistry of brain melanin and attempted to relate this information to the degenerative changes in the substantia nigra pigmented cells which occur in Parkinson's disease.

STRUCTURE OF NEUROMELANIN

Electron Microscopy

Duffy and Tennyson (1) and Moses et al. (2) have described the structural similarities of the neuronal melanin granule to lipofuscin whereas d'Agnostino and Luse (3) stress the structural similarities between neuronal and cutaneous melanin granules. Neuromelanin, lipofuscin, and cutaneous melanin granules all have certain similarities, such as the presence of the polymer melanin (4) and acid phosphatase activity (5–7). Lysosomes are known to be particularly rich in acid phosphatase (8), and there is increasing evidence to suggest that lipofuscin is formed within lysosomes (9–11). Because of certain similarities in their fine structure and their acid phosphatase activities, the neuronal melanin granule, the cutaneous melanin granule, and the lipofuscin granule might all be derived from altered lysosomes. The quantity of melanin in each organelle and the ultrastructural details of each of these pigment granules are different and are summarized in Table 1. The cutaneous melanin granule contains a large quantity of high electron-dense melanin which eventually completely fills the particle (12). There is no visible lipid component in the cutaneous melanin granule. The neuromelanin granule contains both high and low electron-dense melanin fractions and a small lipid globule (1, 2). The lipofuscin granule consists of a large lipid fraction with only a small, low electron-dense component (1, 6). The degree of electron density may depend on both the intensity of melanization and

TABLE 1.

Property (refs.)	Neuromelanin granule	Cutaneous melanin granule	Lipofuscin granule
Ultrastructure (1, 2, 5, 6, 7, 12)	Acid phosphatase Small lipid globule High and low electron density melanin	Acid phosphatase No lipid globule High electron density melanin	Acid phosphatase Large lipid globule Low electron density melanin
Histochemistry (13–18)	Lipid stains − PAS − Acid fast − H_2O_2 + $AgNO_3$ + Thionine − yellow Pyrroles − Nile blue − green	Lipid stains − PAS − Acid fast − H_2O_2 + $AgNO_3$ ++ Thionine − green Pyrroles +	Lipid stains + PAS + Acid fast + H_2O_2 − $AgNO_3$ − Nile blue − blue
UV fluorescence (4)	−	−	+

the amount of metals (e.g., copper) chelated to the melanin in each organelle.

The major ultrastructural difference between the three pigment granules appears to be due to a varying ratio of melanin to lipid in each organelle.

Histochemical Reactions

Table 1 also summarizes the histochemical similarities and differences between neuronal melanin, cutaneous melanin and lipofuscin. Histochemically, lipofuscin is characterized by positive lipid stains, PAS staining, and acid fast staining with carbol fuschin; neuronal and cutaneous melanin granules do not react with these stains (13, 14). Neuronal and cutaneous melanins are bleached with hydrogen peroxide; lipofuscin is not (15). The large lipid component of lipofuscin gives the granule its distinctive histochemistry and may obscure staining reactions with its smaller melanin component. Neuronal melanin is histochemically different from cutaneous melanin in its reactivity to thionine, silver nitrate, and the p-dimethylamino-benzaldehyde reaction for pyrroles (15–18).

Only lipofuscin fluoresces when activated at a wavelength of 365 nm (4), and this is due to the presence of peroxidized polyunsaturated lipids (19). If the lipid fraction is removed from the lipofuscin granule by chloroform–methanol (2:1, v/v) extraction, the residual brown pigment granule does not fluoresce when exposed to ultraviolet light (4).

The histochemical data suggest that neuromelanin has a slightly different chemical structure than cutaneous melanin. The large lipid component of lipofuscin, observed by electron microscopy, is confirmed by histochemical techniques. It would be of interest to determine if the substantia nigra neurons have less oxidizable lipid or a greater lipase activity than cells where lipofuscin is readily synthesized; this might explain the greater melanin to lipid ratio in the substantia nigra granules as compared to the lipofuscin granule.

Spectroscopy

Figure 1 summarizes the spectroscopic properties of melanin isolated from human substantia nigra melanin granules, melanin granules from an amphibian *(Amphiuma)*, and human cardiac lipofuscin granules (4). In the substantia nigra, neuromelanin granules were separated from lipofuscin granules by density-gradient sucrose solution; lipofuscin has a low density due to its large lipid component and neuromelanin a greater density because of its large quantity of melanin. The melanin was purified by solvent extraction of lipids and acid digestion of protein as previously described (4). Nonpigmented fetal heart, liver, and cerebral tissue, when treated to the same digestive and extraction procedures, did not yield any pigment (20). Melanin has a stable free radical which can be measured by electron paramagnetic resonance (EPR) spectroscopy. EPR spectroscopy is of use in identifying melanins since other isolated biological compounds do not have similar spectra. As seen in Fig. 1, the melanin isolated from all three granules had similar EPR spectra. All these pigments have G values of 2.005 and react to light exposure by an increase in intensity of their signal, which is characteristic of melanins.

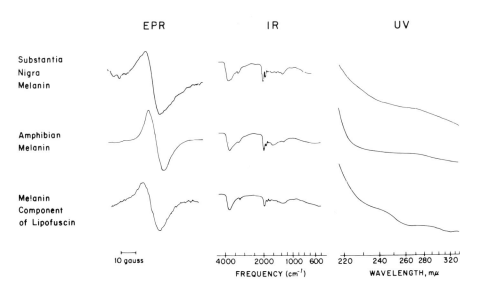

FIG. 1. EPR, IR, and UV spectroscopic comparisons of melanins from substantia nigra, an amphibian, and lipofuscin.

The infrared (IR) spectra were also similar in the melanins isolated from the three different pigment granules (Fig. 1). Mikulski (21) and Maeda and Wegmann (22) also observed that substantia nigra melanin had EPR and IR spectra similar to those of known melanins. The ultraviolet (UV) absorption spectra of all these melanins were similar, but there were no specific absorption peaks (Fig. 1). It is of interest that melanins from mouse melanoma and melanins prepared *in vitro* from L-DOPA, dopamine, and norepinephrine also have similar EPR, IR, and UV spectra (4, 20). Similar spectroscopic studies have been used to identify melanins in the liver of patients with Dubin Johnson's syndrome (23) and in the liver of mutant Corriedale sheep (24) and Howler monkey (25, 26). We have recently isolated and quantified the melanin pigment present in normal human liver and cardiac tissue; the concentrations vary from 0 to 90 mg/100 g wet weight (27). A liver with brown atrophy contained 210 mg of melanin/100 g wet weight which was consistent with the marked increase in lipofuscin granules observed histochemically, suggesting that the isolated melanin was derived from lipofuscin granules.

POSSIBLE SYNTHETIC PATHWAYS FOR NEUROMELANIN

The mechanism by which the substantia nigra melanin pigment decreases and the pigmented neurons eventually degenerate in Parkinson's disease is not known. Identification of the enzyme and substrates involved in the synthesis of neuromelanin might provide clues to the etiology of Parkinson's disease.

Substantia nigra pigment has sufficient spectroscopic and histochemical similarities to be classified as a melanin. Nevertheless, the ultrastructural and histochemical differences between neuromelanin and cutaneous melanin suggest that they may differ chemically and therefore may be synthesized from different substrates by different enzymes. Although the synthesis of cutaneous melanin has been established in detail, virtually nothing is known about the mechanism of neuromelanin synthesis. Numerous investigators (28–30) have suggested that dopamine is a substrate for neuromelanin since the substantia nigra contains many dopamine-rich neurons (31), and this catecholamine is easily oxidized to form melanin both by auto-oxidation and by several different enzymes. Vander Wende and Spoerlein (28) demonstrated that dopamine could be oxidized to a melanin by rat brain *in vitro*. Furthermore, Bazelon et al. (32) found that the distribution of neuromelanin-containing and catecholamine-containing cell bodies was almost identical in the major areas of the human brain. Neuromelanin and dopamine are found together in the substantia nigra and brainstem reticular formation (33, 34). Neuromelanin and norepinephrine are found together in the locus ceruleus, area postrema, and the dorsal nucleus of the vagus. Enzymes which oxidize phenolic and catechol compounds to form melanin *in vitro* will be considered as to their possible role in the synthesis of neuromelanin.

Tyrosinase

In melanocytes derived from neural crest cells (skin, eyes, and meningeal melanocytes), the enzyme tyrosinase oxidizes tyrosine and DOPA to form melanin. However, we (20), as well as other investigators (35), have been unable to find any tyrosinase activity in the human substantia nigra. The hydroxylation of tyrosine to DOPA in brain is catalyzed by the enzyme tyrosine hydroxylase which is biochemically very different from tyrosinase and does not synthesize melanin (36). Further evidence indicating that tyrosinase does not catalyze neuromelanin synthesis was provided by Foley and Baxter (37) who observed that human albinos, who have deficient tyrosinase activity, have normally pigmented substantia nigra.

Monoamine Oxidase

Monoamine oxidase oxidatively deaminates various catecholamines and indoleamines to their respective aldehydes which can polymerize and form melanins *in vitro* (30). Dopamine forms a dark brown melanin pigment, and norepinephrine and epinephrine form lighter brown melanin pigments in the presence of rat brain mitochondrial preparations containing monoamine oxidase. The addition of a monoamine oxidase inhibitor will prevent melanin formation. In an amphibian brain Kusunoki et al. (38) found that the distribution pattern of nerve cells containing melanin pigment corresponded with the regions containing the greatest monoamine oxidase activity. Côté (39) has demonstrated the synthesis of a melanin by mitochondria from monkey substantia nigra; the melanin synthesis was inhibited by low concentrations of the monoamine oxidase inhibitors iproniazid and tranylcypromine.

However, the probability that monoamine oxidase is responsible for neuromelanin formation is not great since it is a mitochondrial enzyme and neuromelanin appears to be synthesized in lysosomes. In addition, monoamine oxidase activity has been reported to be normal rather than decreased in the parkinsonian brain.

Pseudoperoxidase

Metals such as ferric and cupric ions oxidize catechol and catechol derivatives in the presence of hydrogen peroxide to form melanins. Partially degraded heme compounds are also capable of oxidizing catechols. These nonenzymatic reactions are called pseudoperoxidation and the agents are pseudoperoxidases. The hydrogen peroxide may come from monoamine oxidase, nicotinamide-adenine dinucleotide (NADH) oxidase, or flavoprotein enzyme reactions (40, 41). Barden (5) has proposed that neuromelanin is synthesized by the oxidation of dopamine in the presence of hydrogen peroxide (H_2O_2) and a pseudoperoxidase such as copper. Goldfisher et al. (42) had hypothesized a similar metal- or heme-catalyzed pseudoperoxidation of catechol derivatives and lipids for the formation of lipofuscin in lysosomes of the human liver.

Peroxidase

The enzyme peroxidase has also been demonstrated to oxidize L-tyrosine and catechols to form a melanin pigment *in vitro* (43–45). By use of the benzidine histochemical method, peroxidase has been shown to be present in the guinea pig cortex (46). We have measured the peroxidase activity in various regions of normal brains obtained at autopsy (47). Peroxidase activity was measured spectrophotometrically by the method of Lundquist and Josefsson (48). The human brain was found to contain a peroxidase which had characteristics of an enzyme and distinct from pseudoperoxidase (47). As seen in Table 2, the highest peroxidase activity was found in the substantia nigra and the lowest in the temporal cortex. Preliminary studies indicate that peroxidase activities in the substantia nigra and caudate nucleus are reduced in parkinsonian brains (47).

TABLE 2. *Peroxidase activity in normal brain*

Brain region	Peroxidase activity (μ U/mg protein)
Cortex	
Frontal	295 ± 34
Occipital	447 ± 62
Temporal	238 ± 41
Cerebellum	444 ± 72
Vermis	432 ± 117
Substantia nigra	608 ± 83
Caudate	414 ± 72
Putamen	467 ± 89
Globus pallidus	321 ± 39
Thalamus	377 ± 42
Hypothalamus	496 ± 188
Red nucleus	406 ± 66
Locus coeruleus	349 ± 97

The results are expressed as the mean ± SE of eight brains obtained at autopsy. One unit of peroxidase represents the utilization of 1 μmole of H_2O_2 to oxidize an equimolar amount of O-dianisidine per minute at 37°C. The age range of the patients was 56 to 82 years.

NEUROMELANIN METABOLISM AND PARKINSON'S DISEASE

The significance of neuromelanin synthesis in certain specific neurons in the central nervous system remains unknown. The substantia nigra reaches its greatest size and greatest melanization in primates, culminating in man (49, 50). The presence of melanin in the substantia nigra neurons may be related to a special function of the extrapyramidal system which becomes increasingly important as the relationship to man becomes closer. Marsden (29) has postulated that with the evolutionary development of higher centers in the brain, the need for catecholamines in the primitive brainstem nuclei is reduced, and, therefore, L-tyrosine metabolism is diverted toward the formation of neuromelanin rather than catecholamines.

Our data suggest to us that peroxidase may be the enzyme which oxidizes dopamine and norepinephrine in the presence of hydrogen peroxide to form neuromelanin, and it is possible that the reduction in peroxidase activity in the parkinsonian brain may be related to the observed decrease in neuromelanin in substantia nigra and locus coeruleus in Parkinson's disease.

In the substantia nigra, pigmented and nonpigmented neurons have been shown to be metabolically quite different. The neurons without neuromelanin accumulate lipofuscin with age and histochemically show strong succinic dehydrogenase activity (51). Neuromelanin-containing cells have very little lipofuscin (13) and contain much less succinic dehydrogenase activity (51) and cytochrome oxidase activity (52). Although melanin has generally been thought to be biochemically inert, we have recently demonstrated that it can oxidize NADH; the semiquinone free radical of melanin acts as an electron acceptor (53). Melanin may function as an oxidation-reduction polymer since it can exist in either an oxidized quinoid or a reduced hydroquinoid form. Further investigation of a possible role of neuromelanin in the oxidative metabolism of the pigmented neuron is warranted.

Melanin is also reactive with several drugs, particularly phenothiazine compounds. Chlorpromazine (CPZ) has been demonstrated to have a marked affinity for melanin-containing tissues in animals and man due to the formation of a reversible charge-transfer complex. Forrest et al. (54) found that the melanized iris and choroid had the highest concentrations of CPZ of any tissues at autopsy in patients treated with this tranquilizer. In rabbits ^{35}S-labeled CPZ concentrates 50 times more in the pigmented uveal tract than in other body tissues (55). CPZ is known to inhibit DNA synthesis (56) and several tricarboxylic acid cycle enzymatic reactions (57–59), as well as NADH oxidation by melanin (60). CPZ also reduces the EPR signal of melanin probably by forming a charge-transfer complex (61). Since CPZ can interfere with various metabolic reactions, the accumulation of large concentrations of this drug in melanocytes might be toxic to these cells. As would be expected, the growth rate of mouse melanoma has been shown to be reduced by phenothiazine treatment (62). Furthermore, Forrest et al.

(54) and Christensen et al. (63) have reported that psychiatric patients treated with long-term phenothiazine therapy can develop degeneration of the pigmented substantia nigra neurons. Further investigation is indicated to determine if the chronic and irreversible extrapyramidal side effects of phenothiazines might be etiologically related to the accumulation of toxic levels of these drugs in the melanin-containing substantia nigra neurons.

SUMMARY

The brown pigment in the substantia nigra has the general characteristics of melanin, but there are ultrastructural and histochemical differences in the substantia nigra melanin granules and cutaneous melanin granules. Available evidence suggests that substantia nigra melanin and locus coeruleus melanin may be formed in lysosomes by oxidation of dopamine and nor-epinephrine, respectively, by the enzyme peroxidase. A decrease in peroxidase activity might account for the loss of substantia nigra melanin and subsequent degeneration of these neurons. The major difference between substantia nigra melanin granules and lipofuscin granules seems to be greater melanin-to-lipid ratio in the former.

ACKNOWLEDGMENT

This investigation was supported by U.S. Public Health Service grant NS-07542.

REFERENCES

1. Duffy, P. E., and Tennyson, V. M., *J. Neuropathol. Exp. Neurol.* 24, 398 (1965).
2. Moses, H. L., Ganote, C. E., Beaver, D. L., and Shuffman, S. S., *Anat. Rec.* 155, 167 (1966).
3. d'Agnostino, A. J., and Luse, S. A., *Neurology* 14, 529 (1964).
4. Van Woert, M. H., Prasad, K. N., and Borg, D. C., *J. Neurochem.* 14, 707 (1967).
5. Barden, H., *J. Neuropathol. Exp. Neurol.* 28, 419 (1969).
6. Hirosawa, K., *Z. Zellforsch.* 88, 187 (1968).
7. Seiji, M., and Iwashita, S., *J. Invest. Dermatol.* 45, 305 (1965).
8. de Duve, C., in: *Subcellular Particles*, p. 128, Ronald Press, New York (1959).
9. Samorajski, T., Keefe, J. F., and Ordy, J. M., *J. Gerontol.* 19, 262 (1964).
10. Pallis, C. A., Duckett, S., and Pearse, A. G. E., *Neurology* 17, 381 (1967).
11. Essner, E., and Novikoff, A. B., *J. Ultrastruc. Res.* 3, 374 (1960).
12. Seiji, M., Fitzpatrick, T. B., Simpson, R. T., and Birbeck, M. S. C., *J. Invest. Dermatol.* 36, 243 (1961).
13. Wolf, A., and Pappenheimer, A. M., *J. Neuropathol. Exp. Neurol.* 4, 402 (1945).
14. Lillie, R. D., *Anat. Rec.* 108, 239 (1950).
15. Lillie, R. D., in: *Histopathological and Practical Histochemistry*, McGraw-Hill, New York (1965).
16. Lillie, R. D., *J. Histochem. Cytochem.* 3, 453 (1955).
17. Lillie, R. D., *J. Histochem. Cytochem.* 4, 118 (1956).
18. Lillie, R. D., *J. Histochem. Cytochem.* 5, 325 (1957).
19. Hendley, D. D., Mildvan, A. S., Reporter, M. C., and Strehler, B. L., *J. Gerontol.* 18, 144 (1963).

20. Ambani, L. M., and Van Woert, M. H., *unpublished observations.*
21. Mikulski, T., *Acta Physiol. Polonica* 21, 219 (1970).
22. Maeda, T., and Wegmann, R., *Brain Res.* 14, 673 (1969).
23. Arias, I. M., Bernstein, L., Toffler, R., and Ben-Ezzer, J., *Gastroenterology* 48, 495 (1965).
24. Cornelius, C. E., Arias, I. M., and Osburn, B., *J. Am. Vet. Med. Assoc.* 146, 709 (1965).
25. Maruffo, C. A., Malinow, M. R., Depaoli, J. R., and Katz, S., *Am. J. Pathol.* 49, 455 (1966).
26. Katz, S., Gilardoni, A., Genovese, N., Wilkinski, R. W., Cornelius, C. E., and Malinow, M. R., *Lab. Anim. Care* 18, 626 (1968).
27. Ambani, L. M., Edelstein, L. M., and Van Woert, M. H., *Yale J. Biol. Med. (in press).*
28. Vander Wende, C., and Spoerlein, M. T., *Life Sci.* 6, 386 (1963).
29. Marsden, C. D., *Lancet* II, 475 (1965).
30. Van Woert, M. H., and Cotzias, G. C., in: *Parkinson's Disease,* p. 95, Grune and Stratton, New York (1965).
31. Andén, N., Dahlström, A., Fuxe, K., and Larsson, K., *Am. J. Anat.* 116, 329 (1965).
32. Bazelon, M., Fenichel, G. M., and Randall, J., *Neurology* 17, 512 (1967).
33. Bertler, A., *Acta Physiol. Scand.* 51, 97 (1961).
34. Dahlström, A., and Fuxe, K., *Acta Physiol. Scand.,* 62 suppl 232, 1 (1964).
35. Côté, L. J., and Fahn, S., in: *Progress in Neuro-Genetics,* p. 311, Excerpta Medica, Amsterdam (1969).
36. Nagatsu, T., Levitt, M., and Udenfriend, S., *J. Biol. Chem.* 239, 2910 (1964).
37. Foley, J. M., and Baxter, D., *J. Neuropathol. Exp. Neurol.* 17, 586 (1958).
38. Kusunoki, T., Ishibashi, H., and Masai, H., *J. Hirnforsch.* 9, 63 (1967).
39. Côté, L. J., quoted by Marsden, C. D. in: *Pigments in Pathology,* p. 409, Academic Press, New York (1969).
40. Baehner, R., and Karnovsky, M. L., *Science* 16, 1277 (1969).
41. Mason, H. S., *Adv. Enzymol.* 19, 79 (1957).
42. Goldfischer, S., Villaverde, H., and Forshirm, R., *J. Histochem. Cytochem.* 14, 641 (1966).
43. Mason, H., Onoprienko, I., and Buhler, D., *Biochim. Biophys. Acta* 24, 225 (1957).
44. Patel, R., Okun, M., Edelstein, L., and Epstein, D., *Biochem. J.* 124, 439 (1971).
45. Bayse, G. S., and Morrison, M., *Biochim. Biophys. Acta* 244, 77 (1971).
46. Okun, M. R., Donnellan, B., and Lever, W. F., *Histochemie* 25, 289 (1971).
47. Ambani, L. M., and Van Woert, M. H., *Trans. Am. Neurol. Assoc. (in press).*
48. Lundquist, I., and Josefsson, J., *Anal. Biochem.* 41, 567 (1971).
49. Marsden, C. D., *J. Anat.* 95, 256 (1961).
50. Scherer, J., *J. Comp. Neurol.* 71, 91 (1939).
51. Friede, R. L., *Acta Neuropathol.* 2, 113 (1962).
52. Marinesco, G., *Ann. Anat. Pathol.* 1, 121 (1924).
53. Van Woert, M. H., *Life Sci.* 6, 2605 (1967).
54. Forrest, F. M., Forrest, I. S., and Roizin, L., *Rev. Aggressol.* 4, 259 (1963).
55. Potts, A. M., *Trans. Am. Ophthalmol. Soc.* 60, 517 (1962).
56. Pisciotta, A. V., *J. Lab. Clin. Med.* 65, 240 (1965).
57. Abood, L. G., *Proc. Soc. Exp. Biol. Med.* 88, 688 (1955).
58. Berger, M., *J. Neurochem.* 2, 30 (1957).
59. Dawkins, M. J. R., Judah, J. D., and Rees, K. R., *Biochem. J.* 73, 16 (1959).
60. Van Woert, M. H., *Proc. Soc. Exp. Biol. Med.* 129, 165 (1968).
61. Bolt, A. G., and Forrest, I. S., Amer. Chem. Soc. meeting, New York, Sept. 1966.
62. Van Woert, M. H., and Palmer, S. H., *Cancer Res.* 29, 1952 (1969).
63. Christensen, E., Moller, J. E., and Faurbye, A., *Acta Psychiat. Scand.* 46, 14 (1970).

Advances in Neurology, Vol. 5
Raven Press, New York © 1974

Melanocyte-Stimulating Hormone and the Hypothalamic Hormone Which Inhibits Its Release

Abba J. Kastin, André Barbeau, Rudolph H. Ehrensing,
Nicholas P. Plotnikoff, and Andrew V. Schally

*Endocrinology Section of the Medical Service and Endocrine and Polypeptide Laboratory,
Veterans Administration Hospital, and Department of Medicine, Tulane University School
of Medicine, New Orleans, Louisiana 70146; Department of Neurobiology, Clinical Re-
search Institute of Montreal and University of Montreal, Montreal 130, Quebec, Canada;
Department of Psychiatry, Louisiana State University School of Medicine, New Orleans,
Louisiana 70112; and General Pharmacology Department, Abbott Laboratories, North
Chicago, Illinois 60064*

The influence of melanocyte-stimulating hormone (MSH) on pigmentation has been well described by Lerner and others (1). In lower forms of
vertebrates, such as amphibians, the change in skin color serves an adaptive
function by permitting the organism to blend better with the environment
and thereby escape predators. However, black people have essentially the
same amount of MSH in their blood as white people, and pigmentation in
the human being does not change as rapidly as it does in lower vertebrates.
Therefore, it is likely that the main function of MSH in mammals is not the
control of pigmentation. It is possible that MSH could serve no role at all
in man, or during the course of evolution it could have acquired some extrapigmentary functions.

The main site of action of MSH in animals such as the frog is the melanocyte. Embryologically, the melanocyte is derived from the neural crest. It
would be logical, therefore, to expect that if MSH had an important action
in mammals, the effect would be exerted on cells of neural crest origin. It
also might be assumed that the "new" actions of MSH might produce better
adaptation of the mammal to his environment. Support for these hypotheses
has been provided recently by a series of experiments demonstrating an
effect of MSH on the central nervous system (CNS) of rats and man (2).

In the first study of the effects of MSH on the CNS of man, which we
performed in 1966, high-amplitude, low-frequency changes were seen in the
EEG (3). Similar changes have been demonstrated in the rabbit (4), rat (5),
and frog (6) after injection of MSH, and adrenocorticotropic hormone
(ACTH) has also been reported to produce such changes (7, 8). Starting
with ACTH and then trying substances such as MSH which structurally

resemble ACTH, DeWied and co-workers (9, 10) were able to show an effect on the conditioned avoidance response in rats. We have shown that MSH also affects appetitive responses (11), passive avoidance responses (12, 13), and reversal responses (14, 15). These behavioral effects do not seem to be caused only by hyperactivity (16, 17). The somatosensory-evoked response is increased by MSH administered to the human being; this effect is particularly pronounced under conditions of attention (18). That visual attention may be especially affected was shown by improvement in the Benton visual retention test after MSH (18). Both "psychological stress" and "physical stress" release MSH (19, 20). Thus, the release of endogenous MSH may play some sort of adaptive role in mammals, as the observation of behavioral effects after the administration of exogenous MSH seem to indicate.

If MSH serves an important function in mammals, then its release should be very finely and carefully controlled. A series of studies begun in 1963 has shown this to be the case (21, 22). The most important control comes from the hypothalamus. The hypothalamic influence is primarily inhibitory, although a stimulatory influence probably is also present (19, 23, 24). Inhibition is exerted by one or more substances which can be extracted from hypothalamic tissue (25). At the time this review is being written (March, 1973), two compounds have been isolated from bovine hypothalamic tissue (26, 27) which inhibit the release of MSH when applied directly to the surface of the pituitary gland of a frog which has been darkened by destruction of its hypothalamus (28). These MSH-release inhibiting factors (MIF or MRIH) are small peptides, the most potent of which seems to be Pro-Leu-Gly-NH$_2$ (MRIH-I). This was first shown by Celis and co-workers (29) to be the C-terminal tripeptide of oxytocin, which is cleaved from oxytocin by an enzyme present in hypothalamic tissue. However, the remaining portion of the oxytocin molecule, the cyclic pentapeptide ring called tocinoic acid or its amide tocinamide has been claimed by Bower and co-workers (30) to be the main MRIH.

Regardless of which compound proves to be the principal MRIH, our concept that the primary control of MSH release in mammals is exerted by an inhibitory substance has become firmly established. It also appears that the pineal gland exerts some influence on the release of MSH from the pituitary (31, 32), and that the effects of light and dark on MSH release are mediated through the pineal (33). Higher CNS centers probably act through the hypothalamus. Furthermore, as would be expected for a hormone which might have an important role in man, there is evidence for two types of feedback control of MSH release (34, 35).

Studies with MSH demonstrated that small polypeptides can affect the CNS. MRIH-I, like MSH, occurs naturally in the mammalian body. Although MRIH-I would be expected to act by means of MSH, early studies suggested to us that it might exert direct effects on the brain. The MRIH-I tripeptide (Pro-Leu-Gly-NH$_2$) was therefore tested in several animal systems. It was found to potentiate the behavioral effects of DOPA (36), antagonize the tremors induced by oxotremorine (37), and reverse the sedative effects of deserpidine in mice and monkeys (38). The presence of the pituitary gland did not seem to be necessary for these effects of MRIH-I. The second MRIH (Pro-His-Phe-Arg-Gly-NH$_2$), MSH, and tocinoic acid also had slight activity in the DOPA potentiation test, but not nearly to the extent of MRIH-I (39). Another hypothalamic hormone, thyrotropin-releasing hormone (TRH), had some activity in this test system (40), but was not as potent as MRIH-I.

The animal systems just mentioned are considered by some investigators to be models of Parkinson's disease and mental depression. Accordingly, MRIH-I was tested in a preliminary clinical study. The results are shown in Table 1. Most of the beneficial effects occurred for the symptoms of rigidity and tremor, and less for akinesia (41). Rather than potentiating the effects of L-DOPA, it seemed to reduce the abnormal involuntary movements produced by L-DOPA. The highest dose used in these early studies was 50 mg/day. In view of the lack of side effects, larger doses will be tested. Perhaps further improvement in parkinsonism will occur at higher doses.

TABLE 1. *Low doses of Pro-Leu-Gly-NH$_2$ in parkinsonism*

Route	Duration	Dose (mg)	No. of patients	Tremor	Rigidity	Akinesia
i.v.	1 hr	20	8	sl ↓ 3/5	20% ↓	→ 2/2
p.o.	2 days	30	8	sl ↓ 3/5	20% ↓	→
p.o.	2 months	50	3	38% ↓	40% ↓	30% ↓
p.o.	2 days	50*	5		48% ↓ in dyskinesias	

* + L-DOPA (3.7 g)

After these studies on the effects of MRIH-I in Parkinson's disease were completed, we decided to test MRIH-I in mental depression, as suggested by our animal studies. However, at the time it was more feasible to test TRH in depression. Using a bouble-blind, crossover design, we found some improvement in the symptoms of mental depression in all patients receiving TRH, although the effect was brief and minor in most of them (42). It was later shown in animals (40), as could have been predicted from our studies with MRIH-I (36–38), that the presence of the pituitary gland was not required for the effect of TRH. Thyrotropin-stimulating hormone (TSH) release in response to TRH in the mentally depressed patients was decreased, so it is unlikely that the antidepressant effect of TRH is mediated by TSH and thyroid hormones. Prange and co-workers made essentially the same observations (43). However, their approach was entirely different, since they initially felt that the action of TRH in mental depression would be mediated by way of the release of TSH from the pituitary gland and its stimulation of the thyroid hormone secretions (43). It will be interesting to determine whether MRIH-I is more potent in relieving the symptoms of mental depression than is TRH.

In conclusion, this brief chapter has reviewed three of our concepts: control of MSH release in mammals by an MRIH, extrapigmentary effects of MSH on the CNS of man, and extraendocrine effects of hypothalamic hormones. Although each type of action can occur independently of the others, it is possible that they may all prove to be parts of an integrated response.

REFERENCES

1. Lerner, A. B., in: *Advances in Neurology*, Vol. 5, Raven Press, New York (1974).
2. Kastin, A. J., Miller, L. H., Nockton, R., Sandman, C. A., Schally, A. V., and Stratton, L. O., *Progr. Brain Res.* 93, 468 (1973).
3. Kastin, A. J., Kullander, S., Borglin, N. E., Dyster-Aas, K., Dahlberg, B., Ingvar, D., Krakau, C. E. T., Miller, M. C., Bowers, C. Y., and Schally, A. V., *Lancet* 1, 1007 (1968).
4. Dyster-Aas, H. K., and Krakau, C. E. T., *Acta Endocrinol.* 48, 609 (1965).
5. Sandman, C., Denman, P. M., Miller, L. H., Knott, J. R., Schally, A. V., and Kastin, A. J., *J. Comp. Physiol. Psych.* 76, 103 (1971).
6. Denman, P. M., Miller, L. H., Sandman, C. A., Schally, A. V., and Kastin, A. J., *J. Comp. Physiol. Psych.* 80, 59 (1972).
7. Torda, C., and Wolff, H. G., *Am. J. Physiol.* 168, 406 (1952).
8. Woodbury, D. M., *Pharmacol. Rev.* 10, 257 (1958).
9. DeWied, D., *Intern. J. Neuropharmacol.* 4, 157 (1965).
10. DeWied, D., Bohus, B., and Greven, H. M., in: *Endocrinology and Human Behavior*, p. 188, Oxford University Press, London.
11. Sandman, C. A., Kastin, A. J., and Schally, A. V., *Experientia* 25, 1001 (1969).
12. Sandman, C. A., Kastin, A. J., and Schally, A. V., *Physiol. Behav.* 6, 45 (1971).
13. Dempsey, G. L., Kastin, A. J., and Schally, A. V., *Horm. Behav.* 3, 333 (1972).
14. Sandman, C. A., Miller, L. H., Kastin, A. J., and Schally, A. V., *J. Comp. Physiol. Psych.* 80, 54 (1972).
15. Stratton, L. O., and Kastin, A. J., *Physiol. Behav.* 10, 689 (1973).
16. Kastin, A. J., Miller, M. C., Ferrell, L., and Schally, A. V., *Physiol. Behav.* 10, 399 (1973).
17. Nockton, R., Kastin, A. J., Elder, S. T., and Schally, A. V., *Horm. Behav.* 3, 339 (1972).
18. Kastin, A. J., Miller, L. H., Gonzalez-Barcena, D., Hawley, W. D., Dyster-Aas, K., Schally, A. V., Velasco-Parra, M. L., and Velasco, M., *Physiol. Behav.* 7, 893 (1971).
19. Kastin, A. J., Schally, A. V., Viosca, S., and Miller, M. C., *Endocrinology* 84, 20 (1969).
20. Sandman, C. A., Kastin, A. J., Schally, A. V., Kendall, J. W., and Miller, L. H., *J. Comp. Physiol. Psych.* 84, 386 (1973).
21. Kastin, A. J., and Schally, A. V., *Pigmentation: Its Genesis and Biologic Control*, p. 215, Appleton-Century-Crofts, New York (1972).
22. Kastin, A. J., and Schally, A. V., in: *Recent Advances in Endocrinology*, p. 311, Excerpta Medica Int. Congr. Series, Amsterdam 238 (1971).
23. Kastin, A. J., and Schally, A. V., *Gen. Comp. Endocrinol.* 7, 452 (1966).
24. Taleisnik, S., and Orias, R., *Am. J. Physiol.* 208, 293 (1965).
25. Kastin, A. J., Plotnikoff, N. P., Nair, R. M. G., Redding, T. W., and Anderson, M. S., in: *Hypothalamic Hypophysiotropic Hormones: Clinical and Physiological Studies*, p. 159, Excerpta Medica Int. Congr. Series, Amsterdam 263 (1973).
26. Nair, R. M. G., Kastin, A. J., and Schally, A. V., *Biochem. Biophys. Res. Comm.* 43, 1376 (1971).

27. Nair, R. M. G., Kastin, A. J., and Schally, A. V., *Biochem. Biophys. Res. Comm.* 47, 1420 (1972).
28. Kastin, A. J., Schally, A. V., and Viosca, S., *Proc. Soc. Exp. Biol. Med.* 137, 1437 (1971).
29. Celis, M. E., Taleisnik, S., and Walter, R., *Proc. Nat. Acad. Sci.* 68, 1428 (1971).
30. Bower, A., Hadley, M. E., and Hruby, V. J., *Biochem. Biophys. Res. Comm.* 45, 1185 (1971).
31. Kastin, A. J., Redding, T. W., and Schally, A. V., *Proc. Soc. Exp. Biol. Med.* 124, 1275 (1967).
32. Kastin, A. J., Schally, A. V., Viosca, S., Barrett, L., and Redding, T. W., *Proc. Soc. Exp. Biol. Med.* 124, 1275 (1967).
33. Kastin, A. J., Schally, A. V., Viosca, S., Barrett, L., and Redding, T. W., *Neuroendocrinology* 2, 257 (1967).
34. Kastin, A. J., and Schally, A. V., *Nature* 213, 1238 (1967).
35. Kastin, A. J., Arimura, A., Schally, A. V., and Miller, M. C., *Nature* 231, 29 (1971).
36. Plotnikoff, N. P., Kastin, A. J., Anderson, M. S., and Schally, A. V., *Life Sci.* 10, 1279 (1971).
37. Plotnikoff, N. P., Kastin, A. J., Anderson, M. S., and Schally, A. V., *Proc. Soc. Exp. Biol. Med.* 140, 811 (1972).
38. Plotnikoff, N. P., Kastin, A. J., Anderson, M. S., and Schally, A. V., *Neuroendocrinology* 11, 67 (1973).
39. Kastin, A. J., Plotnikoff, N. P., Viosca, S., Anderson, M. S., and Schally, A. V., *Yale J. Biol. Med.* (Dec. 1973).
40. Plotnikoff, N. P., Prange, A. J., Breese, G. R., Anderson, M. S., and Wilson, I. C., *Science* 178, 417 (1972).
41. Kastin, A. J., and Barbeau, A., *Can. Med. Assoc. J.* 107, 1079 (1972).
42. Kastin, A. J., Ehrensing, R. H., Schalch, D. S., and Anderson, M. S., *Lancet* II, 740 (1972).
43. Prange, A. J., Wilson, I. C., Lara, P. P., Alltop, L. B., and Breese, G. R., *Lancet* II, 999 (1972).

DISCUSSION

Dr. Sandler: Regarding Dr. Lerner's last point, Dr. McGee and I, in 1969 at the Val-David meeting, both preferred 6-hydroxydopamine as a possible candidate for this role. Dr. Kastin has reviewed evidence suggesting that there might be an interaction between these hypothalamic peptides and certain biogenic amines. In rats given TRF and MIF with and without L-DOPA, we failed to observe any effect on the metabolism of L-DOPA in rat urine collected over 24 hours. It may very well be that we missed any changes as they may be short term. When we carry out a trial of MIF in human parkinsonism, I hope in the not-too-distant future, we will be able to look at urine samples at closer intervals, and look into this point more carefully.

Dr. Barbeau: Thank you, Dr. Sandler. Preliminary studies with MIF in Parkinson's disease at higher doses than those reported in previous papers now indicate that if an effect occurs, it is mainly on rigidity. We have now given up to 500 milligrams per day without any toxicity and are still increasing doses, following Dr. Cotzias's principle. We would tend to agree that biogenic amines, at least the catecholamines, do not seem to be modified in our preliminary studies of the brain after MIF. We should start looking at other things that may be involved in rigidity, particularly GABA metabolism or serotonin as it applies to tone control.

Dr. Coleman: This is a question for Dr. Lerner or Dr. Van Woert. Nine years ago my research team examined a human brainstem and found that neuromelanin is not in three separate nuclei as originally thought, but rather it is in a continuous column all the way up and down the brainstem. We then noted that this column, with a few minor exceptions, coincided almost exactly with the catecholamine pathway Dr. Fuxe and his group in Sweden described. Since then we have found that the neuromelanin in the substantia nigra probably comes from dopamine-producing cells while the neuromelanin and melanin in the locus ceruleus probably come from norepinephrine-producing cells. My question is: is there any difference in the configuration or in the biochemistry of the neuromelanin in these two separate types of cells? As far as production from separate amines is concerned, is it thought that all neuromelanin comes from dopamine?

Dr. Lerner: I would guess that the biochemical structure would be different. I also would suggest that the experiment be done as follows. The old system that Nicolaus used—involving many years of work degrading the final product and then finding out the nature of the substance—is almost impossible for anyone else to do. Now it can be done with use of the mass spectrograph. Before something goes into the mass spectrograph it is subjected to an electric discharge which breaks the substance down into smaller bits; then in about a week's work you can do everything that Nicolaus did in about 10 years. However, the interpretation of all the information is not so easy. You do get all the molecular weights, and from that one can back-track and tell what some of the polymerizing units are made of. I do not see why one could not collect melanin granules from various parts of the nervous system by a centrifugation technique or some other separation method, and then, working in conjunction with someone who has a mass spectrograph and is interested in determination of the chemical structures by that means, determine what the structure is. I'm sure it is going to be different from the skin melanin and that the dopamine melanin would be different from the norepinephrine melanin.

Dr. Fahn: I wondered if Dr. Lerner or Dr. Van Woert would speculate as to why lower mammals do not have melanin in their substantia nigra. The rat substantia nigra, for example, has plenty of dopamine but no melanin.

Dr. Lerner: No, I have no idea really.

Dr. Coleman: There are three or four papers that show that lower mammals do have neuromelanin. It's just that most mammals studied were either newborn or very young. If you take a 5- or 10-year-old dog or monkey, you will find neuromelanin.

Dr. Roberts: It's well known that there is a group of anion-free radicals that are organic conductors, and I wonder whether these melanins that you've been discussing are either semiconductors or conductors.

Dr. Lerner: People have talked about that point, and as far as I can tell they are semiconductors, but it would really be worth carrying out experiments on that particular point: that is, polymerizing different melanins, putting them out on a sheet, and then determining their conductive properties.

Dr. Barbeau: Dr. Borg is scheduled to talk on this subject.

Dr. Borg: I am going to say something about EPR signals in melanin later, but I want to get into the fray now. The free radical signals that are seen in melanins represent something on the order of 1% of the units, and they seem to be quite randomly scattered. They're an interesting window but I remind you that they're 1% of the units. The first point I want to make is it is relatively clear that all of those free radicals one sees in a mature melanin are indole-type free radicals and not catechol free radicals; they can be distinguished as such. Plant melanins which are catechol melanins look very different on EPR. My second point has to do with the semiconductor properties of melanins, which were invoked by good chemical physicists more than 10 years ago. Without going through the EPR evidence I will cite the individual (another dermatologist), Boyce from Stanford, who looked at this closely with EPR evidence, an important part of the picture. He has concluded rather categorically, and others would agree, that melanins, although you can under some circumstances *in vitro* show a kind of semi-conduction, are not semiconductors. There are not excitation vans that go through the whole polymer. The electrons in the free radical centers are not delocalized through the whole polymer, but they sit very much as they do on free radicals that you see elsewhere in organic chemistry. In short, the free radicals are trapped; the melanin is a random mesh polymer as described and is consistent with the Nicolaus scheme. The semiconductor properties do not seem to be much in vogue now among the physical chemists.

Dr. Kopin: I wonder if there is any evidence that the large doses of DOPA that are being given to parkinsonian patients have any effect on melanin-producing cells as would be indicated from what Dr. Lerner was talking about. Are there instances of anyone developing gray hair or losing pigment cells?

Dr. Lerner: Not that I know of, Dr. Kopin, although that is really what should happen. I know people used to say that when patients are given large amounts of DOPA they should darken. Actually it is just the opposite: they should get gray hair or lighten. But perhaps DOPA has to be given to an individual who is predisposed to that type of change in the first place.

Dr. Forno: I would like to hear more about those possible toxic substances that may develop in the melanin-containing nerve cells. Did Dr. Lerner have 6-hydroxydopamine in mind?

Dr. Lerner: No, we have never used 6-hydroxydopamine in our melanoma cells in culture, and I do not know what the other intermediates are, except the ones I showed from tyrosine to melanin.

Advances in Neurology, Vol. 5
Raven Press, New York © 1974

Manganese and Catecholamines

George C. Cotzias, Paul S. Papavasiliou, Ismael Mena,
Lily C. Tang, and Samuel T. Miller

*The Medical Research Center, Brookhaven National Laboratory, a Clinical Campus,
University of the State of New York at Stony Brook, Upton, L. I., New York 11973*

INTRODUCTION

Mercury, cadmium, and lead are examples of detrimental heavy poly-valent metals which can impair the nervous system by producing either mental aberrations, extrapyramidal symptoms, or both (1). Yet even copper, a metal essential to life, can also cause central nervous system (CNS) damage. It does so both when excessive amounts enter the CNS (as in Wilson's disease) and when its CNS concentrations are deficient (as in swayback) (1, 2). Both Wilson's disease and swayback are linked to geneti-cally controlled predispositions which must be coupled with environmental factors before respective diseases can be induced.

Similarly, the essential trace metal manganese can affect the CNS with both deficiency (2, 3) and excess (4). Genetic factors predisposing to man-ganese deficiency have been discovered thus far only in animals (2). The role of genetic predisposition in the production of human chronic manganese poisonings is only mooted. Environmental factors have been ascertained only qualitatively. Due to its changing roles from a factor essential to life to a cause of disease, manganese has been a challenging investigative sub-ject.

Our earlier experiments with adult animals (5–7), their tissues (8, 9), or their organelles (9–11) have helped us in studying (12, 13) and eventually in treating (14) human chronic manganese poisoning. With the hope of duplicating this success, we have initiated animal experiments at the op-posite extreme of the maturational process, the very young animal. These experiments might hopefully provide a basis for identifying and studying manganese deficiency and excess early in human life. Deficiency might well exist in the midst of plenty, as shown by our earlier studies on rheuma-toid arthritis (15) and by some of the experiments discussed here. Similarly, some of the present experiments indicate that individual susceptibility to excess can depend on both genetic and maturational factors.

PLAN OF PRESENTATION

We will discuss some findings in the adult mouse mutant *pallid*, the young of which are genetically susceptible to the cerebral consequences of manganese deficiency both *in utero* and in early postnatal life (16). Among healthy adult members of the *pallid* strain (also called "manganese" or "neurological" strain), and in the absence of CNS disease, clinically recognizable aberrations have linked the metabolism of manganese to that of exogenous catecholamines (17). Our data link manganese excess with an increase in intrinsic cerebral dopamine in the adult mouse and our findings in adult animals show radical differences between postnatal or neonatal ones. Indeed, the one common denominator pervading these experiments is the concomitant increase of cerebral manganese and of either extrinsic or intrinsic cerebral catecholamines.

METHODS

Turnover studies and organ distributions of the artificial radioactive isotope ^{54}Mn were conducted after injecting the carrier-free tracer intraperitoneally. We measured thereafter its loss from the total body in the intact animals as a function of time or its concentration in tissues after sacrificing and dissecting the animals (18–20). Both the turnover and organ distribution of the radioisotope were willfully and concordantly changed by supplying high, medium, or low manganese diets or by injecting natural manganous salts. The natural metal manganese (^{55}Mn) was measured in tissues by neutron activation analysis. This was conducted with a chemical separation of the ensuing radioactive ^{56}Mn (21, 22) when the manganese concentration was below 20 ng/sample. A new, nondestructive procedure became eminently applicable to tissue samples containing larger amounts of this metal. This procedure, to be detailed elsewhere, permits the analysis of manganese to be followed by analyses of DOPA and of dopamine. Since the validity of the original destructive analysis for manganese had been proven earlier (21, 22), it remained for us to correlate its results with those of the new, nondestructive one. We found with 80 tissue samples (10 to 700 ng of ^{55}Mn per sample), the coefficient of correlation was 0.99.

Behavioral scores were obtained in mice receiving neuroactive drugs by (a) summing several of the effects of the drug after grading each effect in each animal from 0 to 3, and (b) by placing animals in or on an Animex motor activity meter.

Genetic Correlations Between Manganese and L-DOPA

Manganese is absorbed by the intestine as a constant percentile fraction of the metal presented for absorption. Its homeostasis depends, therefore, on its excretion by the bile and by the intestinal mucosa (23). Even in severe deficiency, an obligatory excretion was found among adult animals, and animals burdened with manganese have shown saturation of these excretory pathways. Thus, whenever normal adult mice consuming Purina Chow (30 μg of ^{55}Mn^2 per gram) were earlier injected with ^{54}Mn, the radioactivity accumulated preferentially in the liver and disappeared from that organ and from the intact body at fairly rapid, characteristic rates. Conversely, "normal" mice have always shown a slow but obligatory rate of loss (18), even when placed on a diet severely deficient in manganese (milk, 0.025 μg of Mn/ml). This rate could be willfully accelerated at any time by supplying manganese orally or by injection. When, however, *pallid* mice (pa/pa) were subjected to such maneuvers and were compared to their controls (C$_{57}$ Black/6J, or pa/pa), they showed under a variety of diets the slow turnover and the organ distribution indicative of relative manganese deficiency. This deficiency was confirmed by analyses of some of their tissues for manganese, which showed significantly lower concentrations of the metal in the bone and the brain of *pallid* mice by comparison to Blacks (17).

Tissue concentrations of any metal do not necessarily indicate the presence or absence of functional changes in the tissue analyzed. We therefore sought such changes in bone, in which the well-characterized disease perosis is an accepted criterion for manganese deficiency. We found that three cardinal functional indicators of perosis (high fragility of bone, low density, and low nitrogen content) were present in *pallid* animals by comparison to Blacks (17).

Since low manganese concentration proved to be an indication of functional changes in the bone, the reduced concentrations in brain might indicate functional changes in brain. We therefore tested for such changes by administering L-DOPA to *pallid* and Black mice. We found that *pallid* mice have a remarkable resistance to orally or intraperitoneally administered L-DOPA by comparison to both Blacks and Swiss albino, whether the end point was behavior, cerebral manifestations, or survival (17).

Cerebral effects of L-DOPA have been correlated with cerebral concentrations of DOPA and of dopamine. Brains were therefore analyzed after the i.p. injection of water or L-DOPA (0.4 mg/g). The results indicated that L-DOPA increased the concentrations of both DOPA and dopamine in brain to an impressively lesser degree in *pallid* than in Black mice. The intrinsic cerebral dopamine levels in these healthy *pallid* mice were not different from the Blacks (17), but experiments such as those performed on postnatal Swiss albino mice (see below) have not yet been performed on these *pallids* and Blacks. Concomitant analyses for both manganese and dopamine must be performed on *pallids* and Blacks during the early days of life, because the evidence obtained in postnatal Swiss albinos suggests that the maturation of the dopaminergic apparatus might be manganese dependent.

L-DOPA is a large neutral amino acid whose transportation has similarities to that of other such amino acids. Tryptophan, the precursor of cerebral serotonin, is also a large neutral amino acid. Analyses for serotonin were therefore performed on brains from adult *pallids* and Blacks (0.4 or 0.8 mg/g, i.p.) 30 min before being killed. The lower doses of L-tryptophan used generated significantly less cerebral serotonin in *pallid* than in Black mice, whereas this difference tended to even out with the larger doses. This indicated that transportation of tryptophan from the peritoneum to the brain was also slower in *pallid* mice (17).

Some of the large neutral amino acids, including those tested, are precursors of melanins, and melanin granules are very rich in manganese (24). The melanosomes studied earlier, furthermore, had high manganese uptakes, rivaling those of mitochondria (11). These considerations agree with our present findings in view of the contrast in pigmentation between *pallid* and Black mice.

Taken together, these results indicate that a single gene can influence the transportation of a metal and of two precursors of biogenic amines in the same direction, strengthening the possibility that analyses conducted early in life might show delays in the maturation of the dopaminergic apparatus in these mutants.

Manganese Intake and Its Effects on Manganese and Dopamine in the Brain

Groups of adult Swiss albino mice were placed either on milk (0.025 μg of ^{55}Mn/ml), on milk containing 10 μg of ^{55}Mn/ml, or on milk containing 1.0 mg/ml. The first of these diets is a severely manganese-deficient one, supplying 0.4 μg of Mn/animal/day; the second supplies the same amounts as does Purina Chow (100 μg/day), whereas the third supplies a large excess of metal (10.000 μg/day). The animals were sacrificed over the next 160 days in groups of three and at intervals of 7 to 14 days. Their brains, livers, and diaphragms were analyzed for manganese. The mice receiving manganese intakes similar to those of the Purina Chow on which they had been reared showed steady tissue concentrations over the entire period of observation, with a mean and standard error of 1.85 ± 0.03 μg/g dry brain. By contrast, those receiving only milk showed first a rapid and then a slower decline of their brain manganese concentrations, reaching over the last 45 days of the experiment a mean and standard error of 0.87 ± 0.03 μg of manganese per gram dry brain ($p < 0.01$). Within a week, the ones receiving the high intakes of manganese reached dry brain manganese concentrations with a mean and standard error of 5.86 ± 0.16 μg ($p < 0.01$ from both the above values). This level was maintained for 44 days and declined slowly thereafter, reaching 4.16 ± 0.14 μg/g on the 90th day. This new level remained steady up to the completion of this experiment. The difference between the first and second levels in the high manganese group was significant ($p < 0.01$), and so were the differences among all groups. Among the organs analyzed, however, only the brain showed a decline in the manganese concentration on the high manganese diet, although the other tissues showed increases of the same magnitude as those of brain.

Dopamine analyses have thus far been completed in sufficient numbers only up to the 80th day of these experiments. Still, a remarkable finding was the significant elevation of cerebral dopamine from 0.47 ± 0.02 μg of dopamine per brain to 0.80 ± 0.07 μg ($p < 0.01$) encountered just prior to the decline of the cerebral manganese concentration. This rise in dopamine might be interesting if the subsequent decline in cerebral manganese should prove to be associated with cerebral damage from chronic manganese poisoning. The neurological phase of this poisoning is preceded by a psychiatric phase in man (4), whereas the neurological phase is associated with a decline of striatal dopamine in the monkey (25).

Manganese and Dopamine in the Postnatal and Neonatal Mouse

Despite their surprising results, these studies were initiated to determine whether the obligatory loss of manganese occurring during deficiency in adult Swiss albino mice might be of such magnitude in postnatal animals as to explain their high susceptibility to the cerebral consequences of manganese deficiency.

We injected initially carrier-free ^{54}MnCl$_2$ intraperitoneally into postnatal Swiss albino mice and measured the changes in the isotope's concentration in their whole bodies as a function of time, with a method presented earlier (18–20). To our surprise, instead of the expected obligatory loss, we found a total absence of elimination of the radioisotope over the first 16 to 18 days of life. This is the only example of naturally occurring absence of elimination encountered hitherto by us in all our studies of animals and man. Indeed, the only earlier such example had been artificially induced by our ligating the anus in rats and mice with a pursestring around a plug of cotton, to prove that urinary output of manganese is minimal indeed (20, 23).

The neonatal mice initiated spontaneous elimination of manganese at approximately the 18th day of life, at a rate which was from the outset similar to that of adult Swiss albino mice reared on Purina Chow. Purina Chow was the diet eaten by the mothers of these neonatal mice. Thus far the only method by which we could initiate loss of this isotope from intact neonatal mice prior to the 18th day of life was by injecting 25 μg of natural manganese on the 10th day. This amount of manganese is approximately 10 times the total body concentration of natural manganese at that age in these mice. Since ACTH had accelerated the loss of manganese from the whole bodies of adult mice, this hormone was injected into these neonatal ones (120 ng/mouse, s.c.) but without effect on the turnover of manganese.

It appeared, therefore, that accumulation of natural manganese was triggering the metal's elimination. Analyses were therefore performed for natural manganese (^{55}Mn) on tissues from young of various ages, kept with their mothers in cages containing Purina Chow.

These analyses showed that during the first day of life, the mean and standard error of the manganese concentration in liver was 1.7 ± 0.2 μg/g dry weight, and this fell on the third day to 0.65 ± 0.03 ($p < 0.01$). Despite the animal's growth, this low level prevailed until the 12th day and rose sharply thereafter to reach 11.6 ± 0.8 μg/g dry weight on days 17 to 19. With the initiation of the elimination of manganese on days 17 to 19, this concentration fell, reaching on day 35 the level of 3.0 ± 0.2 μg/g dry weight, which is the adult level for Purina-fed Swiss albino mice.

A similar rise in tissue manganese but without a marked fall was also exhibited by the brain, the mean and standard error being 0.9 ± 0.21 μg/g dry weight at 1 to 3 days, 0.71 ± 0.26 μg/g dry weight at 10 to 13 days, 1.53 ± 0.06 μg/g dry weight at 15 to 21 days, and 1.16 ± 0.04 μg/g dry weight at 35 to 231 days.

In view of the fact that the increase in the weight of the liver as a function of time continued in these mice after the brain had virtually ceased growing, the above data were expressed also as micrograms per total organ. Thus, it was found that both organs showed a rise in manganese content, reaching a maximum at 15 days in the brain and at 17 to 19 days in the liver.

By analogy to milk from other species, which contains only traces of manganese (2), we assumed the same for mouse's milk. We therefore wondered about the source of this metal in these neonatal animals We found that in addition to their mother's milk, these animals began consuming some of the Purina Chow at approximately the 12th day of life, whereas weaning occurred on approximately the 30th day. When we precluded their eating Purina Chow by making the latter available only to the mothers, we eliminated the steep rise of the metal in the liver (the chief excretory organ for this metal), affecting only the rate, and not the timing, of the elimination of radioactive manganese. This experiment indicated that the accumulation in the tissues of neonatal mice of dietary manganese is dissociated from the initiation of its excretion.

The immediate uptake of injected radiomanganese by the brain could not be compared quantitatively between neonatal and adult mice because of the negligible amounts of radioactivity entering the adult brain over short periods of time. Instead, we injected animals of different ages with ^{54}Mn and sacrificed them 18 days after the onset of turnover. Thus, we found that the percent of isotope given and recovered in brain was 10 times higher in animals tagged on the seventh day of life than in those tagged on the 28th day and 20 times higher than in those tagged during the second month of life. These experiments indicated that manganese enters the neonatal brain at much more rapid rates than it enters the adult brain, raising questions regarding the susceptibility of the brains of these animals to this metal. Indeed, whereas adult animals had been consuming for 155 days approximately 10 mg of manganese per day without deaths, 30 μg/day were lethal over 1 week when given with milk orally to neonatal mice.

In view of the previously discussed correlations between cerebral dopamine and cerebral manganese concentrations in adult mice, brains of young animals were analyzed for changes in dopamine concentration as a function of age. The results, expressed as both micrograms per brain and micrograms per gram, are shown in Table 1. Under identical dietary conditions, the dopamine concentration increased with age roughly in the same manner as did the manganese concentration. Indeed, when the results (micrograms of manganese per brain) from all analyses were plotted against the micrograms of dopamine per brain, the data were fitted by a single straight line with an intercept at 0.016 μg of manganese, a slope of 0.25 (steep toward the dopamine axis), and a coefficient of correlation of 0.935. Expressing these data on a molar basis decreased the slope of this line to approximately 1 without affecting the other parameters.

TABLE 1. *Whole brain dopamine*

	Days postpartum	n	μg/brain mean SE	μg/g mean SE
A	6	6	0.05 $\pm$ 0.005	0.32 $\pm$ 0.012
B	9	1	0.04	0.13
C	13	1	0.118	0.44
D	16	6	0.28 $\pm$ 0.013	0.89 $\pm$ 0.029
E	30	7	0.48 $\pm$ 0.02	1.2 $\pm$ 0.04
F	45	6	0.46 $\pm$ 0.02	1.22 $\pm$ 0.02
G	60	8	0.47 $\pm$ 0.02	1.19 $\pm$ 0.04

p values of A versus D, A versus E, A versus F, A versus G, D versus E, D versus F, and D versus G are < 0.0001, whereas the other permutations showed no differences.

DISCUSSION

The sum of these experiments indicates that whenever genetic, environmental, or maturational factors increased the manganese concentrations in brain, either the cerebral dopamine synthesized from exogenous L-DOPA or the intrinsically synthesized amine was also increased. Although this parallelism is not yet amenable to a single unifying explanation, it indicates some priorities which our experiments must follow. Highest among them is to determine whether the maturation and the function of the dopaminergic apparatus are manganese dependent and, if so, to what extent and how. This must be studied in both normal animals and the manganese or *pallid* mutants, which are uniquely susceptible during early life to the cerebral consequences of manganese deficiency. Our placing this emphasis on early life is strengthened by the precedents of some degenerative diseases, which begin early in life although their manifestations can be delayed even up to maturity.

A more immediate dividend of these experiments comes from the realization of the radical differences in manganese metabolism in postnatal or neonatal versus adult animals. These rodents showed postnatally an inability to eliminate dietary manganese from their bodies, coupled with a high capacity for absorbing this metal and for delivering the absorbed metal into the brain. If the same mechanisms should exist also in higher mammals, one would be led to assume that man might also be susceptible to the vagaries of manganese intake (or even inhalation) early in life. We understand, for example, that industry plans to substitute manganese compounds for the tetraethyl lead in gasolines and in some other fuels. In addition to some economic reasons for this change, one which appeals medically is that lead is known to be toxic to the nervous system, whereas manganese is known to be essential to the normal function of the brain. Whereas the present experiments cannot refute this argument, they do question the possible consequences of exposing young children to the excesses of manganese that can build up, particularly in poorly ventilated microenvironments such as garages, tunnels, and even some city streets. Determination of the requirements for manganese early in life is therefore as necessary as is the definition of the consequences of the metal's paucity and excess. Such work must take under consideration the marked individual differences discussed here, some of which are genetically controlled.

SUMMARY

The diminished cerebral manganese concentrations in the mouse mutant *pallid* were associated with diminished production of dopamine from exogenous, systemically administered L-DOPA. Increasing the cerebral concentration of manganese with excess dietary metal has increased the endogenous levels of this amine in the adult Swiss albino mouse. In the neonatal Swiss albino mouse, furthermore, gradual increases of both cerebral manganese and of cerebral dopamine levels were demonstrated to proceed as a function of age and with a high statistical correlation with each other.

These experiments indicate that one must determine whether the maturation and the function of the dopaminergic apparatus are manganese dependent, while they provide methodology, protocols, and animal models by which such studies can proceed.

ACKNOWLEDGMENTS

This work was supported by the U.S. Atomic Energy Commission, the National Institutes of Health (grant NS 09492–03), the Charles E. Merrill Trust, and Mrs. Katherine Rodgers Denckla.

REFERENCES

1. Cumings, J. N., *Heavy Metals and the Brain,* Charles C. Thomas, Springfield, Ill., 1958.
2. Underwood, E. J., *Trace Elements in Human and Animal Nutrition,* Academic Press, New York and London, 1962.
3. Hurley, L. S., and Everson, G. J., *Proc. Soc. Exptl. Biol. Med.* 102, 360 (1959).
4. Mena, I., Marin, O., Fuenzalida, S., and Cotzias, G. C., *Neurology* 17, 128 (1967).
5. Cotzias, G. C., *Physiol. Rev.* 38, 503 (1958).
6. Cotzias, G. C., in: *Mineral Metabolism: An Advanced Treatise,* edited by C. L. Comar and F. Bronner, Academic Press, New York, 1962, p. 403.
7. Cotzias, G. C., *Proc. Sixth Intnl. Cong. Nutrition,* Edinburgh, 1964.
8. Cotzias, G. C., and Papavasiliou, P. S., *Nature* 201, 828 (1964).
9. Maynard, L. S., and Cotzias, G. C., *J. Biol. Chem.* 214, 489 (1955).
10. Prasad, K. N., Johnson, H. A., and Cotzias, G. C., *Nature* 205, 525 (1965).
11. Van Woert, M. H., Nicholson, A., and Cotzias, G. C., *Comp. Biochem. Physiol.* 22, 477 (1967).
12. Cotzias, G. C., Horiuchi, K., Fuenzalida, S., and Mena, I., *Neurology* 18, 376 (1968).
13. Mena, I., Horiuchi, K., Burke, K., and Cotzias, G. C., *Neurology* 19, 1000 (1969).
14. Mena, I., Court, J., Fuenzalida, S., Papavasiliou, P. S., and Cotzias, G. C., *New Engl. J. Med.* 282, 5 (1970).
15. Cotzias, G. C., Papavasiliou, P. S., Hughes, E. R., Tang, L., and Borg, D. C., *J. Clin. Invest.* 47, 992 (1968).
16. Erway, L., Hurley, L. S., and Fraser, A., *Science* 152, 1766 (1966).
17. Cotzias, G. C., Tang, L. C., Miller, S. T., Sladic-Simic, D., and Hurley, L. S., *Science* 176, 410 (1972).
18. Britton, A. A., and Cotzias, G. C., *Am. J. Physiol.* 211, 203 (1966).
19. Hughes, E. R., Miller, S. T., and Cotzias, G. C., *Am. J. Physiol.* 211, 207 (1966).
20. Papavasiliou, P. S., Miller, S. T., and Cotzias, G. C., *Am. J. Physiol.* 211, 211 (1966).
21. Papavasiliou, P. S., and Cotzias, G. C., *J. Biol. Chem.* 236, 2365 (1961).
22. Cotzias, G. C., Miller, S. T., and Edwards, J., *J. Lab. Clin. Med.* 67, 836 (1966).
23. Bertinchamps, A. J., Miller, S. T., and Cotzias, G. C., *Am. J. Physiol.* 211, 217 (1966).
24. Cotzias, G. C., Papavasiliou, P. S., and Miller, S. T., *Nature* 201, 1228 (1964).
25. Neff, N. H., Barrett, R. E., and Costa, E., *Experientia* 25, 1140 (1969).

Advances in Neurology, Vol. 5
Raven Press, New York © 1974

Trace Metals and Biogenic Amines in Rat Brain

J. Donaldson, T. Cloutier, J. L. Minnich, and A. Barbeau

Department of Neurobiology, Clinical Research Institute of Montreal, Montreal 130, Quebec, Canada

INTRODUCTION

Although trace metals in peripheral tissues have received detailed study, only fragmentary data are available on the distribution of trace elements in neural tissue. In view of rapidly accumulating evidence that metals may play a role in transport, storage, or uptake processes of biogenic amines (1–4), it is important that the interrelation between trace metals and neurotransmitters in the CNS be further clarified.

In an attempt to unravel some of the neurochemical intricacies of the role of certain trace metals in the brain, a study was made of the regional content of the inorganic elements copper, zinc, and manganese in rat brain under normal conditions and also during conditions in which neurotransmitter levels were altered by administration of L-DOPA and reserpine. In addition, the behavioral effects evoked in rats injected intraventricularly with manganese salts were also examined.

METHODS

Analysis for copper, zinc, and manganese in various regions of rat brain was conducted by atomic absorption spectroscopy using methods previously outlined (5). The treatment protocol employed was as follows. L-DOPA was administered chronically to rats for a 5-day period following which brain regional metal content was estimated. Twenty male 250-g Sprague-Dawley albino rats were also given the DOPA decarboxylase inhibitor Ro 4–4602 (50 mg/kg) 1 hr before L-DOPA. Both drugs were given by gastric tube. Sixteen control rats received Ro 4–4602 only. The control animals received saline 1 hr following the DOPA decarboxylase inhibitor. Test and control rats were killed 1 hr after the last dose of L-DOPA on the fifth day.

The effect of reserpine on rat brain trace metals was examined by injecting (i.p.) 30 rats daily for 5 days with 5 mg/kg of reserpine. Twenty control rats received saline injections for the same period. Both groups of animals were sacrificed 24 hr after the final injection on the fifth day.

The effect of exogenous metal administration on rat behavior was determined by injecting cannulated rats (6) into the left lateral ventricle with the chloride salt of manganese, at the doses indicated in the text.

RESULTS

Effect of L-DOPA Loading on Rat Brain Metals

As shown in Table 1, Cu^{++} levels increased significantly ($p < 0.05$) in the midbrain region of rats subjected to prolonged treatment with L-DOPA. Zinc levels were significantly decreased in the cerebellum ($p < 0.01$) after L-DOPA compared to control rats.

No significant changes in the level of Mn^{++} were noted in any of the brain regions examined.

Effect of Reserpine on Rat Brain Metals

The effect of chronic treatment with reserpine on rat brain regional content of Cu^{++}, Zn^{++}, and Mn^{++} is shown in Table 2. In contrast to the results obtained with L-DOPA, Cu^{++} levels decreased significantly ($p < 0.05$) in the midbrain region after reserpine treatment. It is of considerable interest that Zn^{++} levels increased in the cerebellum which is the same brain region

TABLE 1. *Effect of L-DOPA administration on rat brain regional Cu^{++}, Zn^{++}, and Mn^{++}*

Region	Cu^{++} ($\mu g/g$)	Zn^{++} ($\mu g/g$)	Mn^{++} ($\mu g/g$)
Medulla (C)	8.4 ($\pm$ 0.4)	32.6 ($\pm$ 2.6)	2.20 ($\pm$ 0.09)
Medulla (T)	9.4 ($\pm$ 0.3)	33.6 ($\pm$ 0.4)	2.18 ($\pm$ 0.08)
Cerebellum (C)	14.7 ($\pm$ 2.0)	60.4 ($\pm$ 1.8)[a]	2.20 ($\pm$ 0.04)
Cerebellum (T)	13.9 ($\pm$ 0.4)	55.7 ($\pm$ 0.5)[a]	2.40 ($\pm$ 0.08)
Striatum (C)	11.9 ($\pm$ 1.2)	56.6 ($\pm$ 1.2)	2.16 ($\pm$ 0.03)
Striatum (T)	14.5 ($\pm$ 1.1)	57.6 ($\pm$ 2.0)	2.22 ($\pm$ 0.05)
Cortex (C)	11.7 ($\pm$ 1.1)	66.5 ($\pm$ 1.9)	1.86 ($\pm$ 0.15)
Cortex (T)	13.0 ($\pm$ 0.8)	70.4 ($\pm$ 2.5)	2.03 ($\pm$ 0.10)
Hippocampus (C)	13.3 ($\pm$ 0.5)	74.1 ($\pm$ 0.5)	1.83 ($\pm$ 0.15)
Hippocampus (T)	14.0 ($\pm$ 0.8)	76.2 ($\pm$ 2.4)	2.05 ($\pm$ 0.20)
Hypothalamus (C)	14.0 ($\pm$ 2.4)	56.7 ($\pm$ 1.9)	3.15 ($\pm$ 0.52)
Hypothalamus (T)	17.3 ($\pm$ 1.7)	54.6 ($\pm$ 1.8)	4.04 ($\pm$ 0.40)
Midbrain (C)	10.6 ($\pm$ 0.5)[b]	41.8 ($\pm$ 3.9)	2.43 ($\pm$ 0.19)
Midbrain (T)	12.5 ($\pm$ 0.4)[b]	44.9 ($\pm$ 1.4)	2.61 ($\pm$ 0.12)
Olfactory bulb (C)	19.0 ($\pm$ 0.9)	67.3 ($\pm$ 2.3)	—
Olfactory bulb (T)	17.8 ($\pm$ 0.7)	63.4 ($\pm$ 2.9)	—

C = Control; T = Test (DOPA); N = 3 for control rats, 5 for test rats. Figures in parentheses = SEM.
[a] $p < 0.01$.
[b] $p < 0.05$.

TABLE 2. *Effect of reserpine on Cu^{++}, Zn^{++}, and Mn^{++} in rat brain regions*

Region	Cu^{++} ($\mu g/g$)	Zn^{++} ($\mu g/g$)	Mn^{++} ($\mu g/g$)
Medulla (C)	9.4 ($\pm$ 0.38)	31.0 ($\pm$ 0.57)	2.47 ($\pm$ 0.10)
Medulla (T)	9.1 ($\pm$ 0.24)	30.6 ($\pm$ 0.82)	2.36 ($\pm$ 0.07)
Cerebellum (C)	11.2 ($\pm$ 0.12)	49.3 ($\pm$ 1.80)	2.34 ($\pm$ 0.07)
Cerebellum (T)	12.4 ($\pm$ 0.36)	53.5 ($\pm$ 0.76)[a]	2.33 ($\pm$ 0.04)
Striatum (C)	15.5 ($\pm$ 1.0)	60.7 ($\pm$ 1.62)	2.19 ($\pm$ 0.20)
Striatum (T)	14.1 ($\pm$ 1.2)	56.9 ($\pm$ 1.20)	1.70 ($\pm$ 0.11)[a]
Cortex (C)	12.5 ($\pm$ 0.11)	67.9 ($\pm$ 3.72)	2.03 ($\pm$ 0.04)
Cortex (T)	13.8 ($\pm$ 0.73)	71.9 ($\pm$ 2.11)	2.06 ($\pm$ 0.04)
Hippocampus (C)	13.2 ($\pm$ 0.47)	70.8 ($\pm$ 1.95)	2.68 ($\pm$ 0.06)
Hippocampus (T)	13.1 ($\pm$ 0.36)	69.0 ($\pm$ 0.92)	2.65 ($\pm$ 0.08)
Hypothalamus (C)	17.7 ($\pm$ 0.45)	57.3 ($\pm$ 0.98)	4.77 ($\pm$ 0.47)
Hypothalamus (T)	21.4 ($\pm$ 1.0)[a]	60.2 ($\pm$ 2.00)	4.44 ($\pm$ 0.64)
Midbrain (C)	14.0 ($\pm$ 0.40)	45.1 ($\pm$ 1.52)	3.04 ($\pm$ 0.05)
Midbrain (T)	12.8 ($\pm$ 0.23)[a]	42.5 ($\pm$ 0.83)	3.11 ($\pm$ 0.13)
Olfactory bulb (C)	18.0 ($\pm$ 1.31)	63.7 ($\pm$ 0.94)	3.61 ($\pm$ 0.64)
Olfactory bulb (T)	18.2 ($\pm$ 0.85)	66.2 ($\pm$ 1.60)	5.07 ($\pm$ 1.25)

C = Control; T = Test (reserpine); N = 4 for control rats and 7 for test. Figures in parentheses = SEM.

[a] $p < 0.05$.

where Zn^{++} content decreased after L-DOPA treatment. Mn^{++} content in the striatum was also significantly decreased in reserpine-treated animals compared to controls.

Effect of Intraventricular Injections of Mn^{++} on Rat Behavior

As shown in Fig. 1, injection of 25 μg of Mn^{++} into the left lateral ventricle of cannulated rats resulted in a number of behavioral alterations. Of particular interest, however, is the circling which occurred in a contralateral direction to the site of injection.

Somnolence and hypersensitivity were also evident in the Mn^{++}-treated animals. None of these symptoms was observed in animals given saline by the intraventricular route.

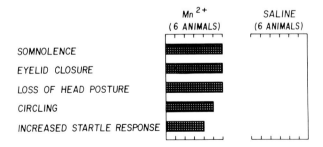

FIG. 1. Effect of Mn^{++} on rat behavior. Rats (six) received 25 μg of Mn^{++} into the left lateral ventricle. Control animals received saline by the same route.

DISCUSSION

Altered Cu^{++} and Zn^{++} Concentrations in Rat Brain Regions after L-DOPA

In order to determine if changes in metal concentrations were related to altered neurotransmitter levels, experiments were carried out with L-DOPA and with a potent amine depletor, reserpine. In rats treated with a peripheral DOPA decarboxylase inhibitor and L-DOPA, conditions which result in a marked accumulation of brain dopamine, there was an enhancement of Cu^{++} in the midbrain region. In addition to dopamine enhancement there is a tendency for the level of serotonin to fall in animals injected with large amounts of L-DOPA (7). Since both dopamine and serotonin are decarboxylated by a similar enzyme, L-aromatic amino acid decarboxylase (8), it is possible that Cu^{++} could play a role in an enzymatic conversion process of DOPA. DOPA may also enhance the level of cerruloplasmin, the Cu^{++} transport protein, or, alternatively, impair the ability of cerruloplasmin to remove excess Cu^{++} from the brain. In this regard DOPA has been shown under *in vitro* conditions to affect the oxidative activity of cerruloplasmin (9). Sass-Kortsak et al. (10) have suggested that Cu^{++} transport is intimately linked to amino acid transport. Addition of amino acids to rat liver slices markedly accelerated the uptake of Cu^{++} into the slices. If a similar situation prevails *in vivo,* the present finding of increased Cu^{++} in rat midbrain after DOPA loading may be explicable in terms of accelerated uptake and transport of the ion mediated by this amino acid. Interestingly, Papavasiliou et al. (11) have found that Mn^{++} is increased in the livers of mice consuming L-DOPA. In patients with parkinsonism undergoing DOPA therapy, some of the side effects encountered at high doses of the amino acid include hypotension, nausea, vomiting, hypotonia, and production of abnormal movements (12). If increased Cu^{++} levels occur in the human in particular brain regions in a fashion similar to that demonstrated in the present study in the rat, it could have a striking effect on the brain's capacity to coordinate and regulate bodily movement, since Cu^{++} is a potent inhibitor of Na^+,K^+-ATPase (6). Conceivably the abnormal movements in parkinsonian patients undergoing long-term DOPA treatment could result from an impaired Cu^{++} metabolism with resultant dysfunction of transport ATPase in discrete brain regions involved with movement coordination.

The levels of Zn^{++} also decreased in the cerebellum after DOPA loading in rats. Since this region is a major center for volitional control and coordination of movement, it is also possible that the Zn^{++}-depressing effect of L-DOPA may result in atypical movement due to faulty regulation of Zn^{++}-dependent enzymes involved in the neurophysiological control of movement. A recent effect ascribed to L-DOPA loading in rats was a reduction in the levels of vitamin B_6 and glutamic acid decarboxylase (GAD) in the brain of animals receiving high doses of the amino acid (13). Pyridoxal kinase, which converts pyridoxal to pyridoxal-5'-phosphate, the active coenzyme of B_6, is also reported to decrease after administration of L-DOPA (14). A reduction in pyridoxal kinase after L-DOPA treatment could be explicable on the basis of the present results where Zn^{++} levels were found to fall in the cerebellum. Pyridoxal kinase is activated in the brain by Zn^{++}. Additionally, GAD in brain tissue is believed by Wu (15) to be regulated by Zn^{++}. Accordingly, the DOPA-induced diminution in Zn^{++} found in the present study could possibly explain the reduction in pyridoxal kinase and thus B_6, and GAD, found after DOPA treatment, since both pyridoxal kinase and GAD are strongly influenced by Zn^{++}. Prolonged administration of L-DOPA has been reported to lead to a deficiency of B_6 in parkinsonian patients undergoing L-DOPA therapy (16), and dietary deficiency of B_6 in rats leads also to diminished levels of brain GAD and gamma-aminobutyric acid (GABA) (17). If a deficiency in this vitamin occurs in the brain of patients undergoing therapy for parkinsonism with L-DOPA, it could perhaps play a role in the pathophysiology of some of the side effects encountered in some patients undergoing long-term L-DOPA therapy.

Since GABA is believed to be an inhibitory transmitter in the CNS, particularly in cerebellar Purkinje cells (17), a derangement in cerebellar GABA metabolism evoked by Zn^{++}-induced GAD deficiency may contribute to the abnormal movements and hypotonia observed in some patients undergoing DOPA treatment.

Altered Cu^{++}, Zn^{++}, and Mn^{++} in Rat Brain Regions after Reserpine Treatment

The possible implications of altered cerebellar Zn^{++} content in relation to a dysfunction of GABA metabolism were noted previously during the discussion of L-DOPA loading in rats. Reserpine administration also led to altered (increased) cerebellar Zn^{++} content, albeit in the opposite direction to that induced by L-DOPA. It is of interest that phenothiazines and reserpine can elicit a hyperkinetic syndrome which is similar to the L-DOPA-induced abnormal movements (19), whereas other investigators have reported an enhanced uptake of ^{65}Zn in rat brain after phenothiazine treatment (20). However, it cannot be concluded from the present evidence whether a common biochemical mechanism exists which involves an effect by these drugs on the metabolism of brain Zn^{++}, thus altering the activity of a Zn^{++}-dependent enzyme in the CNS and producing a dysfunction in cerebral neurotransmission manifested by hyperkinesia. Nonetheless, reserpine increases the activity of the Zn^{++}-activated enzyme pyridoxal kinase, whereas DOPA administration results in a diminishment of this enzyme (14). Conditions which alter the availability of pyridoxal kinase, and thus pyridoxal-5-phosphate, could lead to a dysfunction of regulatory enzymes (principally the decarboxylases) involved in excitatory and inhibitory neurotransmission. In the present experiments it is possible that reserpine may have altered the biosynthesis of Zn^{++}-dependent enzymes involved in neurotransmission, resulting in an increased requirement for this divalent cation. In contrast to the results obtained with DOPA, Cu^{++} levels in the midbrain region decreased after reserpine.

A significantly decreased striatal Mn^{++} was found in rats also after chronic reserpine treatment. This is of particular interest since the striatum is rich in dopaminergic neurons and is especially susceptible to depletion of its endogenous dopamine stores by this drug. Reserpine is also known to reduce the concentration of 3-methoxytyramine in rabbit basal ganglia (22). Formation of 3-methoxytyramine from dopamine is catalyzed by catechol-O-methyltransferase (COMT) which transfers the active methyl group from S-adenosylmethionine to the *m*-hydroxyl group of catecholamines. This reaction under *in vitro* conditions is absolutely dependent on the presence of Mg^{++} or Mn^{++} (23). Although normal COMT activity *in vitro* requires either one of these cations, the situation *in vivo* in certain brain compartments may not be similar and the Mn^{++} requirement could be mandatory. If such were the case, the ability of reserpine to lower striatal Mn^{++} could influence normal transmethylation reactions in this region. Since 3-methoxytyramine is diminished in the basal ganglia of reserpine-treated rabbits (22), reserpine may not only influence O-methylation by depletion of precursor dopamine but also exhibit secondary effects by tying up the available striatal Mn^{++} required for maintenance of normal COMT activity. Substituted tropolones are specific inhibitors of O-transmethylation, and their inhibitory effects have been correlated with their metal-binding properties (24). Reserpine, in the present experiments, also increased the level of Cu^{++} in the rat hypothalamus. Since reserpine administration in animals results in alteration of prolactin secretion and in stimulation of ACTH release (25), the ability of reserpine to influence Cu^{++} levels in this region may indicate that Cu^{++} subserves a role related to processes connected with control of neuroendocrine release mechanisms. Support for this concept comes also from recent investigations which indicate that trace metals can stimulate the release *in vitro* of anterior pituitary hormones (26).

Effect of exogenous Mn^{++} Administration on Rat Behavior

An explanation for the circling behavior observed after injection of Mn^{++} into the left lateral ventricle of treated rats could involve an effect of this cation upon dopaminergic neurons. It has in fact been established that unilateral lesions in the corpus striatum of rats can induce an imbalance in dopamine release so that the rats rotate toward the lesioned side (27). The injection of dopamine into rat striatum also produces contralateral rotation to the injection side (27). Accordingly, the rats tend to move toward the side where less dopamine is available. The ability of Mn^{++} to induce contralateral circling may be due to the ability of this ion to stimulate the release of dopamine in rat striatum. It may also influence the availability of Ca^{++}. Goldstein et al. (28) have shown that the synthesis of ^{14}C-dopamine from ^{14}C-tyrosine, especially in rat striatum, is regulated by Ca^{++} ions. Also, the ability of Mn^{++} to block Ca^{++}-mediated processes at the neuromuscular junction has been found to be 20-fold greater than Mg^{++}, thus indicating that Ca^{++} and Mn^{++} may be competing for a similar site on the presynaptic membrane (29). Somnolence was also quite evident after injection of Mn^{++}. We have found previously that intraventricular injection of Zn^{++} produces yawning and stretching (30). Manganese has been shown to stimulate the release of growth hormone *in vitro* (31). Since we have observed that Mn^{++} is in especially high concentration (endogenously) in the hypothalamus (5), and in particular within the median eminence, it seems conceivable that Mn^{++} can also subserve a role related to neuroendocrine function. The Mn^{++}-activated release of growth hormone observed by many investigators (31) and the somnolence effect observed in the present investigation might be explained by the observation of others (32) that nocturnal growth hormone release is related to the onset of deep sleep in man. Yawning and stretching behavior can probably be considered as an effect of the body to delay the onset of sleep or to reinforce wakefulness after sleep. The possibility that metal ions are somehow involved in the mechanism of sleep via a neuroendocrine relationship is supported by the investigations of Ferrari and collaborators (33). These workers first reported that yawning and stretching could be induced in experimental animals after injection of adrenocorticotropic hormone (ACTH) and melanocyte-stimulating hormone (MSH). We have confirmed their work and have in addition observed that lipotropic-stimulating hormone (LPH) will also produce the yawning-stretching syndrome (30).

   In conclusion, the experiments recorded here clearly indicate that drugs capable of influencing neurotransmitter processes (storage, uptake, or release) also produce alterations in the endogenous content of trace metals in discrete regions of rat brain. Conversely, introduction of trace metals into the brain of cannulated rats produces behavioral effects possibly due to a direct effect on the release mechanisms governing secretion of peptide hormones in the hypothalamus or by indirectly altering biogenic amines involved in brain function. The data reported here also lend considerable support to the hypothesis advanced by some investigators (1–4) of a role for trace metal ions in the mechanism of catecholamine binding, storage, and transport.

ACKNOWLEDGMENTS

   The studies reported in this paper were supported in part by grants from the Medical Research Council of Canada (MA-4938), the Department of

National Health and Welfare, Canada (604-7-812), the United Parkinson Foundation, and the W. Garfield Weston Foundation.

REFERENCES

1. Colburn, R. W., and Maas, J. W., *Nature* 208, 37 (1965).
2. Maas, J. W., and Colburn, R. W., *Nature* 208, 41 (1965).
3. Rajan, K. S., Davis, J. M., and Colburn, R. W., *J. Neurochem.* 18, 345 (1971).
4. Rajan, K. S., Davis, J. M., Colburn, R. W., and Jarke, F. H., *J. Neurochem.* 19, 1099 (1972).
5. Donaldson, J., St.-Pierre, T., Minnich, J., and Barbeau, A., *Can. J. Biochem.* 51, 87 (1973).
6. Donaldson, J., St.-Pierre, T., Minnich, J., and Barbeau, A., *Can. J. Biochem.* 49, 1217 (1971).
7. Goldstein, M., and Frenkel, R., *Nature–New Biology* 233, 179 (1971).
8. Goldstein, M., Anagnoste, B., Battista, A. F., Nakatani, S., and Ogawa, M., *Ann. Meeting Assoc. for Res. in Nervous and Mental Disease* (1972).
9. Nanson, K. M., Austin, D. C., and Aprison, M. H., *J. App. Physiol.* 14, 363 (1971).
10. Sass-Kortsak, A., Clarke, R., Harris, D. I. M., Neumann, P. Z., and Sarkar, B., in: *Progress in Neurogenetics*, Vol. 1, edited by A. Barbeau and J. R. Brunette, Excerpta Medica, Amsterdam, 1969, p. 625.
11. Papavasiliou, P. S., Miller, S. T., and Cotzias, G. C., *Nature* 220, 74 (1968).
12. Barbeau, A., Mars, H., and Gillo-Joffroy, L., in: *Recent Advances in Parkinson's Disease*, edited by F. H. McDowell and C. H. Markham, F. A. Davis, Philadelphia, 1971, p. 204.
13. Kurtz, D. J., and Kanfer, J. N., *J. Neurochem.* 18, 2235 (1971).
14. Ebadi, M. S., Russell, R. L., and McCoy, E. E., *J. Neurochem.* 15, 659 (1968).
15. Wu, J. Y., *Trans. Am. Soc. for Neurochem.* 3, 40 (1972).
16. Mawatari, S., Izumi, K., and Kuroiwa, Y., *Personal communication.*
17. Bayoumi, R. A., Kirwan, J. R., and Smith, W. R. D., *J. Neurochem.* 19, 569 (1972).
18. Roberts, E., and Kuriyama, K., *Brain Res.*, 8, 1 (1968).
19. Carlsson, A., in: *Recent Advances in Parkinson's Disease*, edited by F. H. McDowell and C. H. Markham, F. A. Davis, Philadelphia, 1971, p. 1.
20. Czerniak, P., and Haim, D. B., *Arch. Neurol.* 24, 555 (1971).
21. Jameson, H. D., *J. Am. Med. Assoc.* 211, 1700 (1970).
22. Tagliamonte, A., Tagliamonte, P., and Gessa, G. L., *J. Neurochem.* 17, 733 (1970).
23. Axelrod, J., and Tomchick, R., *J. Biol. Chem.*, 233, 702 (1958).
24. D'Iorio, A., and Mavrides, C., *Biochem. Pharm.* 12, 1307 (1963).
25. Shore, P. A., in: *Handbook of Neurochemistry*, Vol. 6, edited by A. Lajtha, Plenum Press, New York, 1971, p. 349.
26. Labella, F., *Personal communication.*
27. Ungerstedt, U., Butcher, L. L., Butcher, S. G., Andén, N.-E., and Fuxe, K., *Brain Res.* 14, 461 (1969).
28. Goldstein, M., Backstrom, T., Ohi, Y., and Frenkel, R., *Life Sci.* 9, 919 (1970).
29. Meiri, U., and Rahamimoff, R., *Science* 176, 308 (1972).
30. Izumi, K., Donaldson, J., and Barbeau, A., *Life Sci.* 12, 203 (1973).
31. Gautvik, K. M., and Tashjian, H., *Endocrinology* 92, 573 (1973).
32. Takahashi, Y. D., Kipnis, M., and Daughaday, W. H., *J. Clin. Invest.* 47, 2079 (1968).
33. Ferrari, W., Gessa, G. L., and Vargiu, L., *Ann. N.Y. Acad. Sci.* 104, 330 (1965).

Advances in Neurology, Vol. 5
Raven Press, New York © 1974

Effects of Iron and Copper Deficiencies on Monoamine Metabolism

Theodore L. Sourkes, Maryka Quik, and Michel Falardeau

Laboratory of Chemical Neurobiology, Department of Psychiatry, and Department of Biochemistry, McGill University, Montreal, Quebec, Canada

When a metal is a known component of an enzyme system, the essentiality of this constituent can sometimes be demonstrated by preparing animals that are nutritionally deficient in the metal, and then demonstrating that the particular enzyme reaction requiring it now proceeds at a much reduced rate. Other consequences of the enzyme deficiency may be measured. This is the case with deficiency of copper, a metal that is a component of dopamine-beta-hydroxylase. By treating animals with certain chelating agents, it had been shown that the activity of this enzyme in the tissues of various species can be reduced. However, it is always necessary to exclude nonspecific biochemical-pharmacological actions of drugs, including these chelators, and we therefore undertook to make rats deficient in copper simply by lowering the concentration of this metal in their diet. The results demonstrated clearly that copper-deficient rats of two different strains convert labeled dopamine to norepinephrine more slowly than do controls receiving the same diet, with the exception of some added copper sulfate (1). This particular subject has been reviewed recently (2).

The experiments with nutritional deficiency of copper demonstrate that an important enzyme in the pathway of biosynthesis of catecholamines can be affected by simple lack of an essential nutrient in the diet. In other cases, the consequences of a metal deficiency may not be as predictable.

Some years ago when there had been a suggestion that copper is involved in the action of monoamine oxidase (MAO), studies in this laboratory demonstrated successively that copper could not be considered a constituent of a highly purified preparation of this enzyme obtained from rat liver mitochondria (3); that copper deficiency has absolutely no effect on the oxidation of monoamines by rat-liver preparations in vitro (4); and that the deficiency does not affect the metabolism of a typical aliphatic monoamine substrate *in vivo* (5). Thus, several different experimental modes yielded results consistent with the now accepted view that mitochondrial MAO is not a cuproenzyme.

At the time of these experiments we had been studying single and conjoint effects of copper and iron deficiencies in another context (6), but we decided to test some of the iron-deficient rats under the same conditions as those described above. MAO prepared from liver of the deficient rats had subnormal activity (4). Furthermore, *n*-amylamine was oxidized *in vivo* at a subnormal rate (5).

Purified preparations of MAO from rat liver (3) and pig liver (7) contain iron. Nevertheless, our experiments yielded thoroughly unexpected and unpredictable results. Where iron is needed in the action of MAO is not clear. It may be that this metal is required in the biosynthesis of the enzyme. A possible site of action of iron is in the oxidation of the 8-alpha-methyl group of FAD in preparation for the covalent bonding to the peptide chain of the apoenzyme (*cf.* 2).

More recently, because of many suggestions that iron is a constituent of tyrosine hydroxylase or, at least, important for its activity, we have investigated the activity of this enzyme in the adrenal glands and brain of iron-deficient rats. Although there is little change in enzymic activity in cerebral tissue, tyrosine hydroxylase activity of the adrenal glands undergoes significant increases as the rats become anemic (Table 1), and this is evident as early as 15 days after substituting the iron-deficient diet for the nutritionally complete one.

These results are incompatible with the concept of tyrosine hydroxylase as an iron-containing enzyme, but the decision about that matter ultimately

TABLE 1. *Effect of nutritional iron deficiency on the tyrosine hydroxylase activity of rat adrenal glands*

Exp.	Duration (days)	Iron in diet	Body weight (g)	Concn. of Hb (g%)	Organ weight (mg)	No. of det'ns	Total activity[a]	Activity per mg
A[b]	20–34	+	214	12.4	27.8	9[c]	22.2	0.85
		−	134	4.0	24.0	6	28.0	1.18
B	15	+	170	13.8	9.3	11[d]	38.8	4.19
		−	135	6.7	10.3	12	51.9	5.05
C	15	+	126	10.4	16	3[c]	57.3	3.64
		−	93	4.6	18	4	70.4	4.08
	23	+	171	11.9	21	3	56.3	2.85
		−	108	5.4	21	3	81.3	3.83
	35	+	246	14.4	25.5	4	94.6	3.7
		−	138	4.9	20.2	5	113.2	5.7

[a] nmoles DOPA formed per hr
[b] Two replicates (20–25 days and 34 days in duration, respectively) were combined for presentation of results; in each replicate there was an increased enzyme activity in the iron-deficient animals.
[c] Pairs of adrenals
[d] Single adrenals

awaits purification studies. Moreover, we require more data on the iron content of the adrenals in anemic rats of this type. We are also interested in establishing the origin and nature of the increase. An obvious question is whether the increase is central in origin. Experiments designed to answer this question are currently under way. One might point to the diminished growth rate of the animals on the deficient diet. In regard to the latter point, we have sought some effect of starvation; if there is one, it is a decrease of adrenal tyrosine hydroxylase.

ACKNOWLEDGMENTS

This and other current research in the senior author's laboratory is supported by a grant of the Medical Research Council (Canada). M. Q. is the holder of a M.R.C. Studentship. M. F. is the holder of a Studentship of the National Research Council (Canada).

REFERENCES

1. Missala, K., Lloyd, K., Gregoriadis, G., and Sourkes, T. L., *Eur. J. Pharmacol.* 1, 6 (1967).
2. Sourkes, T. L., *Pharmacol. Rev.* 24, 349 (1972).
3. Youdim, M. B. H., and Sourkes, T. L., *Can. J. Biochem.* 44, 1397 (1966).
4. Symes, A. L., Sourkes, T. L., Youdim, M. B. H., Gregoriadis, G., and Birnbaum, H., *Can. J. Biochem.* 47, 999 (1969).
5. Symes, A. L., Missala, K., and Sourkes, T. L., *Science* 174, 153 (1971).
6. Sourkes, T. L., Lloyd, K., and Birnbaum, H., *Can. J. Biochem.* 46, 267 (1968).
7. Oreland, L., *Arch. Biochem. Biophys.* 146, 410 (1971).

DISCUSSION

Dr. Krnjević: There is a point about manganese which perhaps everyone is not aware of. It has been found in recent years that manganese is exceptionally effective as a blocker of calcium movements across membranes. This may or may not be significant in this context.

Dr. Donaldson: Dr. Krnjević, that's an excellent point for two reasons. It is well known that manganese can displace calcium, and Meer and Rashamanoff have found fairly recently that the secretion of acetylcholine at the neuromuscular junction is blocked by manganese and activated by calcium. It has been thought for many years that the most important blocker-antagonist of calcium was magnesium, but it now turns out that manganese has 20 times the potency as a deblocker as calcium.

Dr. Yahr: Dr. Cotzias, have you looked at the brain morphology of the animals with varying manganese intake since birth, and who have had hyperactive behavior?

Dr. Cotzias: Only a very few brain slices have been examined, Dr. Yahr, and there seems to be damage. But I cannot say anything more because the data are not yet fully analyzed.

Dr. Carlsson: Dr. Sourkes reported a very interesting observation concerning iron deficiency. There was quite an unexpected effect on the adrenaline tyrosine hydroxylase: instead of decreasing it, it went up. I wonder if this could be due to a neurogenic activation of the adrenal medulla, as a consequence perhaps of anemia.

Dr. Sourkes: We have some experiments going on in animals with the splanchnic nerve cut, but the results are still very messy.

Dr. Barbeau: Dr. McCann, would you care to comment on the relationship between trace metals and releasing factors?

Dr. McCann: I would like to comment about manganese in this regard. I think it is more likely that manganese is related to the large concentrations of dopamine in that region rather than to releasing factors *per se*. From what Dr. Cotzias said, it seems that there is a parallelism between the manganese and dopamine, and dopamine is located in the median eminence region.

Dr. Barbeau: As you know, dopamine is related to some of these releasing factors, but it is difficult at this stage to say which comes first in this cycle.

Dr. Mars. Just a comment in response to the question that was posed a while ago. We have just completed examination on a patient with severe manganese toxicity. We studied his growth hormone stimulation by DOPA, hypoglycemia, and glycine, and it was intact.

Dr. Borg: Dr. Cotzias, I would like to ask about the form in which manganese is administered. You have not talked about that, and you mentioned at the end of your talk that it looks as if the gasoline companies may be turning to a manganese additive in some form. Is this that same hydrocarbon-bound manganese that they entertained years ago and that seems to behave very differently from other manganese? What can you say about the form in which manganese is offered to the body?

Dr. Cotzias: Well, manganese intoxication occurs usually as a consequence of swallowing, not inhaling as the books say, but swallowing manganic oxide. The compound that the gasoline companies have in mind is the carbonyl which combusts immediately into manganic oxide, and will deliver something of the order of 20 to 40 micrograms of manganese per cubic meter. One dose of about 15 micrograms to neonatal mice was lethal within a week. We have no information about humans. Since we have one species of animal that does not put the manganese out, absorbs it madly, puts a lot of it into the brain, and dies easily from it, I believe it behooves us to conduct some more experiments before substituting an essential metal for a noxious one in gasolines.

Advances in Neurology, Vol. 5
Raven Press, New York © 1974

Some Anomalies in the L-DOPA Response: Recent Biochemical Studies

M. Sandler

Bernhard Baron Memorial Research Laboratories & Institute of Obstetrics & Gynaecology, Queen Charlotte's Maternity Hospital, London W6 OXG, England

When we set out to design a new antiparkinsonian drug, the likelihood, at the present time, is that we synthesize a compound producing a set of pharmacological responses which we interpret as stimulation of a central dopamine receptor. The conceptual model of parkinsonism which most of us carry, in fact, is one characterized by a state of insufficient stimulation of this receptor, whilst the condition itself is thought to derive in some way from degenerative changes in the cells which deliver dopamine, on suitable stimulus, to its site of action. In the light of certain clinical and experimental observations, such a concept is likely to be a considerable oversimplification.

Let us, for instance, consider the drug trivastal (ET-495), which is known to exert a significant stimulatory action (1) on the supersensitive rat central dopamine receptor preparation (2). One might have predicted from this finding that the drug would play a useful role in the treatment of parkinsonism. Yet apart from certain exceptional patients (e.g., refs. 3 and 4) — and it has not yet been possible to identify them in advance on clinical grounds — the drug has proved disappointing during clinical trial. A further example of this type of problem is *m*-tyrosine, which is converted to the pharmacologically active *m*-tyramine by DOPA decarboxylase (5). A good case can be presented as to why this compound *should* be active in parkinsonism (6); and, indeed, in the supersensitive mouse central dopamine receptor preparation, *m*-tyrosine possesses rather better stimulatory ability than L-DOPA (7). When administered together with a peripheral decarboxylase inhibitor, *m*-tyrosine, like L-DOPA, effectively counters experimental tremor in monkeys with unilateral ventromedial tegmental lesions (8) and mimics the action of L-DOPA on the supersensitive rat preparation (8). However, pilot studies of *m*-tyrosine in human parkinsonism, either alone or with L-DOPA, failed to reveal any benefit (9). Nor could improvement be demonstrated when the drug was given with a peripheral decarboxylase inhibitor (10).

Thus, despite their proven ability to stimulate the putative central dopamine receptor, these compounds fall short in the treatment of the human disease. Even the response of parkinsonian patients to L-DOPA is by no means straightforward and can hardly be a matter of simple replacement of lost dopamine, as certain authors would have us believe (11). The delay of days or perhaps weeks before improvement takes hold after drug adminis-tration is at variance with biochemical evidence of dopamine generation in these patients within the hour (see ref. 5). In addition, occasional cases are observed (12) of patients who are refractory to high DOPA dosage yet re-spond to combined DOPA–peripheral decarboxylase inhibitor therapy. Dopamine generation alone can hardly account for such a finding. Some al-ternative qualitative biochemical difference must obviously be sought.

It has recently emerged that major biochemical differences may exist be-tween the metabolism of DOPA in the presence and absence of peripheral decarboxylase inhibition. Far from remaining unchanged in the circulation before crossing the blood-brain barrier for central decarboxylation, when L-DOPA is denied access to peripheral decarboxylase, it is metabolized to a major extent by transamination (13). Large amounts of 4-hydroxy-3-methoxyphenyllactic acid, presumably deriving from the corresponding pyruvic acid, are excreted in the urine; some, at least, presumably derives from transamination of L-DOPA itself rather than of 3-O-methyldopa. It is of interest that the immediate transamination product of L-DOPA, 3,4-di-hydroxyphenylpyruvic acid, is a good substrate for p-hydroxyphenyl-pyruvate oxidase (14). The resulting trihydroxy acid, 3,4,6-trihydroxy-phenylacetic acid, attracts attention on at least two counts. Such a substi-tution pattern is associated with maximal psychotomimetic activity (15). It might be informative to plot the production of this compound against ad-verse psychiatric reactions to therapy. In addition, 6-hydroxydopamine, which brings about degeneration of neurons in which it accumulates (16), possesses just such a distribution of hydroxyl groups on its ring. The pres-ence of compounds of this type should be sought in patients in whom quali-tatively different adverse reactions to those observed in the initial phase of treatment supervene late during therapy. Even without further metabolism to trihydroxy derivatives, the presence of relatively high concentrations of a carbonyl agent such as 3,4-dihydroxyphenylpyruvic acid is interesting for a further reason: compounds falling into this group are highly reactive chemi-cally. They combine, for instance, with primary amines to form Schiff bases which, depending on their nature, may cyclize (Pictet-Spengler condensa-tion) to form pharmacologically active alkaloids (17). There has lately been much speculation about a possible role of compounds of this type in the therapeutic benefit achieved by L-DOPA in parkinsonism.

Because of evidence outlined above that a simple dopamine replacement hypothesis of L-DOPA action in parkinsonism may no longer be tenable, the view has gradually emerged (see ref. 5) that quantitatively minor metabolic pathways of DOPA metabolism are also likely to make a contribution, per-haps acting synergistically with dopamine. One such candidate for this role, proposed by Sourkes (18, 19) on theoretical grounds, is the Schiff base derivative tetrahydropapaveroline (THP), or a closely related compound. THP forms with great facility *in vitro* from the nonenzymatic Pictet-Spengler condensation of one molecule of dopamine with the aldehyde formed from the oxidative deamination of another molecule. Recently there has been considerable discussion (20) about the possibility of this compound and of another tetrahydroisoquinoline, salsolinol, similarly formed from the non-enzymatic reaction of dopamine with acetaldehyde, being "alcohol addictive metabolites." Ethanol is known to promote the formation of these compounds *in vitro*. The suggestion is that certain individuals, perhaps because of genetic predisposition, form larger amounts of these potentially addictive alkaloids than subjects who can ingest alcohol without becoming addicted. This hypothesis has not yet been tested.

The molecule of THP is somewhat similar to that of one of the morphine derivatives, apomorphine. It was because of this resemblance and the fact that apomorphine produces beneficial effects in parkinsonism (21) that Sourkes (18, 19) proposed it as a candidate for the dopamine adjuvant, the unknown minor metabolite, the existence of which has been invoked to account for some of the anomalies in the DOPA response, mentioned earlier. Apomorphine tends to exert its maximum therapeutic effect on tremor (22) in contrast to L-DOPA which initially alleviates akinesia; tremor tends to respond after a longer interval. This pattern is, on the surface, compatible with a slow build-up of an apomorphine-like substance from L-DOPA, THP perhaps, or a closely related compound.

THP itself is known to be a β-adrenergic agonist (20). It has been known for many years to cause a fall in blood pressure (23) and thus might conceivably contribute to the hypotension which sometimes accompanies L-DOPA therapy. The generation of a β-agonist of this type may explain why L-DOPA causes an increase in rat pineal melatonin content (24); β-adrenergic compounds such as isoproterenol are known to foster the production of melatonin by stimulating the N-acetyltransferase responsible for the acetylation of its amino group (25, 26). The simpler tetrahydroiso-quinoline, salsolinol, may under certain circumstances be taken up and stored in catecholamine-binding sites and released by stimuli which normally liberate catecholamines (27). Any *in vivo* role these alkaloids may possess lay in the realms of speculation until recently when my colleagues and I were able to identify them in the urine of parkinsonian patients during treatment with L-DOPA (28). Using gas chromatography–mass spectrometry, both THP and salsolinol were identified unequivocally, salsolinol output being significantly increased after alcohol ingestion. Using deuterated internal standards for precise quantification (29), we have now been able to detect a daily output of salsolinol of approximately 20 μg per 24 hr in normal subjects. Such a finding opens up many new possibilities. It is just conceivable, for instance, that this compound may act as a transmitter in the central nervous system rather than as a false transmitter, as envisaged by Greenberg and Cohen (27).

A search for compounds of this type in brains from parkinsonian patients who have died during L-DOPA therapy is in progress. Their presence as a transmitter might help to explain the otherwise puzzling ability of pyridoxine to neutralize the beneficial effect of L-DOPA (for full discussion, see ref. 5). The Schiff base derivative formed by the reaction of dopamine with pyridoxal (30) might conceivably act as false transmitter in place of the tetrahydroisoquinoline transmitter. Nor need the pyridoxine neutralization effect be unique: it is conceivable that it is, rather, the prototype of a general reaction. Dopamine may react with carbonyl agents coming intermittently from the diet, forming Schiff base derivatives which would similarly act as false transmitters. This sequence of events might provide an insight into the mysterious "on and off" phenomenon (31) for which no ready explanation has been forthcoming. Such an interpretation is not incompatible with the view that this newly recognized adverse reaction represents an exaggeration or a perversion of a periodicity in the clinical signs of parkinsonism which has hitherto gone unrecognized. There are precedents for this conjecture; certain cases of juvenile familial parkinsonism are on record in whom diurnal fluctuation in severity of neurological signs has been a prominent feature of the disease (32, 33).

REFERENCES

1. Corrodi, H., Fuxe, K., and Ungerstedt, U., *J. Pharm. Pharmacol.* 23, 989 (1971).
2. Andén, N.-E., Dahlström, A., Fuxe, K., Larsson, K., *Acta Pharmacol. Toxicol.* 24, 263 (1966).
3. Vakil, S. D., Calne, D. B., Reid, J. L., Jestico, J. V., and Petrie, A., *S. Afr. Med. J.* Suppl., *in press.*
4. Sacks, N., *Personal communication.*
5. Sandler, M., in: *Handbook of Experimental Pharmacology. Catecholamines,* Vol. 33, p. 845. Springer, Berlin (1972).
6. Sandler, M., Goodwin, B. L., Ruthven, C. R. J., and Calne, D. B., *Nature* 229, 414 (1971).
7. Stone, C. A., *Personal communication.*
8. Ungerstedt, U., Fuxe, K., Goldstein, M., Battista, A., Ogawa, M., and Anagnoste, B., *Europ. J. Pharmacol.* 21, 230 (1973).
9. Sandler, M., Corne, S. J., Stephens, R., Shaw, K. M., Hunter, K. R., and Stern, G. M., *Lancet* ii, 605 (1972).
10. Cotzias, G. C., Papavasiliou, P. S., and Mena, I., *J. Amer. Med. Ass.* 223, 83 (1973).
11. Hornykiewicz, O., in: *Parkinson's Disease. Rigidity. Akinesia. Behavior,* Vol. 1, p. 127. Huber, Bern (1972).
12. Markham, C. H., *Personal communication.*
13. Sandler, M., Johnson, R. D., Ruthven, C. R. J., Reid, J. L., and Calne, D. B., *Nature (in press).*
14. Fellman, J. H., Fujita, T. S., and Roth, E. S., *Biochim. Biophys. Acta* 268, 601 (1972).
15. Shulgin, A. T., Sargent, T., and Naranjo, C., *Nature* 221, 537 (1969).
16. Thoenen, H., in: *Handbook of Experimental Pharmacology. Catecholamines,* Vol. 33, p. 813. Springer, Berlin (1972).

17. Whaley, W. M., and Govindachari, T. R., in: *Organic Reactions,* Vol. 6, p. 151. Wiley, New York (1951).
18. Sourkes, T. L., *Biochem. Med.* 3, 321 (1970).
19. Sourkes, T. L., *Nature* 229, 413 (1971).
20. *Lancet* ii, 24 (1972).
21. Schwab, R. S., Amador, L. V., and Lettvin, J. Y., *Trans. Amer. Neurol. Ass.* 76, 251 (1951).
22. Strian, F., Micheler, E., and Benkert, O., *Pharmakopsychiat. Neuro-psychopharmakol.* 5, 198 (1972).
23. Laidlaw, P. P., *J. Physiol.* 40, 480 (1910).
24. Lynch, H. J., Wang, P., and Wurtman, R. J., *Life Sci.* 12, 145 (1973).
25. Deguchi, T., and Axelrod, J., *Proc. Nat. Acad. Sci.* 69, 2208 (1972).
26. Deguchi, T., and Axelrod, J., *Proc. Nat. Acad. Sci.* 69, 2547 (1972).
27. Greenberg, R. S., and Cohen, G., *J. Pharmacol. Exp. Ther.,* 184, 119 (1973).
28. Sandler, M., Bonham Carter, S., Hunter, K. R., and Stern, G. M., *Nature* 241, 439 (1973).
29. Gaffney, T. E., Hammar, C.-G., Holmstedt, B., and McMahon, R. E., *Analyt. Chem.,* 43, 307 (1971).
30. Schott, H. F., and Clark, W. G., *J. Biol. Chem.* 196, 449 (1952).
31. Barbeau, A., in: *Parkinson's Disease. Rigidity. Akinesia. Behavior,* Vol. 1, p. 151, Huber, Bern (1972).
32. Nasu, H., Aoyama, T., and Morisada, A., *Psychiat. Neurol. Jap.* 60, 178 (1958).
33. Yamamura, Y., Sobue, I., Ando, K., Iida, M., Yanagi, T., and Kono, C., *Neurology* 23, 239 (1973).

Advances in Neurology, Vol. 5
Raven Press, New York © 1974

A New Biosynthetic Pathway
to Catecholamines via *m*-Tyrosine

A. D'Iorio, N. L. Benoiton, J. H. Tong, and S. Sharma

Department of Biochemistry, University of Ottawa, Ottawa, Canada

INTRODUCTION

In the last 20 years, many authors have reported the presence of *m*-hydroxyphenyl acids (1–4) and *m*-tyramine (5, 6) in human urine. All of these compounds could have been derived from *m*-tyrosine, which has never been found in the mammalian organism. Coulson, Henson, and Jepson (7), however, reported that *m*-tyramine was formed following incubation of phenylalanine in the presence of rat liver homogenate.

The possibility that *m*-tyrosine is a precursor of catecholamines was first suggested by the work of Sourkes, Murphy, and Rabinovitch (8), who found that the administration of DL-*m*-tyrosine to rats led to an increased excretion of dopamine.

The above findings prompted us to undertake an investigation of the biosynthesis and metabolism of *m*-tyrosine. We were especially interested in finding out whether the latter compound was a possible intermediate in an alternative pathway for catecholamine metabolism.

HYDROXYLATION OF L-PHENYLALANINE TO *m*-TYROSINE

Hydroxylation of phenylalanine to tyrosine is the more common pathway and is mediated by phenylalanine hydroxylase (9). In the present series, we have incubated L-phenylalanine-^{14}C (V) in the presence of tyrosine hydroxylase from beef adrenal medulla (10). The products of the reaction were separated and identified using an amino acid analyzer equipped with a flow-cell scintillation detector (10).

The results of this incubation are reported in Table 1 and indicate that the conversion of phenylalanine to *m*-tyrosine and tyrosine is an enzymatic reaction. The data in Table 1 also show the absolute requirement of DMPH$_4$. As is the case for tyrosine hydroxylase, the formation of *m*-tyrosine is inhibited by α-methyltyrosine and 3-iodotyrosine. The enzymatic preparation also contains DOPA decarboxylase activity, since addition of NSD-1055 increases the formation of *m*-tyrosine.

TABLE 1. *Conversion of L-phenylalanine-¹⁴C to m-tyrosine and tyrosine by beef adrenal medulla enzyme*

Modification to incubation medium	Radioactivity, d.p.m./mg protein	
	m-Tyrosine	Tyrosine
Complete system*	864	4370
Boiled enzyme	17	10
+ 2 μmoles NADPH	823	4312
+ 0.5 μmole FeSO₄	831	4409
− NSD-1055	580	4080
− DMPH₄	34	335
+ 2 μmoles α-methyltyrosine	12	29
+ 2 μmoles 3-iodotyrosine	14	61

* Assay system: 1 μC of L-phenylalanine-¹⁴C (U), 2 μmoles of DMPH₄ (6,7-dimethyl-5,6,7,8-tetrahydropterine · HCl), 2 μmoles of NSD-1055 (3-bromo-4-hydroxybenzyloxyamino phosphate), 100 μmoles of mercaptoethanol, 0.2 ml of N citrate buffer pH 6.0, 0.5 ml of enzyme preparation, final volume 2 ml.

HYDROXYLATION OF *m*-TYROSINE

Although Sourkes et al. (8) had noticed an increased excretion of dopamine in rats and humans after ingestion of *m*-tyrosine, Kaufman (11) and Udenfriend (12) could not detect any hydroxylation of *m*-tyrosine to DOPA when using highly purified tyrosine hydroxylase.

Since the conversion of *m*-tyrosine to DOPA would require the hydroxylation in the *para* position, it was felt that phenylalanine hydroxylase would be a more appropriate enzyme.

m-Hydroxy-DL-phenylalanine was prepared by the condensation of *m*-hydroxybenzyl chloride and ethyl acetamidocyanoacetate and subsequent hydrolysis. The racemate was resolved by the stereospecific action of α-chymotrypsin on the amino acid ethyl ester at pH 5.0. This procedure, described elsewhere for *o*-tyrosine (13), yielded pure L and D isomers of *m*-tyrosine.

Phenylalanine hydroxylase from rat liver was purified according to the procedure described by Kaufman (11). The hydroxylating activity was measured at three stages of fractionation of the enzyme: (a) 22,000 × *g* supernatant, 29.2 mg protein/ml; (b) 10 to 21% ethanol precipitate, 30 mg protein/ml; and (c) ammonium sulfate precipitate, 5 to 4 mg protein/ml. These various fractions were all capable of hydroxylating phenylalanine to tyrosine.

Table 2 summarizes the observations when using *m*-tyrosine as substrate. The formation of DOPA was measured using the amino acid analyzer.

It can be seen that the formation of DOPA is enzymatic, since the boiled enzyme gives rise to no detectable product; furthermore, D-*m*-tyrosine is not converted to DOPA, indicating that we are dealing with an enzymatic

TABLE 2. *Hydroxylation of m-tyrosine to DOPA, nanomoles formed per milligram protein after 3 hr at 37°C*

Substrate	Modification to incubation medium*	Rat liver fractionation**		
		A	B	C
L-*m*-tyrosine	–	42.1	86.6	193
L-*m*-tyrosine	– NSD-1055	0	2.8	178
L-*m*-tyrosine	– DMPH₄	21.7	8.9	0
L-*m*-tyrosine	– NADPH	42.0	87.0	193
L-*m*-tyrosine	boiled enzyme	0	0	0
L-*m*-tyrosine	+ 2 μmoles D-*m*-tyrosine	41.0	–	–
D-*m*-tyrosine		0	0	0
L-*o*-tyrosine		0	0	0
L-tyrosine		0	0	0

*Incubation medium: 2 μmoles of NADPH, 2 μmoles of DMPH₄, 2 μmoles of NSD-1055, 100 μmoles of mercaptoethanol, 0.5 ml of enzyme preparation suspended in 0.005 M phosphate buffer pH 7.0, 0.2 ml of N phosphate buffer pH 7.0, total volume 2 ml.

** *Rat liver*

Fraction A: Supernatant following centrifugation of the liver homogenate at 22,000 × g for 1 hr.

Fraction B: Precipitate of second ethanol fraction 10 to 21%.

Fraction C: Precipitate of first ammonium sulfate fraction 20 to 25%.

reaction. Fractions A and B still contain appreciable DOPA decarboxylase activity, since the omission of NSD-1055 will apparently inhibit formation of DOPA. The pteridine cofactor DMPH₄, conversely, is more important to the highly purified fraction C. NADPH does not appear to be required for the hydroxylation reaction. Similarly, the addition of D-*m*-tyrosine has no effect on the rate of the reaction.

The data thus obtained indicated that an enzyme similar to phenylalanine hydroxylase could convert *m*-tyrosine to a substance which in the amino acid analyzer was undistinguishable from DOPA. This amino acid, when separated by paper chromatography in three different solvent systems, also migrated exactly like DOPA. Furthermore, its fluorescence spectrum coincided with that of DOPA, with an activation peak at 285 nm and an emission peak at 320 nm.

FORMATION OF 3-O-METHYL-DOPA

To ascertain further that the compound formed was 3,4-dihydroxyphenylalanine, the following experiment was conducted. The 22,000 × g supernatant from rat liver homogenate was incubated in the presence of L-*m*-tyrosine and S-adenosylmethionine-methyl-[14]C. If DOPA was formed, it could be further O-methylated in the 3 position, and the product, 3-O-methyl-DOPA, could easily be separated and identified. Table 3 shows the radioactivity of the isolated 3-O-methyl-DOPA. As can be seen, L-*m*-

TABLE 3. *The formation of 3-O-methyl-DOPA from* L-*m-tyrosine by rat liver**

Substrate	Radioactivity of 3-O-methyl-DOPA
	$10^{-2} \times$ d.p.m./mg protein 12 hr
—	4.43
L-*m*-tyrosine	57.10
L-*m*-tyrosine less Mg^{++}	7.43
D-*m*-tyrosine	4.56
L-tyrosine	9.21
L-*o*-tyrosine	4.50
L-phenylalanine	4.87

* Incubation medium: 0.5 μ C of S-adenosyl-L-methionine-methyl-^{14}C, 4 μmoles of L-*m*-tyrosine, 2 μmoles of NSD-1055, 20 μmoles of MgCl$_2$, 0.2 ml of 0.5 M phosphate buffer pH 8.0, and 0.5 ml rat liver preparation (22,000 $\times$ g supernatant).

tyrosine in liver is a better precursor for 3-O-methyl-DOPA than are phenylalanine and tyrosine. In all probability, these substances are more actively metabolized to other products.

METABOLISM OF L-*m*-TYROSINE-2-^{14}C

As an additional proof for the conversion of *m*-tyrosine to catecholamines, radioactive L-*m*-tyrosine-2-^{14}C was prepared (13) and its metabolism studied *in vivo* and *in vitro*. The specific activity of the radioactive compound was 118 μC/mmole. Incubations of L-*m*-tyrosine-2-^{14}C were carried out with partially purified preparations of rat liver and brain (15) and the whole homogenate of adrenal glands under the conditions described in Table 2. Following incubation, the sample was deproteinized with sulfosalicylic acid and the product isolated by chromatography on a 50-cm Aminex AA-15 resin column. Using this method, the amount of DOPA in micromoles per gram of wet tissue produced in 30 min was found to be 0.019 for brain, 0.270 for the adrenal gland, and 0.806 for liver.

Two preliminary experiments have been conducted *in vivo*. Two mice were each injected with 5 mg of L-*m*-tyrosine-2-^{14}C. One hour later they were killed by decapitation and the whole body homogenized in the presence of nine volumes of cold 0.4 N perchloric acid. The clear supernatant was brought to pH 4 and treated with 5 g of alumina, pH 8.8. The alumina was then washed with sodium acetate solution until no further radioactivity was found in the washings.

The adsorbed material was then eluted by treating the alumina three times with 5 ml of 1 N acetic acid. The concentrated eluate was then chromatographed on precoated silica gel plates in a butanol/acetic acid/water,

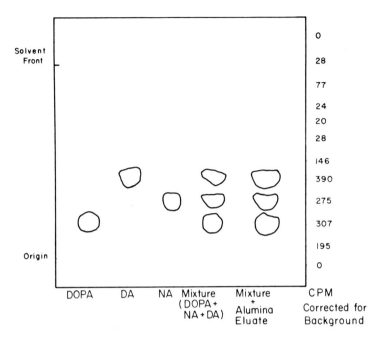

FIG. 1. Chromatography of the alumina-adsorbed fraction obtained from the whole homogenate of mice injected with L-*m*-tyrosine-2¹⁴C.

15:3:5 solvent system. The chromatogram was sprayed with ethylene diamine and the fluorescent spots localized under an ultraviolet lamp. One section of the chromatogram was cut in 1-cm strips, which were extracted with 1.5 ml of 0.5 N acetic acid. The radioactivity of the extracts was determined in a liquid scintillation counter using Aquasol as the scintillation fluid.

The results of this experiment are summarized in Fig. 1, which shows the relative position of the various catecholamines when separated on thin-layer chromatography and the distribution of the radioactivity. It can be seen that the largest amount of radioactivity is associated with the areas of dopamine noradrenaline and DOPA.

CONCLUSION

The data presented above, together with the already published data (10), clearly demonstrate that a preparation of beef adrenal medulla can convert phenylalanine to *m*-tyrosine. The fact that α-methyltyrosine and 3-iodotyrosine inhibit this reaction would indicate that tyrosine hydroxylase is involved in the formation of *m*-tyrosine from phenylalanine.

L-*m*-Tyrosine can in turn be converted to DOPA both *in vitro* and *in vivo*.

These two reactions thus indicate that in the mammalian organism there exists an alternative pathway for the biosynthesis of catecholamines, as was suggested by earlier findings (8). It appears that this pathway is possible with the existing hydroxylating enzymes except that *m*-hydroxylation would occur before *p*-hydroxylation.

The physiological significance of this pathway is not clear, and further experimentation is needed to establish its quantitative contribution to the formation of catecholamines.

ACKNOWLEDGMENTS

This work was supported by a grant from the Medical Research Council of Canada.

REFERENCES

1. Boyland, E., Manson, D., Solomon, J. B., and Wilshire, G. H., *Biochem. J.* 53, 429 (1953).
2. Boscott, R. J., and Bickell, H., *Scand. J. Clin. Lab. Invest.* 5, 380 (1953).
3. Armstrong, M. D., Wall, P. E., and Parke, V. J., *J. Biol. Chem.* 218, 921 (1956).
4. Armstrong, M. D., Shaw, K. N. F., and Wall, P. E., *J. Biol. Chem.* 218, 293 (1956).
5. Jepson, J. B., Lovenberg, W., Zaltzman, P., Oates, J. A., Sjoerdsma, A., and Udenfriend, S., *Biochem. J.* 74, 5P (1960).
6. Perry, T. L., Shaw, K. N. F., Walker, D., and Redlich, D., *Pediatrics* 30, 576 (1962).
7. Coulson, W. F., Henson, G., and Jepson, J. B., *Biochim. Biophys. Acta* 156, 135 (1968).
8. Sourkes, T. L., Murphy, G. F., and Rabinovitch, A., *Nature* 189, 577 (1961).
9. Udenfriend, S., and Cooper, J. R., *J. Biol. Chem.* 194, 503 (1952).
10. Tong, J. H., D'Iorio, A., and Benoiton, N. L., *Biochem. Biophys. Res. Comm.* 44, 229 (1971).
11. Kaufman, S., in: *Methods in Enzymology*, Vol. V, edited by C. H. W. Hirs, Academic Press, New York, 1962, p. 809.
12. Udenfriend, S., *Pharmacol. Rev.* 18, 43 (1966).
13. Petitclerc, C., D'Iorio, A., and Benoiton, N. L., *J. Labelled Comp.* 5, 265 (1969).
14. Tong, J. H., D'Iorio, A., and Benoiton, N. L., *Biochem. Biophys. Res. Comm.* 43, 819 (1971).
15. Nagatsu, T., Levitt, M., and Udenfriend, S., *J. Biol. Chem.* 239, 2910 (1964).

Advances in Neurology, Vol. 5
Raven Press, New York © 1974

Acidic Metabolites of Dopamine and Serotonin in Cerebrospinal Fluid

Theodore L. Sourkes

Departments of Psychiatry and Biochemistry, McGill University, Montreal, Quebec, Canada

The mean concentrations of homovanillic acid (HVA) and 5-hydroxy-indoleacetic acid (5-HIAA) are highest in the ventricular compartment of the cerebrospinal fluid (CSF). By a mechanism of active transport that is sensitive to probenecid, a substantial fraction of these acidic metabolites in the CSF circulating down through the ventricular system seems to be removed at the cisternal level. The cisternolumbar gradient is also quite steep. We have measured the concentrations of these metabolites of dopamine and serotonin in these various compartments, as well as in CSF removed for pneumoencephalography. The injection of air during the latter procedure causes some mixing of CSF in various compartments, so that values for HVA in the fluid that is removed are intermediate between cisternal and lumbar concentrations. In contrast, the values for 5-HIAA are closer to the lumbar concentration (1, 2).

Several groups have recently questioned the assumption that the concentrations of the acidic metabolites in CSF obtained by lumbar puncture reflect the state of the parent amines, or even of the metabolites themselves, in the brain. Bulat and Živković (3) showed that 5-HIAA in the lumbar CSF may come entirely, or at least in large part, from the corresponding regions of the spinal cord in cat. Curzon, Gumpert, and Sharpe (4) reported clinical cases with complete or nearly complete block of the circulation of the CSF at the cervical level: their results indicated that an intact circulation of CSF is necessary to provide the HVA found in the lumbar compartment. This dependence was sometimes apparent in the case of 5-HIAA, but not always. Post, Goodwin, Gordon, and Watkin (5) have shown that in cases of block of CSF circulation owing to transection of the spinal cord, the concentrations of 5-HIAA and 3-methoxy-4-hydroxyphenylglycol are not affected (as compared to cases without CSF block), but the HVA is extremely low in concentration.

In our cases there was blockade of CSF circulation at various levels. When the cisternal transport mechanism is affected in a natural condition (Table 1, Case No. 2), the concentrations of the two metabolites are very high in both lumbar and mixed compartments of CSF. Qualitatively, this is

TABLE 1. *Concentrations of HVA and 5-HIAA (ng/ml) in CSF of patients with obstruction of circulation of the CSF*

Case no.	Site of the block	HVA		5-HIAA	
		Mixed	Lumbar	Mixed	Lumbar
1	Both foramina of Monro (complete)	<10	19	35	26
2	Between ventricular and subarachnoid compartments	266	177	106	83
3	At thoracic level (complete)	188[a]		86[a]	32
4	At thoracic level (complete)	46[a]	<5	80[a]	36
	Normal	65	47	35	31

Cases 1–3 from (1); Case 4, Young, Lal, Martin, Ford, and Sourkes, *in preparation*. The normal values are weighted means estimated from data in the literature summarized by Garelis and Sourkes (1).
[a] Cisternal CSF

the type of effect brought about by administering probenecid to animals or humans. In the other cases, including one with a complete block of the foramina of Monro and others with blockade at the thoracic level, the HVA concentrations are sharply diminished, but the concentrations of 5-HIAA are not really affected. These, as well as the other cases reported by Garelis and Sourkes (1), provide abundant evidence that HVA enters the CSF entirely, or virtually entirely, at the level of the lateral ventricles. Assessment of the various parameters of dopamine and HVA production and of the rate of secretion of CSF (taken from clinical-neurochemical, as well as some animal-experimental investigations) leads to the conclusion that a considerable portion of the caudate nuclei may be involved in delivering HVA to the ventricular CSF (Sourkes, *in preparation*). In fact, the rate found by Portig and Vogt (6) for the HVA production in perfused ventricles seems to be of the same order as in man.

On the other hand, the data in Table 1 for 5-HIAA, along with the other reports cited, make it clear that 5-HIAA has multiple origins within the CNS. Our previous calculations led us to think that as much as 40% of the 5-HIAA in the lumbar CSF is contributed by the spinal cord, the remainder from above. As this estimate depends to a great extent on the concentrations found in the cisternal CSF, it may have to be modified as more values for CSF of this compartment become available. In any case the results in cases of complete block of CSF circulation, without neuronal damage, suggest that much more than 40% of the 5-HIAA in the CSF may be of proximal origin. These data, then, caution against too facile interpretation of concentrations of this metabolite in the lumbar CSF of patients with psychiatric and other disorders.

In the case of HVA, although the lumbar value is only about 10% of the concentration in the ventricles, i.e., the point where HVA is delivered from the caudate nucleus to the CSF, at least we have the assurance that this is coming from the brain and not the spinal cord. The concentration of HVA in the lumbar CSF represents a balance between rate of delivery of this compound into the lateral ventricles, circulation of the CSF downwards, and rate of removal of HVA. Recently we have observed a negative correlation between the concentration of HVA in lumbar CSF and the hydrostatic pressure of this fluid (Garelis and Sourkes, *in preparation*).

ACKNOWLEDGMENT

Research in the author's laboratory is supported by a grant of the Medical Research Council (Canada).

REFERENCES

1. Garelis, E., and Sourkes, T. L., *J. Neurol. Neurosurg. Psychiat.* 36, 625 (1973).
2. Sourkes, T. L., in: *The Treatment of Parkinson's Disease — The Role of Dopa Decarboxylase Inhibitors,* edited by M. D. Yahr. Raven Press, New York (1973).
3. Bulat, M., and Živković, B., *Science* 173, 738 (1971).
4. Curzon, G., Gumpert, E. J. W., and Sharpe, D. M., *Nature, New Biol.* 231, 189 (1971).
5. Post, R. M., Goodwin, F. K., Gordon, E., and Watkin, D. M., *Science* 179, 897 (1973).
6. Portig, P. J., and Vogt, M., *J. Physiol.* 204, 687 (1969).

DISCUSSION

Dr. Brossi: I would like to caution Dr. Sandler a bit regarding his generalizations about tetrahydropapavernoline. From tetrahydropapaverolinol you go to aporphines and from aporphines, you may go even to morphine. The fact is that understanding the stereochemistry of these alkaloids is essential. During the past several months we have studied about 50 aporphine alkaloids, those which have stereochemistry similar to aporphine, a synthetic compound prepared from morphine. These are all very potent compounds. All the aporphine alkaloids which correspond, for instance, to bulbocapnine — which has a hydrogen in an alpha position — are absolutely inactive. In considering these stereochemical speculations, I think one has to take that into account. Second, I would like to mention salsolinol and its O-methyl-esters which are also potential metabolites. I would like to see these compounds isolated, and not only on pieces of paper and represented by all kinds of curves, but unmixed with isomers and other substances. Another point: there is no need to have ethanol present in order to make these methyl compounds. It is well known that the cactus alkaloids, mescaline, for instance, originated from pyruvate and that pyruvate is abundantly available. In the case of tetrahydropapaveroline and the salsolinols, I think pyruvate and corresponding keto acids could do as well to make the corresponding tetrahydroxyquinolines.

Dr. Sandler: Of course, we are beginners in this game, and I will be cautious, but we found these compounds. Knowing of Antoine D'Iorio's work, we looked very carefully for evidence of DOPA production when we gave metatyrosine to our parkinsonian patients. In man we were unable to find evidence of this transformation *in vivo.*

Dr. Goldstein: Dr. Sandler, what are the clinical effects of the combination of ethanol *with* DOPA? Did you see improvement in your patients?

Dr. Sandler: No, unfortunately we did not look into this carefully at the time; in retrospect, we should have, but there were no dramatic changes.

Dr. Boulton: Dr. Sandler, did you exclude the gut in looking at the excretion of these Schiff bases, because I think it quite possible.

Dr. Sandler: No, we have not done that. I suppose we ought to give the patients neomycin and look again.

Advances in Neurology, Vol. 5
Raven Press, New York © 1974

Free Radicals in the Human Nervous System

Donald C. Borg

Medical Research Center, Brookhaven National Laboratory, Upton, New York 11973

Within the framework of this volume, the aim of this chapter is not to report new data but rather to remind the reader of a highly reactive molecular form that can be produced from many biochemicals, including some neurotransmitters and a number of drugs active in the nervous system. I have in mind, as the title indicates, free radicals. Experimental evidence has established as a reality the existence of reactive free radical forms of many biologically important molecules (1). Their participation in neuronal or other biological functions of special interest to the reader of this volume is another matter. I shall not be able to provide hard evidence of a clinically meaningful involvement of free radicals in neurophysiology or neuropharmacology, but I will highlight a few instances that may intrigue researchers in Parkinson's disease.

First, I will refresh the recollection of the reader regarding what a free radical is; next, I will say a few words about the most important method used in their detection; and then I will present a partial list of biological subjects that *are* known to involve free radicals to remind the reader of the potentially far-ranging importance of free radical biochemistry. I will conclude with three examples: (a) a clinical correlation with the conformation of cationic free radicals of phenothiazine drugs; (b) involvement of free radical intermediates in the formation of model melanin chromophores; and (c) a provocative indication that free radicals *may* play a role in brain and neuromuscular excitation.

A reminder of some of the salient features of free radicals is given by Table 1. In essence, a free radical is a molecule with an unreacted or "free" valence or bonding electron (2). This is in contradistinction to most biological and other organic molecules which have even numbers of electrons that fill the available molecular energy levels in pairs. It can be said as a generality that the odd electron configuration is unstable and that free radicals tend to undergo reactions wherein the odd electron is lost (oxidation) or an orbital partner is gained (reduction), thereby producing a diamagnetic or electron-paired product. As a result, free radicals are characteristically highly reactive chemical species, and hence in reactions in which they are

TABLE 1. *Properties of free radicals (F.R.)*

F.R. = A molecule with one unpaired valence electron.
Most organic compounds have even numbers of spin-paired electrons.

Odd electrons of F.R. are readily lost or paired up.
  F.R., therefore, are usually chemically aggressive and short-lived.
  F.R. are essentially half-oxidized, half-reduced species.
    Oxidation = electron loss.
    Reduction = electron gain.
      Combustion and respiration are examples of oxido-reductions.
  High reactivities of F.R. keep their concentrations low.
    Transient F.R. are difficult to detect experimentally.
Breadth, utility, and value of F.R. reactions are enormous.
  F.R. concept touches many chemical problems:
    Oxidation-reduction, substitutions, additions, polymerizations, photochemistry, radiation chemistry.
  F.R. are important industrially:
    Plastics, synthetics, catalysis, etc.
Many vital life processes involve F.R. intermediates.

---

present as intermediates their concentrations are apt to be very low, making their detection difficult. Experimentally this is an important consideration (1–3), but it will not be developed further here. As indicated by Table 1, free radicals are important in many kinds of reactions, but for the present purpose it suffices to emphasize that many vital life processes involve free radical intermediates, especially oxidation-reduction processes such as respiration.

A word must be said about electron paramagnetic resonance (EPR), also known as electron spin resonance (ESR), because this method has been so important in experimental research on free radical chemistry and biochemistry. Simplified phenomenological introductions to EPR are available (2, 3), so only a few points need be emphasized here in order to provide sufficient orientation to allow comprehension of the figures that follow.

Free radical molecules are paramagnetic because of the net unpaired electronic magnetic moments of their odd electrons. Since the bulk of organic molecules are spin-paired and diamagnetic, it is possible to utilize this magnetic property to detect dilute paramagnetic species in a complex matrix of diamagnetic molecules—even within living systems. This is an advantage that few other spectroscopies possess. In the EPR experiment, it is possible to align the electronic moments of individual free radical molecules by holding a sample between the poles of an electromagnet; under these conditions, simultaneous exposure to an electromagnetic field of appropriate frequency (usually in the microwave region) will give rise to a resonance condition wherein quanta of energy are exchanged between the microwave field and the aligned assembly of paramagnets (2, 3). Initially, there will be a net absorption of energy, whose detection provides the basis of EPR measurements. The net absorption of energy increases with the field and frequency at which resonance occurs (usual experimental frequencies are in the radar range: X-band at approximately 9.5 GHz or, less commonly, Q-band at approximately 35 GHz, for example), but the energy exchanged at resonance is always trivial, chemically speaking, and therefore signal-to-noise problems are often limiting in free radical biochemical research.

To improve the sensitivity of detection, phase-sensitive methods usually are used, and this results in EPR spectra that closely approximate the first derivative of the microwave energy absorbed. In other words, as exemplified by Fig. 2, free radical spectra are usually presented as the first derivative of microwave power absorbed plotted against the independent variable, which is the DC magnetic field. Typical free radical spectra have widths on the order of a few to several tens of gauss, usually centered about the region of 3,400 gauss for X-band EPR and approximately 12,500 gauss for Q-band EPR (3).

Although there is much information that can be analyzed from a detailed EPR spectrum, it suffices for this chapter to point out that under appropriate conditions EPR spectra can manifest complex shapes that are susceptible to interpretation. One important component of spectral shape, hyperfine structure, is due largely to the interaction of the unpaired electron with magnetic nuclei in the free radical molecule, and this hyperfine structure (see Fig. 1, for example) can be a powerful aid in identifying and analyzing free radicals (1–3).

For the present purpose, a partial listing of biomedical subjects known to involve free radicals is in order. Table 2 presents several such examples. One case from each category which is of some special relevance to parkinsonism or to CNS neurophysiology and pharmacology will be discussed in more detail: free radical effects in brain and neuromuscular transmission from (A) (the parenthetical insertion in this instance denotes the fact that this role for free radicals is only speculative), some aspects of model studies on melanin chromophores from (B), and from category (C) one point concerning a new clinical insight correlated with an EPR analysis of free radical forms of certain drugs.

It can be seen from Table 2 that many important biological processes are known to involve free radical intermediates, but characteristically the free radicals are short-lived, and experimentation has been difficult. It is not surprising that enzyme actions requiring electron transfer involve free radicals, and one of these, dopamine β-hydroxylase (4), is of some special interest with regard to the biosynthesis of neurohumors.

In a smaller number of cases, generally of less sweeping biological importance, stable free radicals are found in biological materials (Table 2,B). In these cases, the potentially reactive molecular sites on the free radical entities tend to be sterically shielded from reaction partners, or else the free radicals are trapped in relatively inert environments which isolate them.

TABLE 2. *Biomedical subjects involving free radicals*

A. Biological processes associated with F.R. activity
   Normal respiratory metabolism
   Mitochondrial electron transport
   Mechanisms of enzyme action
   Oxidases (including microsomal mixed-function hydroxylases and reductases that detoxify and/or activate many drugs, carcinogens, and other xenobiotics), peroxidases, superoxide dismutase, dopamine β-hydroxylase, ferroxidase (ceruloplasmin), flavoenzymes (flavoproteins and metalloflavins), ascorbic acid oxidase, lipoxidase, etc.
   Ionizing irradiation damage
   All target materials, including biomacromolecules
   Photosynthesis
   Chlorophyll and bacteriochlorophyll, quinones, etc.
   (F.R. effects on the brain and neuromuscular system brain: EEG arousal, phenylhydrazine inhibition)

B. Biological materials containing relatively stable F.R.
   Tissues, in general
   Fresh, frozen, or lyophilized (as opposed to actively metabolizing)
   Melanins (and age pigments)
   Natural pigments (chromophoric components only), synthetic melanins (autooxidation, chemical or enzymatic oxidation)
   Stressed bone, nerve, and collagen
   Crystal defects in bone, ferromagnetic inclusions in nerves, ruptured bonds in collagen
   Woody plants (lignins)

C. Biochemicals in which F.R. have been produced
   Hormones
   Catecholamines (epinephrine, norepinephrine, DOPA, dopamine), histamine, indoleamines (serotonin, adrenochromes), estrogens (steroids, synthetics), insulin
   Vitamins
   A, C, E, K, Q
   Drugs
   Tranquilizers and neuroleptics (including all phenothiazines), stimulants and energizers (imipramine, ephedrine), salicylates, etc.
   Enzymes, coenzymes, visual pigments, porphyrins, amino acids, dyes, uncoupling agents, carcinogens and mutagens, pollutants, etc.

It is only fair to point out that in most of the examples in which free radicals have been produced from biochemicals (Table 2,C), the concentrations of reactants are orders of magnitude greater than their biological levels, and frequently the reagents used to produce the radicals are not biological materials. Nonetheless, these studies are important because direct measurements of the free radicals *in vivo* usually are far beyond the reach of experimental techniques (1), and hence the scientists investigating the roles of free radical intermediates must characterize the chemical properties of the radicals in order to determine if they are compatible with the biological and biochemical situations under study. For example, EPR is seldom able to make useful measurements of radical concentrations below approximately 10^{-8} M in an aqueous environment (1, 3), yet reactive biochemicals such as some hormones and drugs are effective when their biological concentrations are in the picomolar or nanomolar range. Clearly any reaction mechanisms that would at any given instant convert only small fractions of these total amounts to the free radical form would be orders of magnitude below the present limits of detection. Although the possible biological significance cannot be reviewed here, Table 2 (C) shows that transient free radicals are known from several classes of neurotransmitter substances that are being discussed in this volume (1, 5).

To give a better feeling for the possible utility of EPR in biological investigations of interest to readers of this volume, one point will be made regarding some EPR studies of free radical forms of phenothiazine drugs. These drugs are well known as powerful neuroleptics and tranquilizers, but they also have a wide range of other pharmacological properties, including parkinsonian manifestations as a toxic effect. For some years, a number of investigators have concluded that the electron-donor propensities of these drug molecules underlie many of their actions (see the citations in ref. 1, for example). Nevertheless, when attempts have been made to correlate the electron-donor abilities of these drugs with their antipsychotic effects (as opposed to, for example, antihistamine, antiemetic, sedative, anti-parkinsonian effects), no good one-to-one correspondence could be made (6). However, detailed analyses of EPR spectra from the cation radical forms of phenothiazine drugs have allowed Fenner (7, 8) to make a correlation that may be of some clinical utility, one which also tends to confirm that free radical properties may underlie a number of the CNS pharmacological effects of phenothiazine drugs.

By analyzing the hyperfine structures from EPR spectra of radicals of chloropromazine and related compounds, Fenner (8) has been able to determine that phenothiazine free radicals in solution tend to exist in either one of two conformations in terms of inversion at the ring nitrogen: either a quasi-equatorial conformation in which the substituted amine side chain is roughly co-planar with the phenothiazine nucleus, or a quasi-axial conformation (which is favored by branched or bulky side chains). Significant from the clinical point of view is that the quasi-axial conformation of the side chain in solution appears to be associated with antidepressant activity of the drugs, whereas the quasi-equatorial species correlate with neuroleptic potential. In other words, the drugs possess two components of activity, and the different stereochemical properties of the free radical forms direct the predominance of one or the other of the components in terms of clinical effect (7). One may speculate that this is due to the fact that the two conformations of the free radicals do not fit equally well with different membrane receptors.

An example of a biological material containing relatively stable free radicals is melanin. For many years, melanins have been known to contain paramagnetic centers, and EPR studies have played a significant role in our present understanding of the random nature of melanin polymers (9, 10). Although biological roles for melanin other than light screening remain moot (11), neuromelanins are well known, and their depigmentation is associated with parkinsonism (11, 12). There has been some speculation that neuro-melanin may be a by-product of norepinephrine and dopamine metabolism that accumulates in adrenergic neurons (13); however, the melanization of the dorsal motor nucleus, the locus ceruleus, and the substantia nigra during early childhood seems to indicate that neuromelanin is the result of an active neurochemical process rather than a waste product of aging (14).

In any case, the chromophoric components of natural melanin pigments strongly resemble certain artificial melanins made by either enzymic or nonenzymic oxidation *in vitro* (10). Free radical reactions have been documented during the formation of the latter pigments, which are more accessible to study during the process of melanogenesis, so they may therefore be regarded as good models for biological melanin formation, especially because there is evidence that melanogenesis *in vivo* may be mediated by peroxidases (15), enzymes well known to produce free radical forms of many electron-donor substrates (1).

An example of free radical involvement in the formation of a model melanin-like pigment is shown in Fig. 1. The relatively detailed EPR spectrum from the transient free radical anion of L-DOPA [recorded with the use of a fast-flow apparatus for obtaining EPR from transient radical species (3)] is superimposed upon the weaker (note the lowered signal-to-noise) but still interpretable spectrum obtained from the resulting reaction mixture 15 min later, as the solution begins to turn brown. From analysis of the hyperfine structure of such spectra, the nature of the free radicals giving rise to them can often be determined (16), but the only point that need be made here is that as oxidative polymerization begins in these model compounds,

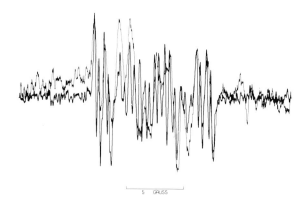

5   GAUSS

FIG. 1. L-DOPA oxidized by Ce (IV) at pH 12.7. Bold line indicates transient free radical during flow. Lighter line indicates 15 min after flow.

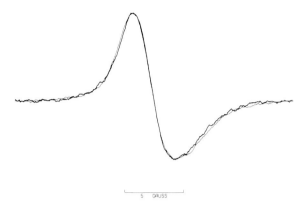

FIG. 2. Pre-melanin from L-DOPA oxidized in air. Bold line indicates air oxidation at pH 8.6. Lighter line indicates tyrosinase oxidation at pH 10.1.

the hyperfine structure begins to change but is still recognizable. Although different precursor substrates for melanogenesis show characteristically different EPR spectra at this stage (1), the spectral detail disappears and a slightly asymmetric EPR singlet is obtained as insoluble melanin-like precipitates form (Fig. 2). Occasionally there are small differences in signal width due to pH effects, but essentially identical EPR singlets are obtained by X-band EPR from various catecholamine and indole precursors or from natural melanins, including neuromelanins (9, 12).

Using Q-band, a higher but less commonly employed EPR frequency, the spectrum of natural melanins can be seen to have a more complex structure than that observed at X-band. This structure changes with pH (10), and at alkaline pH a biphasic shape is found (Fig. 3). This shape is characteristic of indole-like melanins, whether produced from indole precursors or by oxidative indolization of catecholamines (10). For example, as seen in Fig. 3, the typical Q-band EPR spectrum of an alkaline melanin suspension is

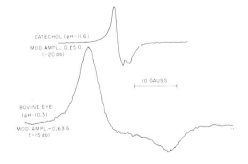

FIG. 3. Melanins (Q-band).

readily distinguished from the melanin-like pigments made from catechols or from plant melanins, which are catechol-like.

The point to be emphasized is that even under Q-band EPR conditions, where melanin EPR spectra have structure, both natural and artificial melanins have similar character (10), so it is likely that the free radical reaction paths demonstrated to occur in chemical melanogenesis may apply also to biological melanogensis *in vivo*. This is especially likely, as noted before, in light of the finding of Okun et al. (15) that mammalian peroxidase, a free radical-forming enzyme, mediates the formation of melanin from tyrosine in mast cell granules, eosinophil granules, and melanosomes. Furthermore, indole pathways of melanin formation are present in human blood serum, where soluble melanin-like pigments ("rheomelanins") form after incubation of epinephrine, adrenochrome, or adrenolutin for some hours (17). In fact, further incubation can give rise to insoluble melanin precipitates which show the characteristic asymmetric EPR singlet at X-band (Fig. 4).

The final example of free radicals related to the nervous system concerns provocative but inconclusive evidence that free radicals may be associated with neuronal and/or neuromuscular transmission. By incubating a number of peptides or proteins with an inorganic free radical, nitrosyl disulfonate, Polis and his colleagues (18) have been able to produce so-called "free radical peptides" which are relatively stable. Polis has shown that intravenous administration of free radical proteins or peptides into rabbits implanted with chronic cranial electrodes and sedated with pentobarbital causes sudden EEG arousal accompanied by activity indicative of brain excitation (18). Enhancement of the free radical content of the administered material by illumination prior to infusion markedly increases the effects, whereas untreated peptides or inorganic free radicals are inactive. The findings suggest the involvement of free radical structures in energy transfer in nervous tissue (18).

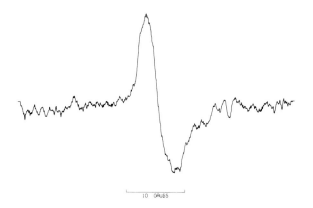

10   GAUSS

FIG. 4. Pre-melanin from L-DOPA after 20 hr in plasma + oxygen.

Tyrosine or tryptophan residues are required for proteins to be converted into the free radical species, implicating these residues as primary sites for free radical formation, presumably with resonance stabilization of the amino acid radicals in the peptide structure. A short latent period between intravenous administration and arousal plus the inability of the carrier peptides to cross the blood-brain barrier suggest the formation of an intermediate that transfers the excitatory action to the brain (18). Polis points out that since treatment with serotonin *in vitro* increases both the EPR signal and the brain arousal capacity of free radical albumin whereas norepinephrine quenches them, the blood-brain transfer may involve these known neurohumors. If this is so, one might further speculate that since free radicals from these neurotransmitter substances are already known (1, 5), it is possible that similar free radical reactions at neuronal receptor sites may be a part of the normal action of these substances at synaptic junctions, thereby initiating intracellular 3′,5′-cyclic AMP stimulation or other subsequent events of neuronal excitation.

Some further indication that transmission of neuromuscular excitation may involve free radical carriers is given by studies on phenylhydrazine inhibition of neurally evoked contractions in insect, frog, and turtle muscle. Typically, free radicals react readily with other free radicals and are thereby scavenged. Hence free radical forms of phenylhydrazine might be expected to suppress free radical processes mediated by neurohumors. In this light, the findings of McDonald (19) regarding phenylhydrazine inhibition are most intriguing: neither unchanged phenylhydrazine nor its fully oxidized products are inhibitory, and the neuromuscular effects observed apparently are induced only by free radical intermediates of phenylhydrazine oxidation that form in the test media (19).

In conclusion, it is my view that although several disconnected examples have been presented regarding free radical reactions of possible relevance to the nervous system, the time has not yet come for researchers in Parkinson's disease to rush out and buy EPR spectrometers. However, it is clear from the reminders I have presented that free radicals are ubiquitous in life processes, so it still might be worthwhile to keep a weather-eye on what is happening over the horizon of free radical research.

REFERENCES

1. Borg, D. C., in: *Biological Applications of Electron Spin Resonance*, p. 265, Wiley-Interscience, New York (1972).
2. Borg, D. C., *Do Free Radicals Control Our Lives? Free Radicals in Biology and Medicine*. BNL 50294. Nat. Tech. Info. Service (1971).
3. Swartz, H. M., Bolton, J. R., and Borg, D. C., in: *Biological Applications of Electron Spin Resonance*, p. 1, Wiley-Interscience, New York (1972).
4. Blumberg, W. E., Goldstein, M., Lauber, E., and Peisach, J., *Biochim. Biophys. Acta* 99, 187 (1965).
5. Borg, D. C., *Proc. Nat. Acad. Sci.* 53, 633 (1965).

6. Matthysse, S., *Fed. Proc.* 32, 200 (1973).
7. Fenner, H., *Pharmako. Neuro-Psychopharm.* 3, 332 (1970).
8. Fenner, H., and Möckel, H., *Tetrahedron Lett.* 2815 (1969).
9. Blois, M. J., Jr., in: *Solid State Biophysics,* p. 244. McGraw-Hill, New York (1969).
10. Grady, F. J., and Borg, D. C., *J. Am. Chem. Soc.* 90, 2949 (1968).
11. Luckiewicz, S., *Folia Histochem. Cytochem.* 10, 93 (1972).
12. Van Woert, M. H., Prasad, K. N., and Borg, D. C., *J. Neurochem.* 14, 707 (1967).
13. Bazelon, M., Fenichel, G. M., and Randall, J., *Neurology* 17, 512 (1967).
14. Fenichel, G. M., and Bazelon, M., *Neurology* 18, 817 (1968).
15. Okun, M., Edelstein, L., Or, N., Hamada, G., and Donnellan, B., *Life Sci.* 9(II), 491 (1970).
16. Borg, D. C., and Elmore, J. J., Jr., in: *Magnetic Resonance in Biological Systems,* p. 341, Pergamon, Oxford (1967).
17. Hegedus, Z. L., and Altschule, M. D., *Arch. Biochem. Biophys.* 126, 388 (1968).
18. Polis, B. D., Wyeth, J., Goldstein, L., and Graedon, J., *Proc. Nat. Acad. Sci.* 64, 755 (1969).
19. McDonald, T. J., *Comp. Gen. Pharmac.* 3, 319 (1972).

DISCUSSION

Dr. Roberts: In this Polis work, is it ruled out that free radicals could react with a sulfhydryl groups on endothelial cells and alter the permeability of the blood vessels?

Dr. Borg: No, I don't think it is ruled out. Polis does not know; he is speculating. And my last speculation is speculation built on speculation.

Dr. Roberts: Would you care to comment about some of the convulsive activities of hydrazine and hydrazides; what would be the free radical forms of those? Supposing you take phenylhydrazine and so on, what is the free radical form and what is it doing?

Dr. Borg: Well, I do not know offhand, but I know free radicals have been studied in the chemical substance phenylhydrazine and other hydrazines. They have not been studied in a biological environment but only as chemical entities.

There is, as you know, a great deal of work in physical organic chemistry. I recall having seen reports on phenylhydrazine and other hydrazine free radicals, but I do not recall what the radical species were.

Dr. Cotzias: There is a recent article in *Lancet,* which I cannot quote at the moment, that reports a theory of parkinsonism on the basis of melanins, in which the fundamental premise is that melanins can release dopamine, in other words, become sources of dopamine. Is there any evidence of such a thing as a melanase? When I was a medical student, there was no lactase and no coagulase—so is there perhaps a melanase?

Dr. Borg: Recently I have seen it stated positively that melanin formation seems to go only in the forward direction. However, melanin can be digested. Mel Van Woert is using oxidative methods for getting some fragments from melanins. Nicolaus also did this some years ago, as Dr. Lerner mentioned. You can pull melanins apart if you try hard enough. I do not think that melanins are very interesting functionally. The presence of neuromelanin may only show that catecholamine metabolism is going on and that a little leak of some of the reaction intermediates has occurred. I think that accumulation of age pigment shows the combination of this plus the fact that lipoperoxy radicals have been around—in other words, age pigment is simply the garbage left by a history of oxidative metabolism. But maybe I'm wrong and there *is* some reactivity to the free radical centers in melanins. I didn't point it out in my presentation, but the very fact that with bovine eye melanin you can see EPR changes as a function of pH means that a significant fraction of the free radical sites, which appear to be distributed pretty randomly throughout the bulk of melanin, is interacting with solvent. This indicates that the meshwork of most of the melanin polymer is loose enough to exchange protons with solvent. Hence, too, melanins can serve as very good ion exchangers as diffusing metal cations compete with protons at the exchangeable sites. The metal ions have much higher binding affinities, so once they get to the sites, they will tend to stick; but some ions probably find their way deep into melanin. In the laboratory one can show by EPR and color changes reaction of melanin with copper, as well as with strong oxidants and reductants. I suppose you could make a case from all of this evidence that melanins need not be chemically inert in the body, but I'm not impressed that they do anything.

Dr. Lerner: Dr. Borg, I am sure that you would agree melanin is very important, not only from a social standpoint but also from an ultraviolet light standpoint.

Dr. Borg: That's right. I should not have implied that melanins are unimportant. I would not say that melanin has no function, but rather no demonstrated biochemical redox function; that is what I had in mind.

Dr. Lerner: With regard to the melanase, melanin is removed by going into other cells in the skin, into the keratinocytes, and taken off from the surface. It is also taken up by macrophages and by lymph nodes. There are many internal organs in animals where there is a great deal of melanin and no pigment cells. Whether or not there is a melanase is a rather important point, and as far as I know there have not been any really detailed studies on it.

Dr. Borg: Isn't there some evidence also that melanin granules can be transferred intercellularly?

Dr. Lerner: Usually the whole dendrite goes into another cell and the tip of the dendrite gets chopped off. This is the way that transfer of melanin from one cell to another usually occurs.

Dr. Goldberg: I use a lot of dopamine that turns black very quickly, especially if I put it in an isolated bath with oxygen; I can prevent this with sodium metabisulfite. Now the question is: when I inject this dopamine into the blood, how do I know it's not acting by its conversion to dopachrome?

Dr. Borg: I don't think you do. In fact there are some reports on this point. Mark Altshule in Boston has invented the term "rheomelanin." He says that plasma with normal oxygen potential has the capability of allowing this sort of polymerization to go on through adrenochromes and on into what I call pre-melanins. This change certainly does happen, but it happens over long periods of time. I don't know of any evidence to suggest that if you take care to preserve dopamine before you administer it that it's going to be changed to dopachrome within minutes.

Dr. Goldberg: Will injected dopamine change immediately into this dopachrome in the blood?

Dr. Borg: I honestly don't know. I almost showed you a slide of work done some years ago where Harmon and Piette used very large innocula of a number of compounds, including noradrenaline, ascorbate, thyroxin, and many easily oxidizable amines in concentration orders of magnitude greater than their physiological one. They wanted to determine if the potential for forming free radicals exists in blood serum. When they used such high concentrations they could see EPR signals; but I don't know what happens when you have a trace of materials, most of which is probably carried on some serum protein.

Dr. D'Iorio: If I remember correctly, this question as to whether there was dopachrome or adrenochrome in circulation was discussed years ago. This was brought up I think by Hoffer and his group in Canada as a possible cause for schizophrenia. I believe Axelrod's group was unable to find any evidence that there was such a substance.

Dr. Borg: Well, there's one other case where the possible occurrence of adrenochrome in the blood has been brought up. There is a very strange hemolysis following massive trauma (some of you may have known of this) where blood just seems to disappear; it is not seen as a bile pigment either. And there is an indication that there is high level of plasma adrenochrome that does funny things to the red cells in this condition. I know adrenochrome can cause hemolysis of red cells, but I don't think the evidence that adrenochromes cause hemolysis in blood "loss" following massive trauma is very good.

Dr. Van Loon: One possible speculative point here. I really don't believe in it at all, but a few years ago when we were studying the possible effect of dopamine on release of hormones from the pituitary, we used a medium that we had previously accumulated from incubated pituitaries, that was, as far as we knew, cell free. We incubated that again with fairly high concentrations of dopamine, and then re-assayed the medium for the hormone and found that we no longer had any hormone.

Dr. Roberts: When you administer a number of these substances, they can be converted into epoxides or free radicals by cytochrome P450 in the liver, so that you have a fantastic potential for generating them.

Dr. Borg: You have just touched upon the subject of an important part of my current research. Mixed function oxidases containing cytochrome P450 appear to play critical roles in both the activation and detoxification of many chemical carcinogens. The critical question is whether the final combining form of carcinogens and some mutagens as they form adducts with DNA (if that is the ultimate carcinogenic act) is an epoxide or a cationic free radical. At present the evidence is more in favor of the latter than the former.

Advances in Neurology, Vol. 5
Raven Press, New York © 1974

L-DOPA: Chemical Modifications and Biological Evaluation

A. Brossi,* W. Pool, H. Sheppard, J. J. Burns, A. Kaiser,*
R. Bigler,* G. Bartholini,* and A. Pletscher*

*Chemical Research Department, Hoffmann-La Roche, Inc., Nutley, New Jersey 07110, and *Chemical Research Department, F. Hoffmann-La Roche & Co., AG, Basel, Switzerland*

The naturally occurring amino acid L-3,4-dihydroxyphenylalanine (L-DOPA) is therapeutically useful in the treatment of Parkinson's disease (1). Its efficacy, first observed in 1961, was firmly established by Cotzias and co-workers (2), who showed that high sustained doses were necessary. The study by Langrall and Joseph (3) confirmed the clinical utility of L-DOPA in 1500 patients who received the drug for up to 5 years. Apparently, L-DOPA crosses the blood–brain barrier and is converted into dopamine (2), which acts as a specific transmitter at certain dopaminergic synapses to restore the function of the brain tissues. Prolonged administration of L-DOPA is required for the continued control of parkinsonian symptoms. However, since side effects can be a limiting factor, it was of interest to develop an even more effective and better tolerated drug.

For this purpose and in view of the findings that dopamine does not cross the blood–brain barrier and that D-DOPA cannot replace its optical isomer L-DOPA as an antiparkinsonian agent (4), the Roche research centers at Nutley and Basel prepared and evaluated more than 100 derivatives of L-DOPA (1). Based on the premise that certain derivatives of L-DOPA might act as an *in vivo* source of dopamine, the structure of L-DOPA was modified by the conversion of the phenolic groups into esters or ethers, of the carboxyl function into esters or amides, and of the primary amino group into alkyl or acyl derivatives. Further variations of L-DOPA involved a combination of some of the above as well as substitution in the aromatic ring.

Evaluation of these structural modifications of L-DOPA for antiparkinson-like activity was based mainly on prevention of tremor and hypothermia induced by the administration of oxotremorine and the reversal of ptosis and catatonia induced by reserpine (5). In the former test, oxotremorine (0.5 mg/kg) was injected intraperitoneally in CF-1S male mice 15 min after the oral or subcutaneous administration of the test drug in 5% gum acacia. Tremor was evaluated visually 30 min after the drug was given. Colonic temperatures were measured with a thermistor 15 min after drug administration. Alternatively, 4 hr after the intraperitoneal injection of reserpine (5 mg/kg), the test compound was given either orally or intraperitoneally and the animals checked after 15 to 20 min for ptosis by visual examination and for catatonia by their inability to move from a bizarre positioning on a fixed rubber stopper. In addition, the effect of a few derivatives on catecholamine levels in the rat brain was determined by standard fluorometric procedures.

Utilizing these parameters for the evaluation of dopamimetic agents, neither the phenolic lower aliphatic diesters nor the isomeric mono-O-methyl ethers of L-DOPA were active. Further, the monoethers were without effect in preliminary clinical trials on parkinsonian patients. This was disappointing, since the 3-mono-O-methyl ether and its 4-isomer are the major and minor metabolites, respectively, of L-DOPA accumulating in the brain and other tissues and thus might be expected to act as a precursor pool of dopamine (2).

With regard to modifications involving the primary amino group of L-DOPA, the N-dimethyl, N-benzyl, and N-acetyl derivatives were inactive in the oxotremorine test; the N-methyl derivative did not elevate brain dopamine levels; and the urethane derivative proved to be toxic. Similarly, additional substituents in the aromatic moiety of L-DOPA destroyed the activity. For example, the 2-hydroxy derivative (commonly known as 6-hydroxydopa) was inactive in the oxotremorine test and neither the 2-bromo, 2-methyl, or 3-chloro derivatives elevated catecholamine levels in the rat brain.

On the other hand, although the simple carboxamide of L-DOPA was inactive in the reserpine-induced catatonia and oxotremorine tests, some of the dipeptides with neutral, acidic, or basic amino acids at the C-terminal or N-terminal position were as active as L-DOPA, whereas the tripeptide Gly-Gly-DOPA was found to be superior (6). However, the overall low activity profile of this tripeptide did not warrant clinical study.

In conclusion, none of the described structural modifications of L-DOPA have led to a more useful dopamimetic agent.

REFERENCES

1. Barbeau, A., and McDowell, F. H., L-DOPA and Parkinsonism, F. A. Davis Co., Philadelphia, 1970.

2. Cotzias, G. C., Van Woert, M. H., and Schiffer, L. M., *New Engl. J. Med.* 276, 374 (1967); Cotzias, G. C., Papavasiliou, P. S., and Gellene, R., *ibid.* 280, 337 (1969).
3. Langrall, H. M., and Joseph, C., *Neurology* 22, 1 (1972).
4. Shindo, H., *Ann. Rep. Sankyo Res. Lab. (Japan)*, 24, 46 (1972).
5. Horst, W. D., Pool, W., and Spiegel, H., *Europ. J. Pharmacol. (in press)*.
6. Felix, A. M., Winter, D. P., Wang, S.-S., Kulesha, I. D., Pool, W. R., Hane, D. L., and Sheppard, H., *J. Med. Chem (in press)*.

Advances in Neurology, Vol. 5
Raven Press, New York © 1974

Unexpected Findings with Apomorphine and Their Possible Consequences

George C. Cotzias, Ismael Mena, Paul S. Papavasiliou, and Jorge Mendez

Medical Research Center, Brookhaven National Laboratory, and Clinical Campus, University of New York at Stony Brook, Upton, New York 11973

Dr. Brossi has indicated various avenues that can lead to developing DOPA, dopamine, and apomorphine analogues that are potentially useful in the treatment of parkinsonism and of allied conditions. Supportive of Dr. Brossi's thesis is the discussion by Dr. Papavasiliou elsewhere in this volume of the current clinical potentialities of injected apomorphine. The present chapter will relate some unexpected findings encountered first while studying injected apomorphine and later with the orally administered drug. We will then try to interpret some of these findings by reconsidering the structure of apomorphine, and will indicate some consequences of this consideration.

INJECTED APOMORPHINE

Studies of apomorphine were undertaken because of the well-known findings by others (1, 2) which had indicated that this complex catecholamine has dopaminergic properties on the animal level.

When injected by itself subcutaneously into patients with parkinsonism (1 to 3 mg/patient), apomorphine diminished primarily the tremor and the rigidity (3), whereas it was less effective against akinesia. Since the symptoms responded in the reverse sequence as they had to L-DOPA (4), injections of apomorphine were also given to patients receiving L-DOPA, in the hope of evoking additive therapeutic effects of these two drugs (5). Indeed these drugs did show additive therapeutic effects, as exemplified by the abortion of the "on-off" phenomenon of L-DOPA with apomorphine discussed by Dr. Papavasiliou. Several of the side effects of apomorphine, however, were not additive to those of L-DOPA, although some of them, surprisingly, tended to cancel each other. For example, nausea induced by L-DOPA was repeatedly counteracted in one patient by injected apomorphine; involuntary movements of the extremities induced by L-DOPA were strikingly reduced in 11 patients by apomorphine injections (1 to 3 mg) (5) without diminishing the symptomatic control of parkinsonism; the sedative effects of apomorphine were generally antagonized by L-DOPA; and the "awakening" effects of L-DOPA were antagonized by apomorphine. Apomorphine given alone (1 to 3 mg/patient, s.c.) did induce hypotension, but when injected into patients receiving L-DOPA, the hypotension was either mild or absent with the doses of apomorphine given at that time. Even by itself, apomorphine had some paradoxic effects, namely, emesis versus antiemesis and increased versus decreased salivation (5).

We are now even more impressed by the canceling of some effects of L-DOPA by apomorphine injections. During unpublished experiments, injected apomorphine was increased to higher doses than those previously published (5). Specifically, injections of 5 mg of apomorphine have abolished in two patients the L-DOPA-induced involuntary movements, first in the extremities, then in the trunk and head, and finally in the face, albeit with the induction of some bradycardia and considerable nausea. It therefore appears that the antidyskinetic effect of apomorphine is dose dependent and affects various parts of the brain sequentially.

ORAL APOMORPHINE

We studied thereafter the oral administration of apomorphine (6) because of the differences between the therapeutic spectrum of apomorphine and that of L-DOPA as well as their differing side effects. Among 14 patients participating in these oral tests, two were also receiving L-DOPA, the requirements for which were reduced during the coadministration of apomorphine. Five among the others showed steady improvement with passing time and with slowly increasing doses. The improvement involved tremor, rigidity, and akinesia, resulting in a diminution of the total disability scores by at least 50%. In some of the less improved patients, however, there occurred diminution or loss of tremor.

The lowest doses at which clinical improvement emerged ranged between 150 and 600 mg/day, as compared with the maximal injectable doses of 10 mg allowed for the emetic use of apomorphine by the U.S. Pharmacopoeia. Although oral apomorphine was given only during the day, the rate of improvement continued to be progressive each day. The progressive improvement of the scores was in surprising contrast to the effects of injected apomorphine, where each injection had only short-lived observable effects. Maximal daily doses of oral apomorphine ranged between 660 and 1440 mg given in six equal portions.

Regarding side effects, only one patient showed involuntary movements, and even these were mild and were restricted to the head. Two patients who were very prone to the development of hallucinations, delusions, paranoia, and excitement from L-DOPA failed to develop such manifestations while on apomorphine, although their parkinsonism had been treated with commensurate success.

The classical side effects of injected apomorphine were also totally absent, with the exception of rare, mild, transitory nausea. Not one episode of vomiting occurred with this standard among emetic drugs when it was given orally in very slowly increasing doses. Oral apomorphine, therefore, had apparently induced tachyphylaxis in peripheral receptors without inducing tachyphylaxis within the brain. Since it had followed in this respect the precedents of oral D-L DOPA (7) and oral L-DOPA (4), oral apomorphine looked like a plausible alternative to treatment, except for the following unexpected, limiting complication which has disqualified this drug for oral treatment of parkinsonism.

Three patients developed marked elevation of blood urea nitrogen (BUN) and blood creatinine, almost without any changes in urinalysis or serum electrolytes. This azotemia progressed for 7 to 10 days after discontinuing apomorphine, reaching highest respective levels of 32 to 133 mg% for BUN and 2.3 to 9.5 mg% for creatinine. After stopping apomorphine these levels declined spontaneously over the next 7 to 10 days, during which symptoms of parkinsonism quickly reemerged. Later elevations of BUN and of creatinine were also found in some of the patients receiving lesser doses of apomorphine. We were able to collect indirect evidence suggesting that this azotemia was apparently both dose dependent and extrarenal in origin.

These findings suggested that trials might now be conducted with N-propyl norapomorphine, which in some animal tests has been 30 to 100 times as potent as apomorphine. One might, therefore, expect commensurate decrease in its therapeutic doses by comparison to apomorphine, so that sufficient therapeutic effects might be obtained with doses which might hopefully avoid azotemia. Trials of N-propyl norapomorphine are therefore in progress at Brookhaven, but the results are much too preliminary for discussion at present.

STRUCTURAL COMPONENTS OF APOMORPHINE

The additive therapeutic effects of L-DOPA and apomorphine could be easily understood on the basis of their both having dopaminergic effects and overlapping chemical structures. The nonadditive nature of the side effects, particularly of those that canceled each other, could hardly be explained on the basis of this similarity. We therefore examined the structural formula of apomorphine for the presence of other neuroactive moieties, in addition to the well-known dopaminergic one (1).

Figure 1 shows this essentially planar molecule, coded in a manner displaying the discernible neuroactive moieties imprinted on it. (a) A dopamine-like moiety. Dopamine is known to be a neurotransmitter and, therefore, this moiety might be functional in the therapeutic activation of dopaminergic receptors. (b) A phenylethylamine-like moiety. Phenylethylamine is not a

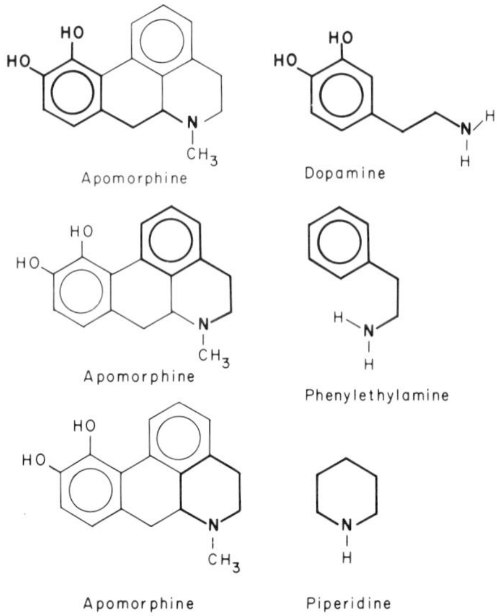

FIG. 1. Neuroactive substances in apomorphine. (Reproduced by permission of the Harvey Society, to which it was first presented on December 14, 1972.)

neurotransmitter but displaces neurotransmitters from various cellular sites (8, 9). Presentation of this moiety of apomorphine to hitherto unspecified receptors might be responsible for the antagonistic effects between L-DOPA and apomorphine. (c) A piperidine-like moiety. Since piperidine is considered as a tranquilizer (10), its presence in apomorphine might account for the sedation induced by this drug, contrasting it to the awakening effects of DOPA and of dopamine.

These considerations might indicate that apomorphine can act like a hybrid drug, provided that one can show that the sum of its parts can equal the effects of the whole in an appropriate pharmacological system: one could perhaps duplicate the behavioral effects of apomorphine on mice with a mixture of drugs which imitates its composition. Such a mixture would be one containing equimolar amounts of dopamine, phenylethylamine, and piperidine. This mixture would imitate the composition of apomorphine only roughly, since it would provide 3 moles of nitrogen for the one provided by apomorphine without providing an N-methyl group (Fig. 1). The two amines included in this mixture, however, are widely considered as almost totally incapable of crossing the blood–brain barrier, by contrast to apomorphine, which readily enters the brain. These two amines are primary and therefore are substrates for monoamine oxidase, whereas apomorphine is a tertiary amine and is not significantly attacked by mono-aminoxidase. We thought, therefore, that the main reason why the primary amines have not entered the brain or have done so very sparsely might be their inactivation by monoaminoxidase on the way to the brain. We therefore pretreated groups of mice with the monoaminoxidase inhibitor nialamide (0.25 or 0.5 mg/g mouse) and administered thereafter to each of these groups either apomorphine or the aforementioned neuroactive moieties, the latter both singly and as an equimolar mixture. Administration of dopamine to nialamide pretreated mice imitated closely the effects of L-DOPA, namely, hyperactivity, rearing, corkscrew tails, gnawing, and stereotyped movements. Administration of phenylethylamine induced head shaking and jerky movements. Administration of piperidine induced sedation. Administration of the equimolar mixture, however, duplicated the behavioral effects of apomorphine, namely, impeded motor activity, head bobbing, gnawing, sedation, and ataxic gait. The effective doses of apomorphine were much smaller than those of the mixture. Similar responses from intraperitoneally injected doses were obtained from $2 \mu g/g$ of apomorphine HCl and from 13 $\mu g/g$ of the equimolar mixture containing its neuroactive subunits.

CONCLUSIONS

The above considerations might perhaps explain how apomorphine can be centrally active, whereas dopamine ordinarily is not (2), and why apomorphine can be synergistic to some actions of L-DOPA and antagonistic to others.

ACKNOWLEDGMENTS

This work was supported by the U.S. Atomic Energy Commission and the National Institutes of Health (grant NS 09492-03), grant OH 00313-08 coordinated by Pan American Health Organization, Project AMRO-4618; by the Charles E. Merrill Trust; and by Mrs. Katherine Rodgers Denckla.

REFERENCES

1. Ernst, A. M., and Smelik, P. G., *Experientia* 22, 837 (1966).
2. Andén, N.-E., Rubenson, A., Fuxe, K., et al, *J. Pharm. Pharmacol.* 19, 627 (1967).
3. Cotzias, G. C., Papavasiliou, P. S., Fehling, C., Kaufman, B., and Mena, I., *New Engl. J. Med.* 282, 31 (1970).
4. Cotzias, G. C., Papavasiliou, P. S., and Gellene, R., *New Engl. J. Med.* 280, 337 (1969).
5. Düby, S. E., Cotzias, G. C., Papavasiliou, P. S., and Lawrence, W. H., *Arch. Neurol.* 27, 474 (1972).
6. Cotzias, G. C., Lawrence, W. H., Papavasiliou, P. S., Düby, S. E., Ginos, J. Z., and Mena, I., *Trans. Am. Neurol. Ass.* 97, 156 (1973).
7. Cotzias, G. C., Van Woert, M. H., and Schiffer, L. M., *New Engl. J. Med.* 276, 374 (1967).
8. Jonsson, J., Grobecker, H., and Holtz, P., *Life Sci.* 5, 2235 (1966).
9. Abelin, J., *Biochem. Z.* 141, 458 (1923).
10. Abood, L. C., Ostfeld, A., and Biel, J. H., *Arch. Int. Pharmacodyn.* 120 (2), 186 (1959).

Advances in Neurology, Vol. 5
Raven Press, New York © 1974

Dihydroxyphenylacetic Acid in the Treatment of Parkinsonism

Arthur Dale Ericsson and Daisy S. McCann*

*Department of Neurology, Baylor College of Medicine, Houston, Texas 77025; and *Department of Medicine, Wayne County General Hospital, Eloise, Michigan 48132, and University of Michigan, Ann Arbor, Michigan 48104*

INTRODUCTION

Ericsson, Wertman, and Duffy (1), in a series of experiments in which the effects of metabolites of L-3,4-dihydroxyphenylalanine (L-DOPA) were investigated in reserpinized rats, demonstrated that dihydroxyphenylacetic acid (DOPAC) and dihydroxymandelic acid (DOMA) are effective in reversing the extrapyramidal syndrome. Further sensitivity studies in the reserpinized rat model indicated that both these metabolites are more effective than L-DOPA in minimizing abnormal involuntary movements (2). For this reason, consideration should be given to the use of these agents in treating parkinsonism in humans.

L-DOPA has proved to be of enormous practical value in the treatment of parkinsonism, but there are a number of dose-related limitations to this form of therapy (3–7):

a. Peripheral side effects, including nausea and vomiting, postural hypotension, tachycardia, and occasionally cardiac dysrhythmia.

b. General side effects, including abnormal induced movements of a choreiform or choreo-athetotic nature, nausea and vomiting, anxiety or lethargy, or both.

c. A peculiar syndrome in parkinsonian patients on long-term L-DOPA therapy manifested by on–off effect, periodic variation of response to L-DOPA, neuropsychological behavioral changes, abnormal induced movements while on progressively decreasing dosages of L-DOPA, and subtle cerebellar features with hypotonia.

A number of investigators have utilized a variety of adjunctive drugs in combination with L-DOPA in an effort to overcome these limitations. The DOPA decarboxylase inhibitors α-methyl-DOPA hydrazine (8–10) and α-methyl-DOPA (11) are the most commonly used drugs. Tissot, Gaillard, Guggisberg, Gauthier, and de Ajuriaguerra (12) reported that these agents increase DOPA delivery to the central nervous system, making it possible to reduce the daily dosage of L-DOPA. However, even though these drugs increase the effectiveness of a given dose of L-DOPA, at the same time toxic central side effects of the drug are potentiated. An alternative approach employing a catechol-O-methyltransferase (COMT) inhibitor (N-butyl gallate, GPA 1714) has been found effective in potentiating L-DOPA therapy (13) and in reducing the central side effects of L-DOPA. Small subcutaneous doses of apomorphine, an analogue of dopamine, also have been found effective (14). All these agents have limitations in potentiating the effect of L-DOPA, however, and a study was begun to select an appropriate means of treating parkinsonism patients. After selective toxicity studies were performed with a number of metabolites of L-DOPA, DOPAC was selected for this investigation.

MATERIAL AND METHOD

Patients with parkinsonism selected for the DOPAC study were of two categories: (a) those who had not previously received L-DOPA; and (b) those taking L-DOPA who had improved only moderately or had developed peripheral or central side effects from L-DOPA.

Specific clinical studies were carried out: (a) effect of DOPAC alone on the symptoms and signs of parkinsonism; (b) effect of DOPAC plus L-DOPA; (c) effect of GPA 1714 plus DOPAC compared with item (a); and (d) effect of DOPAC compared with L-DOPA in short-term alleviation of symptoms of parkinsonism.

DOPAC rapidly becomes hydroxylated nonenzymatically, so that purity of the drug is a necessity. The drug was administered orally in 250-mg capsules in an initial daily dose of 250 mg three times daily. The dosage was gradually increased to 4.0 g per day. Complete blood count, fasting blood sugar, blood urea nitrogen, urinalysis, electrocardiogram, and complete liver function profile were performed every third day, and blood and cerebrospinal fluid samples were drawn for monoamine analysis.

RESULTS

No clinical or biochemical signs of toxicity to DOPAC were noted in any of these patients, but on occasion patients taking 3 to 4 g of DOPAC daily reported having nausea or having a peculiar "dream-like" feeling.

A 0 to 4 point nonweighted system and a 0 to 81 point weighted system were used in scoring the patients. Rigidity, tremor, mentation and speech, posture and gait, cranial nerves, autonomic nervous system, and functional ability were evaluated in each patient. The numerator for each was nonweighted and the denominator was weighted. As the patient's symptoms of parkinsonism improve, the numerator decreases while the denominator increases in total points.

In two unpublished double-blind studies of 30 parkinsonism patients, the mean change while the patient was on placebo was $-0.17 - 1.5/+4.1 - 4.5$. This change represents the standard deviation of this scoring system.

Effect of DOPAC Alone

The mean dose of DOPAC in this group of 13 patients was 1.8 g/day. The mean pre-DOPAC score was 14.2/36.8, and the post-DOPAC score 2 weeks after beginning therapy was 7.3/58.3 (Table 1). The mean change was $-6.9/21.5$ points. Rigidity, speech, posture, gait, and functional ability were improved to a greater extent than tremor and autonomic symptoms. The initial improvement of rigidity following administration of DOPAC, 250 mg three times daily, was accompanied by diminution of bradykinesia.

TABLE 1.

Case no.	Pre-DOPAC	Post-DOPAC	Change	Dosage (g/day)
1	7/37	3/71	−4/+34	2.25
2	14/42	8/58	−6/+16	2.0
3	12/48	6/67	−6/+19	1.5
4	12/51	5/67	−5/+16	2.0
5	17/25	12/42	−5/+17	2.0
6	14/43	6/66	−8/+23	2.25
7	11/51	4/68	−7/+17	2.25
8	16/35	7/59	−9/+24	1.5
9	19/17	10/48	−9/+31	1.5
10	20/17	14/36	−6/+19	2.25
11	14/38	7/61	−7/+23	1.0
12	9/61	6/66	−3/+ 6	1.0
13	19/13	12/49	−7/+36	2.0
Mean	14.2/36.8	7.3/58.3	−6.9/21.5	1.8

Effect of DOPAC and L-DOPA on Parkinsonism

Following concurrent administration of DOPAC plus L-DOPA in four patients with parkinsonism, abnormal induced movements and hypokinesia increased even though a stable dosage of L-DOPA had been achieved prior to starting DOPAC therapy (Table 2). Reduction of L-DOPA dosage from a mean of 4.5 to 2.7 g/day was necessary, but this reduction did not exacerbate the clinical signs of parkinsonism. Improvement was noted in all parameters evaluated. The mean pre-DOPAC score of 12.8/45.5 was improved to 6.5/63.3, or a decrease of $-6.3/+17.8$. The L-DOPA-sparing effect was evident. Addition of pyridoxine (25 mg three times daily) did not inhibit the abnormal induced movements that occurred when DOPAC was given to patients already taking L-DOPA. However, the addition of the COMT inhibitor GPA 1714 to the treatment regimen did provide relief.

TABLE 2. *Effect of L-DOPA and DOPAC*

| | Total score | | Change | Dosage | |
	Pre	Post		Pre	Post
	12/48	11/67	−6/+19	L-DOPA 2.5 g	L-DOPA 1.5 g / DOPAC 2.0 g
	16/35	7/59	−9/+24	L-DOPA 5.0 g	L-DOPA 3.0 g / DOPAC 1.5 g
	14/38	7/61	−7/+23	L-DOPA 4.5 g	L-DOPA 3.5 g / DOPAC 1.0 g
	9/61	6/66	−3/+ 6	L-DOPA 6.0 g	L-DOPA 3.0 g / DOPAC 1.0 g
Mean	12.8/45.5	6.5/63.3	−6.3/17.8	4.5 g	L-DOPA 2.8 g / DOPAC 1.4 g

Effect of DOPAC Plus COMT Inhibitor (GPA 1714)

COMT is the principal means of degradation of DOPAC. The product of this process is homovanillic acid (HVA). The addition of GPA 1714, 500 mg three times daily, by those who are taking DOPAC should further alleviate the signs and symptoms of parkinsonism. In four patients (Table 3) evaluated prior to DOPAC therapy, the mean score was 15.3/36.5. After taking DOPAC in a dosage of 2.25 mg/day, the mean score improved to 7.8/57.3, or a change of −7.5/+20.8. GPA 1714, 2.5 g/day, was added in divided doses, and the mean score became 5.5/65.13, or a change of −2.3/+8.0. Improvement was noted between the pre-DOPAC and the post-DOPAC score and the post-DOPAC plus GPA 1714 score.

TABLE 3. *Pre-DOPAC + DOPAC + GPA 1714*

Case no.	Pre-DOPAC A Score	DOPAC B			GPA 1714 C		
		Score	Change	Dosage	Score	Change	Dosage
1	14/43	6/66	−8/+23	(2.25 g/day)	3/75	−3/+9	1.5 g
2	11/51	4/68	−7/+17	(2.25 g/day)	2/74	−2/+6	1.5 g
3	20/17	14/36	−6/+19	(2.25 g/day)	11/48	−4/+12	1.5 g
4	16/35	7/59	−9/+24	(2.25 g)	6/64	−1/+5	1.5 g
Mean	(15.3/36.5)	7.8/57.3 (−7.5/+20.8)			5.5/65.3 (−2.3/+8.0)		

Comparison of DOPAC and L-DOPA in Same Patients

A single-blind study was performed in four patients (Table 4). Mean changes from the pre-DOPAC score to the post-DOPAC score (2.0 g/day) was −9.0/+33.3. DOPAC was discontinued, and each patient was placed on L-DOPA and the dosage gradually increased to a mean of 4.5 g/day in divided daily doses. The mean change (DOPAC to L-DOPA) was +3.2/−7.5. Although the number of patients in this element of the study is small, the evidence suggests that DOPAC is as effective as L-DOPA.

TABLE 4.

Case no.	Pre-DOPAC Period I	DOPAC (2.0 g) Period II	L-DOPA (4.5 g) Period III
1	17/25	12/42 (−5/+17)	15/34 (+3/−12)
2	19/17	10/48 (−9/+31)	15/41 (+5/−7)
3	14/42	8/58 (−6/+16)	9/56 (+1/−2)
4	19/13	12/49 (−7/+36)	16/27 (+4/−9)
Mean		(−9/+33.3)	(+3.2/−7.5)

DISCUSSION

DOPAC given intravenously in two patients and orally in 14 patients with parkinsonism had the remarkable effect of partially reversing signs and symptoms of the disease without producing the central or peripheral toxic effects that occur with L-DOPA therapy. Biochemical alterations in DOPAC, HVA, 3-O-methyl-DOPA in cerebrospinal fluid, and urinary secretion of these metabolites in patients with parkinsonism who are taking L-DOPA have been evaluated by Szpunar, Ericsson, and McCann (15), Ericsson, Sharpless, Honos, Szpunar, and McCann (16), Sharpless, Ericsson, and McCann (17), and Sharpless and McCann (18).

The specific effects of treatment with DOPAC alone, DOPAC versus L-DOPA, and DOPAC plus L-DOPA demonstrate the efficacy and need for further controlled trials with this drug in patients with parkinsonism.

SUMMARY

Dihydroxyphenylacetic acid (DOPAC) was given to 14 patients with Parkinson's disease. A comparative study of the effect of DOPAC alone, DOPAC versus L-3,4-dihydroxyphenylalanine (L-DOPA), and DOPAC plus L-DOPA demonstrated the effectiveness of DOPAC in treatment of patients with the signs and symptoms of Parkinson's disease. Remarkably few toxic side effects were noted. DOPAC used in combination with L-DOPA has an L-DOPA-sparing action.

ACKNOWLEDGMENTS

The drug GPA 1714 used in this study was kindly supplied by Geigy Pharmaceuticals.

REFERENCES

1. Ericsson, A. D., Wertman, B. G., and Duffy, K. M., *Neurology* 21, 1023 (1971).
2. Ericsson, A. D., and Wertman, B. G., *Neurology* 21, 1129 (1971).
3. Barbeau, A., *Can. Med. Ass. J.* 101, 791 (1969).
4. Van Woert, M. H., and Weintraub, M. I., *Lancet* 1, 1015 (1971).
5. Cotzias, G. C., Papavasiliou, P. S., Ginos, J., Steck, A., and Düby, S., *Ann. Rev. Med.* 22, 305 (1971).
6. Martin, W. E., *J. Am. Med. Ass.* 216, 1979 (1971).
7. Muenter, M. D., and Tyce, G. M., *Mayo Clin. Proc.* 46, 231 (1971).
8. Yahr, M. D., Duvoisin, R. C., Mendoza, M. R., Shear, M. J., and Barrett, R. E., *Trans. Am. Neurol. Ass.* 96, 55 (1971).
9. Yahr, M. D., and Duvoisin, R. C., *J. Am. Med. Ass.* 216, 2141 (1971).
10. Cotzias, G. C., Tang, L., Ginos, J. Z., Nicholson, A. R., Jr., and Papavasiliou, P. S., *Nature* 231, 533 (1971).
11. Sweet, R., Lee, J., and McDowell, F., *Trans. Am. Neurol. Ass.* 96, 59 (1971).
12. Tissot, R., Gaillard, J. M., Guggisberg, M., Gauthier, G., and de Ajuriaguerra, J., *Presse Med.* 77, 619 (1969).
13. Ericsson, A. D., *J. Neurol. Sci.* 14, 193 (1971).
14. Feature Article, *Med. World News,* May 7, 1971.
15. Szpunar, W. E., Ericsson, A. D., and McCann, D. S., *Clin. Chem. Acta* 35, 209 (1971).
16. Ericsson, A. D., Sharpless, N. S., Honos, E., Szpunar, W. E., and McCann, D. S., in: L-*DOPA and Parkinsonism,* F. A. Davis, Philadelphia, 1970, p. 217.
17. Sharpless, N. S., Ericsson, A. D., and McCann, D. S., *Neurology* 21, 540 (1971).
18. Sharpless, N. S., and McCann, D. S., *Clin. Chem. Acta* 31, 155 (1971).

Advances in Neurology, Vol. 5
Raven Press, New York © 1974

Apomorphine Derivatives and Dopaminergic Activity

Samarthji Lal and Theodore L. Sourkes

Laboratory of Chemical Neurobiology, Department of Psychiatry, McGill University, Montreal, Quebec, Canada

Interest has centered around apomorphine as a tool to explore the role of dopaminergic mechanisms in extrapyramidal disorders (1, 2) and in anterior pituitary hormone release (3). Apomorphine has also been tested as a potential agent in the treatment of Parkinson's disease (1, 4–7).

Apomorphine has certain advantages over L-DOPA in that it does not have to be metabolized to another compound to be effective. It crosses the blood-brain barrier readily and acts directly on dopamine receptor sites (8–11). However, the compound is poorly absorbed from the gut and its duration of action is short. In the rat a dose of 10 mg/kg induces stereotyped behavior lasting 65 min, and the duration is proportional to the logarithm of the dose (12). The duration can be prolonged by interference with the metabolic degradation of apomorphine by catechol-O-methyltransferase inhibitors and by drugs which themselves undergo glucuronidation (13), but large doses of these drugs must be administered to double the duration of action.

An alternative approach has been to search for a long-acting dopaminergic drug. Various authors have investigated a variety of aporphine alkaloids as possible candidates (14–16). Lal et al. (16) used induction of stereotyped behavior, reversal of the reserpine syndrome, and reduction of the concentration of HVA in the rat as screening methods for potential dopaminergic action. Of the series of 11 compounds tested, only apocodeine and methylenedioxyaporphine were active on these tests but were very much less potent than apomorphine. Koch and Cannon (17) have investigated various N-alkyl and N-allyl derivatives of apomorphine for their effects on gnawing potency in mice, pecking potency in pigeons, and emesis in pigeons and dogs. Of the 11 compounds tested, N-ethylnorapomorphine was about three times more potent than apomorphine in inducing gnawing in mice and pecking in pigeons, but also three times as potent in inducing emesis in dogs. N-(*n*-Propyl)-norapomorphine had a potency similar to that of apomorphine, but the other compounds were all less effective in inducing compulsive behavior in mouse and pigeon.

ACKNOWLEDGMENT

The work in the authors' laboratories is supported by grants from the Medical Research Council (Canada).

REFERENCES

1. Cotzias, G. C., Papavasiliou, P. A., Fehling, C., Kaufman, G., and Mena, I., *New Engl. J. Med.* 282, 31 (1970).
2. Lal, S., de la Vega, C. E., Garelis, E. V., and Sourkes, T. L., *Psychiat. Neurolog. Neurochirurg.* 76, 113 (1973).
3. Lal, S., de la Vega, C. E., Sourkes, T. L., and Friesen, H. G., *Lancet* 2, 661 (1972).
4. Schwab, R. S., Amador, L. V., and Lettvin, J. Y., *Trans. Amer. Neurol. Ass.* 76, 251 (1951).
5. Braham, J., Sarova-Pinhas, I., and Goldhammer, Y., *Brit. Med. J.,* 3, 768 (1970).
6. Struppler, A., and Von Uexküll, T., *Zeit. klin. Med.* 152, 46 (1953).
7. Von Uexküll, T., *Verhandl. Deutsch. Gesellsch. Inn. Med.* 59, 104 (1953).
8. Andén, N.-E., Rubenson, A., Fuxe, K., and Hökfelt, T., *J. Pharm. Pharmacol.* 19, 627 (1967).
9. Butcher, L. L., and Andén, N.-E., *Europ. J. Pharmacol.* 6, 255 (1969).
10. Ernst, A. M., *Psychopharmacologia* 10, 316 (1967).
11. Roos, B. E., *J. Pharm. Pharmacol.* 21, 263 (1969).
12. Lal, S., and Sourkes, T. L., *Arch. Int. Pharmacodyn.* 202, 171 (1972).
13. Missala, K., Lal, S., and Sourkes, T. L., *Europ. J. Pharmacol.* 22, 54 (1973).
14. Granchelli, F. E., Neumeyer, J. L., Fuxe, K., Ungerstedt, U., and Corrodi, H., *Pharmacologist* 13, 252 (1971).
15. Cannon, J. G., Smith, R. V., Modiri, A., Sood, S. P., Borgman, R. J., and Aleem, M. A., *J. Med. Chem.* 15, 273 (1972).
16. Lal, S., Sourkes, T. L., Missala, K., and Belendiuk, G., *Europ. J. Pharmacol.* 20, 71 (1972).
17. Koch, M. V., and Cannon, J. G., *J. Med. Chem.* 11, 977 (1968).

Advances in Neurology, Vol. 5
Raven Press, New York © 1974

3-O-Methyldopa in Parkinson's Disease

Manfred D. Muenter, Nansie S. Sharpless, and
Gertrude M. Tyce

Mayo Clinic and Mayo Foundation, Rochester, Minnesota 55901

In patients on L-DOPA therapy for Parkinson's disease, clinical improvement consists of two distinct types, long-duration improvement (lasting
3 to 5 days) and short-duration improvement (lasting 1 to 4 hr) (1). Most
patients show a mixture of the two responses. Figure 1 shows data from a
patient, on chronic L-DOPA therapy, with marked short-duration improvement but no long-duration improvement. The disability score prior to treatment with L-DOPA had been 51 (0 is normal and 64 is maximal disability).
The disability score in the fasting state 10 hr after the last previous dose of
L-DOPA was 52, indicating that the patient's condition at this time was as
poor as prior to L-DOPA therapy. After a 1-g dose of L-DOPA, the disability score decreased to 20; within 4 hr it was back to 51, the pretreatment

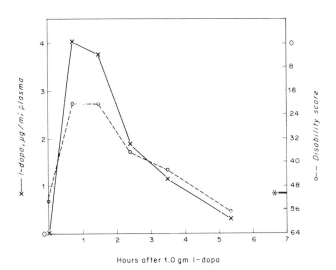

FIG. 1. Lack of difference between fasting disability (first circle) and disability prior to
L-DOPA therapy (*) indicates lack of long-duration improvement. Transient decrease of
disability between examinations 1 and 6, along with a transient increase in plasma concentration of DOPA, indicates marked short-duration improvement.

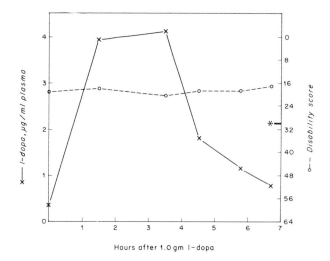

Hours after 1.0 gm l-dopa

FIG. 2. Moderate long-duration improvement is indicated by the decrease of fasting disability (first open circle) as compared with disability prior to L-DOPA therapy (*). The absence of a significant decrease in disability during the period of observation and during the transient increase in concentration of DOPA in plasma indicates lack of short-duration improvement. From (1).

level. The short-duration improvement corresponded in its time course with the transient increase in concentration of DOPA in plasma.

Figure 2 shows data from a patient with long-duration but no short-duration improvement. The pretreatment disability score had been 29; in the fasting state it was 18, indicating, in contrast to the previous patient, that significant improvement was still present 10 hr after the last dose of L-DOPA and when the concentration of DOPA in plasma was insignificant. In contrast to the previous patient, disability remained unchanged after a 1-g dose of L-DOPA although the concentration of DOPA in plasma increased markedly. This type of improvement subsides only 3 to 5 days after L-DOPA therapy is stopped.

OBSERVATIONS

It was in regard to long-duration improvement that we became interested in 3-O-methyldopa (3-OMD), a metabolite of L-DOPA found in plasma of patients on chronic L-DOPA therapy. Its concentrations are higher and more stable than those of DOPA (Fig. 3) (2, 3). Figure 4 shows measurements of disability in the fasting state only (indicating the degree of long-duration improvement compared with the pretreatment disability score of 45). A positive correlation, significant at the 0.001 level, was found between long-duration improvement and concentration of 3-OMD in plasma of each

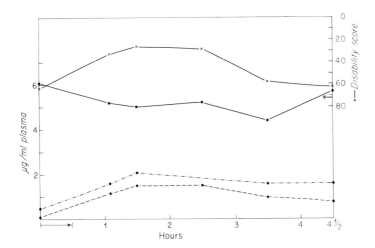

FIG. 3. Plasma concentrations of DOPA (•– – – •), 3-O-methyldopa (•———•), and HVA (•·—·—·—·•) and disability score (x———x) after 11.45 mg/kg dose (arrow) of L-DOPA (750-mg capsule); patient had been on L-DOPA therapy for 18 months. Because of dysphagia, the dose was spread over a 30-min period. Total dose during the preceding 72 hr was 147.97 mg/kg (9.75 g). Pretreatment disability score (*) was 72. Note little long-duration improvement, high fasting concentration of 3-OMD which decreases after the L-DOPA dose, and marked short-duration improvement. From (2).

patient studied (2). However, if the relationship between long-duration improvement and concentration of 3-OMD in plasma is compared between patients, a negative correlation, significant at the 0.02 level, is found – that is, the greater the concentration of 3-OMD in plasma, the lesser the long-duration improvement, and vice versa. Others (4) have reported that 3-OMD may be demethylated *in vivo* to L-DOPA, conceivably providing a store of L-DOPA. The question arose whether the negative correlation between 3-OMD in plasma and long-duration improvement indicated that patients

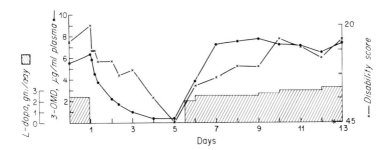

FIG. 4. Plasma concentration of 3-OMD and long-duration improvement after discontinuation and resumption of L-DOPA in patient on chronic L-DOPA therapy. Pretreatment disability score (*) was 45. From (2).

with more active formation of DOPA from 3-OMD, and consequently lower concentrations of 3-OMD, improved more because of the greater amounts of DOPA formed.

To test this hypothesis, we treated patients with Parkinson's disease with 3-OMD (5). In two patients, L-DOPA was replaced by 3-OMD for brief periods (9 and 10 days, respectively) starting on the fourth day after abrupt discontinuation of L-DOPA therapy. The therapeutic response to L-DOPA disappeared after withdrawal of L-DOPA, and, although low levels of L-DOPA could be detected in plasma during 3-OMD therapy, these were insufficient to induce clinical improvement. In two patients who had never received significant therapy for Parkinson's disease previously, 3-OMD was given for 105 and 30 days, respectively. The concentration of DOPA in plasma ranged in most instances from 0.1 to 0.4 µg/ml and was not accompanied by detectable clinical improvement.

Unexpected observations were made in two patients who received 3-OMD in addition to chronic L-DOPA therapy. In the case illustrated in Fig. 5, dosage of L-DOPA was maintained at 3.75 g/day while 3-OMD was added to the regimen. The concentrations of DOPA and 3-OMD in plasma were determined daily in the fasting state and, on several days, also five times at 45- to 60-min intervals after a dose of 3-OMD or L-DOPA (a profile study) (2). The concentration of DOPA during the fasting state remained negligible. Peak concentration of DOPA after a dose was lower after 3-

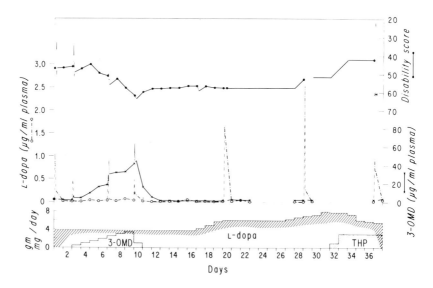

FIG. 5. Combined chronic therapy with L-DOPA and 3-OMD, and effect of trihexyphenidyl (THP). Fasting concentrations of DOPA and 3-OMD in plasma; fasting clinical disability. Profiles (see text) on 1, 3, 7, 10, 20, 29, and 37 are shown in fine lines. Pretreatment disability score shown by *. From (5).

OMD was added. The concentration of 3-OMD in plasma increased to approximately 68 μg/ml. Marked clinical deterioration occurred when 3-OMD was added. The disability score prior to any treatment had been 61. During treatment with L-DOPA only, the disability score in the fasting state was 47, indicating significant long-duration improvement (14 points). This was followed, after each dose of L-DOPA, by short-duration improvement of approximately 11 points. During administration of 3-OMD, the disability score during the fasting state increased gradually to the pretreatment level of 61 and the short-duration response disappeared although the L-DOPA dosage had not been changed. Findings were similar in the second patient treated with L-DOPA and 3-OMD simultaneously.

One is tempted to interpret this phenomenon as due to interference of 3-OMD with absorption of L-DOPA from the gastrointestinal tract. Closer analysis, however, shows that this explanation alone is insufficient. Absence of the therapeutic effect of L-DOPA continued for several days after 3-OMD had been stopped and concentrations of 3-OMD in plasma had decreased to levels as low as those observed prior to administration of 3-OMD. An increase in L-DOPA dosage from 3.75 to 6 g/day failed to induce clinical improvement. The concentration of DOPA in plasma at this time (day 20) was higher than prior to administration of 3-OMD. A partial return of improvement occurred 17 days after 3-OMD had been stopped and only after the dosage of L-DOPA had been increased to 8 g/day. A dramatic and complete return of short- and long-duration improvement was noted within 12 hr after administration of 2 mg of trihexyphenidyl. This increased effectiveness of trihexyphenidyl was observed in five of the six patients treated with 3-OMD alone or in combination with L-DOPA.

Another finding supports the interpretation that the interference of 3-OMD with the therapeutic effect of L-DOPA occurs in the central nervous system rather than in the gastrointestinal tract: if the concentration of DOPA in cerebrospinal fluid is measured during treatment with L-DOPA only and during treatment with L-DOPA combined with 3-OMD, at the time of maximal interference by 3-OMD the concentration of DOPA remains essentially unchanged (5).

Our experience with treatment of Parkinson's disease with 3-OMD, which is very limited in regard to long-term therapy, indicates that this compound is insufficiently effective when used alone, and it interferes with the therapeutic effect of L-DOPA.

INTERPRETATIONS AND MECHANISMS

An interpretation of the role of 3-OMD in the context of L-DOPA therapy of Parkinson's disease has to explain several observations.

1. In patients treated with L-DOPA only, the concentration of 3-OMD in plasma has: (a) a positive correlation with long-duration improvement in

individual patients; (b) a negative correlation with long-duration improvement when compared between different patients; and (c) a transient decrease after a dose of L-DOPA, that has a negative correlation with short-duration improvement.

2. In patients treated with L-DOPA and 3-OMD simultaneously, 3-OMD: (a) cancels the long- and short-duration therapeutic effects of L-DOPA; (b) does this in spite of unchanged concentrations of DOPA in lumbar cerebrospinal fluid; and (c) decreases the peak concentration of DOPA in plasma.

3. In patients treated with 3-OMD alone, 3-OMD: (a) fails to cause significant clinical improvement; and (b) fails to induce therapeutic levels of DOPA in plasma.

Competition for a transport mechanism across the intestinal wall may explain the decrease and delay in peak concentration of DOPA when both compounds are administered simultaneously.

Interference of 3-OMD with transport, storage, or utilization of L-DOPA could take place in the central nervous system at the junction of the capillary and glial membranes, at the junction of the capillary wall and the extracellular parenchymal intracerebral space, at the junction between glial and neuronal membranes, at the junction between the extracellular parenchymal space and neuronal membranes, or at the postsynaptic dopamine-sensitive membranes. This would explain the disappearance of the therapeutic effects of L-DOPA when given together with 3-OMD, the negative correlation between 3-OMD in plasma and long-duration improvement when L-DOPA is given alone, and the negative correlation between transient decrease of 3-OMD in plasma after a dose of L-DOPA and short-duration improvement.

Neither of these mechanisms explains the positive correlation between concentration of 3-OMD in plasma and long-duration improvement in individual patients receiving L-DOPA only. It is unlikely that 3-OMD causes long-duration improvement in patients receiving L-DOPA if, in patients receiving 3-OMD, it is unable to produce that effect when the concentration of 3-OMD in plasma is so much higher. The positive correlation could be due to the formation rather than the presence of 3-OMD; in that case it would be difficult to explain why patients with higher concentrations of 3-OMD have less long-duration improvement while receiving L-DOPA.

Finally, it is possible that the positive correlation between 3-OMD in plasma and long-duration improvement in patients on L-DOPA alone is coincidental. In that case one would have to assume that the primary effect of 3-OMD is to interfere with absorption as well as with the central therapeutic effects of L-DOPA, suggesting that further investigation of catechol-O-methyltransferase inhibitors may be useful.

The mechanisms responsible for short-duration and long-duration improvement remain uncertain. It is possible that long-duration improvement is related to storage of dopamine or one of its precursors, in a form that prevents its immediate metabolic destruction, either in glial cells or in axons and terminals of dopaminergic nigrostriatal neurons. If the primary disease process affecting nigral neurons decreases the ability of the neurons to synthesize DOPA early in the disease process, it is conceivable that accumulation of DOPA in partly impaired dopaminergic axons may temporarily reestablish an approximation of normal function until complete neuronal degeneration interrupts the process. Short-duration improvement, on the other hand, may be due to the direct effect of dopamine formed in those parts of cerebral capillary walls which adjoin the extracellular intracerebral parenchymal space; this dopamine may then diffuse through the extracellular space and act directly on the postsynaptic dopaminergic membranes, which have lost the nigrostriatal neuronal terminal due to complete neuronal degeneration. This would explain why short-duration improvement increases and long-duration improvement decreases as the disease progresses.

It is unclear why the therapeutic response to trihexyphenidyl should be altered in patients receiving 3-OMD.

ACKNOWLEDGMENT

This investigation was supported by U.S. Public Health Service research grants RR-585 and NS-9143, and by a donation from Mrs. Charles S. Lips. Dr. Sharpless has a special traineeship (5F 11 NS-2540) from the National Institute of Neurological Diseases and Stroke.

REFERENCES

1. Muenter, M. D., and Tyce, G. M., *Mayo Clin. Proc.* 46, 231 (1971).
2. Muenter, M. D., Sharpless, N. S., and Tyce, G. M., *Mayo Clin. Proc.* 47, 389 (1972).
3. Sharpless, N. S., Muenter, M. D., Tyce, G. M., and Owen, C. A., Jr., *Clin. Chim. Acta* 37, 359 (1972).
4. Bartholini, G., Kuruma, I., and Pletscher, A., *J. Pharmacol. Exp. Ther.* 183, 65 (1972).
5. Muenter, M. D., Dinapoli, R. P., Sharpless, N. S., and Tyce, G. M., *Mayo Clin. Proc.* 48, 173 (1973).

Advances in Neurology, Vol. 5
Raven Press, New York © 1974

Effect of L-DOPA and Analogues on Central Dopamine and Noradrenaline Mechanisms

Nils-Erik Andén and Jörgen Engel

Department of Pharmacology, University of Göteborg, Göteborg, Sweden

Administration of L-DOPA influences both dopamine and noradrenaline synapses in the central nervous system. It is often desirable to distinguish between the L-DOPA-induced effects on the dopamine and the noradrenaline mechanisms. It is possible to do so, for instance, in the corpus striatum and the spinal cord, whose catecholamine nerve terminals are mainly of the dopamine and noradrenaline type, respectively (1). The catecholamine pathways to these two regions have the advantages that they can be selectively damaged and that their functions can be easily observed.

METHODOLOGY

Corpus Striatum

The dopamine neurons from the substantia nigra to the neostriatum are uncrossed and regulate, among other things, muscle tone. Therefore, a unilateral lesion of this neuron system should cause asymmetries of posture and movement. The pathway can be destroyed in two principal ways: acute removal of the corpus striatum including the neostriatal dopamine nerve terminals (2), or chronic damage of the ascending dopamine axons (2, 3). Surprisingly, these unilateral lesions as such produce no asymmetry or only a slight turning of the head and tail to the operated side in rats. If L-DOPA is given to a rat with the corpus striatum removed on one side, the rat vigorously turns and rotates to the operated side; see Fig. 1 (2). This effect is more pronounced after pretreatment with reserpine, after which L-DOPA induces a turning of the head and tail from the unoperated side (caused by the reserpine treatment) to the operated side. After a chronic lesion of the ascending dopamine axons, the treatment with L-DOPA induces the opposite effect, that is, turning to the unoperated side, in all probability due to denervation supersensitivity of the neostriatal dopamine receptors on the operated side (2, 4). Treatment with the 5-hydroxytryptamine precursor 5-hydroxytryptophan does not cause any asymmetry of unilaterally oper-

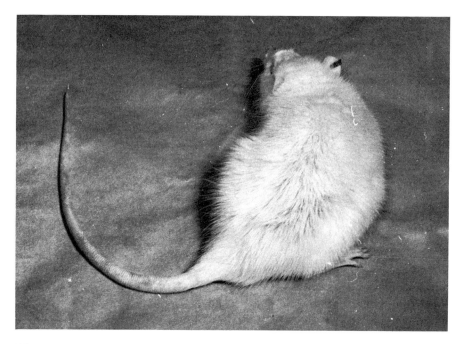

FIG. 1. Effect of L-DOPA on a rat with the corpus striatum removed on the left side. The rat was operated on about 8 hr before, and it was treated with reserpine (10 mg/kg, i.p., 7 hr before), nialamide (100 mg/kg, i.p., $2\frac{1}{2}$ hr before), and L-DOPA (75 mg/kg, i.p., 30 min before).

ated animals, indicating that the 5-hydroxytryptamine and dopamine receptors are different (2).

Spinal Cord

Injection of L-DOPA to acutely spinalized animals induces an enhancement of the flexor reflex activity of the hind legs; see Fig. 2 (5, 6). Treatment with 5-hydroxytryptophan causes a different change in hindlimb reflex activity of spinal animals, indicating that catecholamines and 5-hydroxytryptamine act also on different receptors in this region (7, 8).

DOPA ANALOGUES

The effects of some analogues to L-DOPA have been analyzed in the models described above. Injection of m-tyrosine produces a turning of unilaterally striatotomized rats to the operated side. As after L-DOPA, this effect is markedly potentiated by pretreatment with a monoamine oxidase inhibitor or with a peripheral L-DOPA decarboxylase inhibitor, indicating

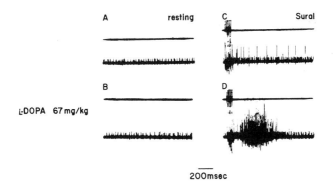

FIG. 2. Discharges in flexor motor neurons before (record A and C) and after (record B and D) an intravenous injection of L-DOPA to a spinal cat. The lower traces in each record are the efferent discharges in a nerve to a flexor muscle (tenuissimus), and the upper traces are from the sciatic nerve (afferent). A and B are resting discharges; an ipsilateral, cutaneous nerve (sural) was stimulated by a train of volleys in C and D. Before treatment with L-DOPA (C), there is an early and short reflex discharge followed by an afterdischarge in both α- and γ-efferents. After treatment with L-DOPA (D), there is a late, massive, and long-lasting discharge in both α- and γ-efferents. Such a discharge is not seen in a nerve to an extensor muscle. (From ref. 5.)

that the effect is mediated via amines formed centrally (9, 10). Also, the hindlimb flexor reflex activity of spinal rats is somewhat facilitated by treatment with m-tyrosine, provided that the endogenous stores of noradrenaline are intact (see below). On the other hand, injection of o-tyrosine does not result in any of the effects seen after treatment with L-DOPA or m-tyrosine. However, changes in spinal reflexes and in gross behavior are seen, as after administration of 5-hydroxytryptophan, indicating stimulation of 5-hydroxytryptamine receptors (11–13). Injection of m-tyrosine produces a quite different behavioral syndrome characterized by sniffing, licking, or gnawing, as after treatment with L-DOPA or apomorphine.

After administration of α-methyl-m-tyrosine to rats pretreated with reserpine, there is no functional change in the striatal and spinal function, as is seen after injection of L-DOPA. Injection of the α-methylated analogue to L-DOPA, α-methyl-DOPA, to rats with the corpus striatum removed unilaterally induces a decrease in the reserpine-induced turning, but does not cause any deviation to the operated side. On the other hand, the hindlimb flexor reflex activity is markedly enhanced after treatment with α-methyl-DOPA, although with a longer latency than after treatment with L-DOPA (9).

The injection of 3-O-methyl-DOPA (L-form) in a dose up to 1000 mg/kg intraperitoneally does not cause any change in the reserpine-induced turning to the unoperated side of unilaterally striatotomized rats. Nor is any effect observed on the flexor reflex activity of spinal rats. Even when combined with an inhibitor of the monoamine oxidase (nialamide, 100 mg/kg, i.p., 1 hr before) or the catechol-O-methyl transferase (α-propyldopace-tamide, 500 mg/kg, i.p., 30 min before) or both, the treatment is inefficient in both models. It should be noted, however, that only acute experiments have been done (13).

The *m*-tyrosine injected is readily decarboxylated to *m*-tyramine, which is subsequently β-hydroxylated to *m*-octopamine in the noradrenaline nerves (9, 11, 13–15). These processes are of about the same order of magnitude as for L-DOPA. The *o*-tyrosine is decarboxylated to *o*-tyramine at a rate which is at least as fast as the decarboxylation of L-DOPA (11, 13, 14). The α-methylated analogues are decarboxylated more slowly, but, since the amine products are resistant to the monoamine oxidase, the β-hydroxylated amines will eventually reach relatively high concentrations (9, 13, 15). After administration of even high doses of 3-O-methyl-DOPA, only slight, if any, increases are found in brain catecholamines (13, 16, 17).

MODE OF ACTION OF L-DOPA AND ANALOGUES

The injection of L-DOPA after inhibition of the peripheral L-DOPA decarboxylase activity produces an increase in hindlimb reflex activity of spinal rats without, but not with, pretreatment with reserpine; see Fig. 3 (6). The formation of catecholamines is about the same in both cases. Therefore, it appears that the dopamine acts by release of noradrenaline from the endogenous stores. Further support for an indirect effect is the finding that repeated doses of L-DOPA produce smaller effects (6, 18). However, after inhibition of the monoamine oxidase, treatment with reserpine plus L-DOPA causes a marked stimulation of flexor reflex activity concomitant with an accumulation of both dopamine and noradrenaline; see Fig. 4 (6). When an inhibitor of the dopamine-β-hydroxylase is added, the L-DOPA effect is somewhat reduced simultaneously with blockade of the noradrenaline formation, indicating that dopamine can stimulate the noradrenaline recep-tors, although more weakly than noradrenaline.

Administration of dopamine directly into the neostriatum on one side results in turning of rats to the contralateral side, showing that the L-DOPA effect after unilateral removal of the corpus striatum is evoked from the dopamine formed in the intact neostriatum (19). Intrastriatal administration of noradrenaline induces only a slight turning of rats pretreated with reser-pine, α-methyltyrosine, and nialamide, indicating that noradrenaline can stimulate the dopamine receptors, although more weakly than dopamine.

The actions induced by *m*-tyrosine have been analyzed as described for DOPA. The finding that pretreatment with reserpine blocks the effect of *m*-tyrosine on hindlimb flexor reflex activity indicates that this noradrenaline receptor stimulation is also indirect (13, 18). The *m*-tyramine and the *m*-octopamine formed from *m*-tyrosine appear to lack effect on the noradrena-line receptors in the spinal cord, to judge from results obtained in experi-

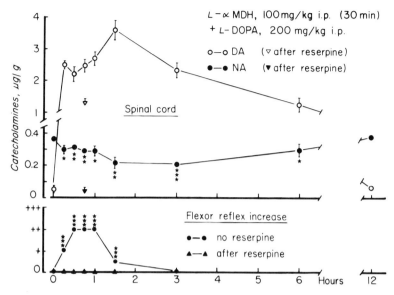

FIG. 3. Effect of L-α-methyl-DOPA hydrazine (L-α-MDH, 100 mg/kg, i.p.) plus L-DOPA (200 mg/kg, i.p., 30 min later) on the concentrations of dopamine (DA) and noradrenaline (NA) in the rat spinal cord (upper panel) and on the flexor reflex activity in the hindlimbs of spinal rats (lower panel). Some animals were pretreated with reserpine (10 mg/kg, i.p., 6 hr prior to the DOPA injection). The concentrations are the means ± SEM (45 min: $N = 5$; reserpine: $N = 4$; all others: $N = 3$). The flexor reflex activities are the medians of 26 (no reserpine) and 18 (reserpine) experiments. The statistical significances of the changes in the NA concentrations are indicated by *** ($p < 0.001$), ** ($p < 0.01$), and *($p < 0.05$) (Student's t test). The statistical significances of the differences in flexor reflex activity between the reserpine-pretreated and untreated groups are indicated by ⋯ ($p < 0.002$; Mann-Whitney U test). (From ref. 6.)

ments with reserpine and nialamide plus m-tyrosine (9). On the other hand, m-tyramine must be able to stimulate the neostriatal dopamine receptors directly, since treatment with m-tyrosine also evokes turning to the operated side in rats pretreated with reserpine, α-methyltyrosine, and nialamide. Furthermore, treatment with m-tyrosine antagonizes the reserpine-induced suppression of locomotor activity and conditioned avoidance response (9, 20, 21).

Treatment with α-methyl-DOPA evokes a marked stimulation of the hindlimb flexor reflex activity even after pretreatment with reserpine and α-methyltyrosine, indicating that the α-methylated amines formed have a direct effect on the spinal noradrenaline receptors (9). The finding that this functional effect, as well as the formation of α-methylnoradrenaline, are blocked by pretreatment with a dopamine-β-hydroxylase inhibitor indicates that α-methylnoradrenaline is the active agent, and that it is as potent as noradrenaline on the noradrenaline receptors. The very weak effect of treatment with α-methyl-DOPA on the neostriatal dopamine receptors

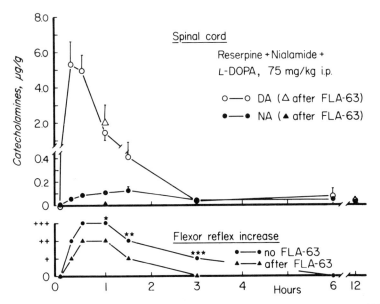

FIG. 4. Effect of L-DOPA (75 mg/kg, i.p.) on the concentrations of dopamine (DA) and noradrenaline (NA) in the rat spinal cord (upper panel) and on the flexor reflex activity in the hindlimbs of spinal rats (lower panel) after pretreatment with reserpine (10 mg/kg, i.p., 10 to 18 hr prior to the DOPA injection) and nialamide (50 mg/kg, i.p., 1 hr prior to DOPA). Some animals were also pretreated with the DA-β-hydroxylase inhibitor FLA-63 (25 mg/kg, i.p., 30 min prior to DOPA). The concentrations at each interval are the means $\pm$ SEM of three experiments. The flexor reflex activities are the medians of 21 (no FLA) and eight (FLA) experiments. The statistical significances of the differences in flexor reflex activity between the FLA-pretreated and untreated groups are indicated by $\cdots$ ($p <$ 0.002), $\cdots$ ($p < 0.02$), and $\cdot$ ($p < 0.05$) (Mann-Whitney U test). (From ref. 6.)

(see above) is, in all probability, due mainly to a slow formation of α-methyl-dopamine, since this amine is almost as efficient as dopamine in inducing turning after intrastriatal administration (13). In agreement with these results on receptor activation, treatment with α-methyl-DOPA only partially reverses the suppression of locomotor activity induced by reserpine plus α-methyltyrosine (9).

AGENTS STIMULATING CATECHOLAMINE RECEPTORS DIRECTLY

Treatment with the dopamine analogue apomorphine produces a turning of unilaterally striatotomized rats from the unoperated to the operated side after pretreatment with reserpine plus α-methyltyrosine (22). No effect is observed on the flexor reflex activity of spinal rats. Recently, piribedil (Trivastal®, ET 495) has been described as producing effects similar to, but more long lasting than those produced by apomorphine, although it seems to have a slight catecholamine-releasing effect as well (23, 24). In contrast, the antihypertensive drug clonidine (Catapres ®, St 155) strongly stimulates the spinal noradrenaline receptors directly without affecting the neostriatal dopamine receptors (25). Injection of amphetamine also produces stimulation of the dopamine and noradrenaline receptors, but these effects are indirect since they are prevented by pretreatment with reserpine plus α-methyltyrosine (22).

CONCLUDING REMARKS

Of various DOPA analogues studied, treatment with m-tyrosine induces a strong stimulation of neostriatal dopamine receptors by its metabolite m-tyramine, whereas treatment with α-methyl-DOPA induces a strong stimulation of central noradrenaline receptors by its metabolite α-methyl-noradrenaline. No catecholamine receptor stimulation is observed after treatment with 3-O-methyl-DOPA, o-tyrosine, or α-methyl-m-tyrosine. The animal models used appear suitable for study of whether and how drugs influence central dopamine and noradrenaline receptors.

ACKNOWLEDGMENTS

The work was partially supported by the Swedish Medical Research Council (B73–04X–502–09B) and the Swedish Board for Technical Development.

REFERENCES

1. Andén, N.-E., Carlsson, A., and Häggendal, J., *Ann. Rev. Pharmacol.* 9, 119 (1969).
2. Andén, N.-E., Dahlström, A., Fuxe, K., and Larsson, K., *Acta Pharmacol. Toxicol.* 24, 263 (1966).
3. Ungerstedt, U., *Europ. J. Pharmacol.* 5, 107 (1968).
4. Ungerstedt, U., *Acta Physiol. Scand.* suppl. 367, 69 (1971).
5. Andén, N.-E., Jukes, M. G. M., Lundberg, A., and Vyklický, L., *Acta Physiol. Scand.* 67, 373 (1966).
6. Andén, N.-E., Engel, J., and Rubenson, A., *Naunyn-Schmiedeberg's Arch. Pharmacol.* 273, 1 (1972).
7. Andén, N.-E., Jukes, M. G. M., and Lundberg, A., *Nature* 202, 1222 (1964).
8. Andén, N.-E., *Adv. Pharmacol.* 6A, 347 (1968).
9. Andén, N.-E., Butcher, S. G., and Engel, J., *J. Pharm. Pharmacol.* 22, 548 (1970).
10. Ungerstedt, U., Fuxe, K., Goldstein, M., Battista, A., Ogawa, M., and Anagnoste, B., *Europ. J. Pharmacol.* 21, 230 (1973).
11. Mitoma, C., Posner, H. S., Bogdanski, D. F., and Udenfriend, S., *J. Pharmacol. Exp. Ther.* 120, 188 (1957).
12. Bogdanski, D. F., Weissbach. H., and Udenfriend, S., *J. Pharmacol. Exp. Ther.* 122, 182 (1958).
13. Andén, N.-E., and Engel, J., *Unpublished results.*
14. Blaschko, H., *Biochim. Biophys. Acta* 4, 130 (1950).
15. Carlsson, A., and Lindqvist, M., *Acta Physiol. Scand.* 54, 87 (1962).
16. Bartholini, G., Kuruma, I., and Pletscher, A., *J. Pharmacol. Exp. Ther.* 183, 65 (1972).
17. Carlsson, A., and Waldeck, B., *Naunyn-Schmiedeberg's Arch. Pharmacol.* 272, 441 (1972).

18. Rubenson, A., *J. Pharm. Pharmacol.* 23, 228 (1971).
19. Ungerstedt, U., Butcher, L. L., Butcher, S. G., Andén, N.-E., and Fuxe, K., *Brain Res.* 14, 461 (1969).
20. Blaschko, H., and Chruściel, T. L., *J. Physiol.* 151, 272 (1960).
21. Engel, J., *Acta Pharmacol. Toxicol.* 30, 278 (1971).
22. Andén, N.-E., Rubenson, A., Fuxe, K., and Hökfelt, T., *J. Pharm. Pharmacol.* 19, 627 (1967).
23. Corrodi, H., Fuxe, K., and Ungerstedt, U., *J. Pharm. Pharmacol.* 23, 989 (1971).
24. Corrodi, H., Farnebo, L.-O., Fuxe, K., Hamberger, B., and Ungerstedt, U., *Europ. J. Pharmacol.* 20, 195 (1972).
25. Andén, N.-E., Corrodi, H., Fuxe, K., Hökfelt, B., Hökfelt, T., Rydin, C., and Svensson, T., *Life Sci.* 9, 513 (1970).

Advances in Neurology, Vol. 5
Raven Press, New York © 1974

Piribedil in Parkinsonism

Donald B. Calne

Department of Medicine (Neurology), Royal Postgraduate Medical School, Hammersmith Hospital, London W12OHS, England

We have investigated piribedil (ET 495, Trivastal®) in a double-blind study involving 21 parkinsonian patients already receiving maximum tolerated doses of L-DOPA. Piribedil was given in maximum tolerated doses of 20 to 240 mg per day for periods ranging from 6 to 12 weeks. Clinical evaluations, timed tests, and measurement of blood pressure were performed every 2 weeks. We find our results difficult to interpret. A statistical analysis of our observations was undertaken when only 15 patients had entered the study, and a significant ($p < 0.05$) therapeutic action emerged. However, after observations on 21 patients, this statistical significance was no longer evident. One of our patients, who incidentally had postencephalitic parkinsonism, displayed an unequivocal and dramatic improvement in tremor when taking piribedil. I am convinced that this was a reliable observation because when the patient was given placebo he telephoned to demand an earlier appointment because of his deterioration. As he requested permission to increase the dose of tablets, he was still manifestly "blind."

I think the most probable explanation for our results is that only a small minority of patients benefit from piribedil, and it is possible for therapeutic activity to be missed in a statistical analysis because improvement of the responders is "diluted" and masked by the large majority of nonresponders. A useful approach to the problem may be a detailed study of selected groups of responders.

The adverse reactions we encountered with piribedil were of interest. All our patients had been titrated to a stable dose of L-DOPA which did not produce side effects. We found that administration of piribedil to these patients commonly precipitated dsykinesia and confusion. In contrast, others who have used piribedil without L-DOPA reported nausea as the dominant dose-limiting factor. Patients who have already developed tachyphylaxis to nausea induced by L-DOPA seem to display tolerance to nausea induced by piribedil. On the other hand, tachyphylaxis does not develop for dyskinesia and confusion induced by L-DOPA, so the observation that piribedil exacerbates these problems is no surprise. Our findings taken together indicate that if piribedil leads to relatively selective dopaminergic activity as has been suggested, then nausea, dyskinesia, and confusion are all more likely to be produced by dopamine rather than any other metabolite of L-DOPA.

Advances in Neurology, Vol. 5
Raven Press, New York © 1974

Demethylation of 3-Methoxy-4-Hydroxyphenylalanine in the Isolated Perfused Rat Liver

Gertrude M. Tyce, Nansie S. Sharpless, and Charles A. Owen, Jr.

Department of Biochemistry, Mayo Clinic and Mayo Foundation, Rochester, Minnesota 55901

3-Methoxy-4-hydroxyphenylalanine (3-O-methyldopa, 3-OMD) accumulates in plasma and cerebrospinal fluid during the treatment of patients with Parkinson's disease with L-DOPA (1, 2). The possibility that demethylation of 3-OMD occurs has attracted considerable interest. This reaction would provide a steady source of L-DOPA and thereby tend to stabilize the DOPA concentration in plasma, which normally fluctuates widely after each dose of L-DOPA.

Demethylation of 3-OMD has been shown to occur in rats (3). Relatively nonspecific demethylases located in liver microsomes may be responsible for this reaction (4). On the other hand, Chalmers and co-workers (5) showed that, in rats with external bile fistulas, there was negligible demethylation of 3-OMD. They concluded that demethylation normally was carried out by gastrointestinal bacteria after the excretion of 3-OMD (or a conjugate) into bile.

In the present experiments the hepatic metabolism of 3-OMD was studied with the isolated perfused rat liver system (6). A particular goal was to separate and identify the biliary metabolites of 3-OMD and to define the extent and location of demethylation.

The isolated rat liver was continuously perfused with warmed, oxygenated rat blood; bile was collected continuously. ^{14}C-L-3-OMD (5 μC) (New England Nuclear), uniformly labeled except in the methoxy carbon, was injected into the perfusate. This resulted in an initial concentration of 3-OMD in the perfusate of almost 15 μg/ml, a concentration only slightly higher than that found in the plasma of patients during L-DOPA treatment (1). Total ^{14}C was measured in samples of whole blood taken at intervals and in samples of plasma and of bile. After 5 hr of perfusion, the liver was removed and total ^{14}C was measured in perchloric acid homogenates of it.

^{14}C-3-OMD and metabolites in perchloric acid extracts of plasma, erythrocytes, bile, and liver were separated by ion-exchange and alumina-adsorption chromatography (7), by solvent extraction, and by paper chromatography (8).

Carlsson and Waldeck (9) have recently shown that some samples of ^{14}C-3-OMD contain trace amounts of ^{14}C-DOPA, which might account for apparent demethylation in some experiments. Therefore we critically examined our ^{14}C-3-OMD for the presence of ^{14}C-DOPA. After addition of carrier-stable DOPA, separations were done in an amino acid analyzer and by paper chromatography with n-butanol–acetic acid–water (12:3:5). We failed to find any DOPA by these methods, which would have detected a contamination of 0.2% or more.

During the 5 hr after the injection of ^{14}C-3-OMD into the perfusate, total ^{14}C decreased to 61% of the dose in whole blood and to 45% in plasma. The difference between ^{14}C in whole blood and ^{14}C in plasma was largely accounted for by ^{14}C in erythrocytes; this fraction represented 30% of the dose after 5 min of perfusion but decreased to 16% after 5 hr. Uptake of ^{14}C by liver was not great; less than 10% of the dose was present in liver at any one time during the perfusion. However, much more was taken up by the liver because the cumulative excretion of ^{14}C into bile accounted for 20% of the dose.

The disappearance of ^{14}C-3-OMD from plasma followed a triphasic course. After only 5 min of perfusion, less than 60% of the dose remained as unmetabolized ^{14}C-3-OMD. This initial rapid loss is largely accounted for by the initial uptake of ^{14}C by liver and erythrocytes. Between 5 min and 2 hr, ^{14}C-3-OMD disappeared less rapidly from plasma, and, after 2 hr, yet more slowly. Two components were defined for the disappearance between 5 min and 5 hr. There was an initial rapid phase, essentially complete by 2 hr, in which the half-life of 3-OMD was 25 min, and a slower component with a half-life of 6 hr. These half-lives are considerably shorter than the half-life of 12 hr previously observed in the intact rat (10). This is probably because, in the intact animal, 3-OMD is stored in extrahepatic tissues and slowly released.

After 5 min of perfusion, 10% of the total ^{14}C present in protein-free extracts of erythrocytes was ^{14}C-DOPA but only 3% of the total ^{14}C in extracts of plasma was ^{14}C-DOPA. The early appearance of ^{14}C-DOPA in the erythrocytes indicated that they were a site of demethylation.

At the end of the perfusion, in plasma 22% of the dose was accounted for by ^{14}C-3-OMD and 2% by the glucuronide of 3-OMD. Known demethylated compounds (DOPA, 3,4-dihydroxyphenylacetic acid [dopac], and dopac-sulfate) accounted for 2.6% of the dose. Vanillactic acid (VLA), present free and as a sulfate conjugate, accounted for 12.3% of the dose, and free and conjugated homovanillic acid (HVA) accounted for 8%. In erythrocytes, 8.5% of the dose was ^{14}C-3-OMD and 1.4% was ^{14}C-DOPA; free and conjugated VLA and HVA accounted for 3.5% of the dose. In bile, only 1.1% of the dose was free ^{14}C-3-OMD and 3.7% was 3-OMD-glucuronide, known demethylated compounds (chiefly the glucuronide of dopamine) accounted for 3.0% of the dose, and free and conjugated VLA and HVA accounted for 12.2%. In liver, ^{14}C-3-OMD accounted for 3.4% of the dose. Smaller amounts of free and conjugated VLA and HVA were also present.

In summary, demethylation occurred in the isolated perfused rat liver, accounting for almost 9% of the dose. The site of demethylation was probably the erythrocytes. Little free 3-OMD was excreted in bile. The chief biliary metabolites were the glucuronides of dopamine and 3-OMD and free and conjugated HVA and VLA.

ACKNOWLEDGMENT

This investigation was supported in part by Research Grant NS–9143 and Special Fellowship 5F 11 NS–2540 (Dr. Sharpless) from the National Institutes of Health, U.S. Public Health Service, and by a donation from Mrs. Charles S. Lips.

REFERENCES

1. Sharpless, N. S., Muenter, M. D., Tyce, G. M., and Owen, C. A., Jr., *Clin. Chim. Acta* 37, 359 (1972).
2. Sharpless, N. S., and McCann, D. S., *Clin. Chim. Acta* 31, 155 (1971).
3. Bartholini, G., Kuruma, I., and Pletscher, A., *J. Pharmacol. Exp. Ther.* 183, 65 (1972).
4. Axelrod, J., *Biochem. J.* 63, 634 (1956).
5. Chalmers, J. P., Draffan, G. H., Reid, J. L., Thorgeirsson, S. S., and Davies, D. S., *Life Sci. [1]* 10, 1243 (1971).
6. Brauer, R. W., Pessotti, R. L., and Pizzolato, P., *Proc. Soc. Exp. Biol. Med.* 78, 174 (1951).
7. Tyce, G. M., Sharpless, N. S., and Owen, C. A., Jr., *Biochem. Pharmacol.* 21, 2409 (1972).
8. Tyce, G. M., *Biochem. Pharmacol.* 20, 3447 (1971).
9. Carlsson, A., and Waldeck, B., *Naunyn-Schmiedeberg's Arch. Pharmacol.* 272, 441 (1972).
10. Bartholini, G., Kuruma, I., and Pletscher, A., *Br. J. Pharmacol.* 40, 461 (1970).

Advances in Neurology, Vol. 5
Raven Press, New York © 1974

The "On–Off" Response to Chronic L-DOPA Treatment of Parkinsonism

Richard D. Sweet and Fletcher H. McDowell

Department of Neurology, Cornell University Medical College, New York, New York 10021

Chronic medical disorders often have a variable course, and parkinsonism is no exception. Changes in motility and tremor with different emotional stimuli and excellent motor performance in an emergency by usually incapacitated patients are common. Nevertheless, motor ability, or lack of it, is predictable from hour to hour and day to day in most patients with parkinsonism.

Consistently good motility is found in many patients starting L-DOPA treatment. Large amounts of DOPA given three or four times a day initially usually provide smooth improvement without interruption.

However, we have found that a number of patients followed on L-DOPA develop variability in response to the medication which cannot be altered by routine changes in dose regimen. Changes in such patients may be dramatic and sudden, leading to the comparison with a light switch and the designation "on–off" effect.

The onset of this variable course is best illustrated by the case history of one of our most dramatically affected patients.

Mrs. A. B., now aged 60, first noticed left-sided tremors and slowness at age 54. Her disability became bilateral within the next few years, and she had difficulty arising, walking, and manipulating the switchboard in her work as a telephone operator. L-DOPA was begun at age 57 with a striking beneficial effect. With her L-DOPA dose stabilized at 5.0 g/day, she returned to a virtually normal life and full-time work. Twenty-four months after starting L-DOPA, she noticed periods of slow walking just before her next dose of DOPA was due, which was corrected by that dose. Dyskinesia became prominent 29 months after starting L-DOPA. Two and one-half years after she started L-DOPA, she returned early from a vacation in Florida complaining of severe, painful dyskinesia alternating with sudden episodes of complete immobility. She appeared quite mobile and dyskinetic, suddenly became very flushed, and within 1 or 2 min became severely akinetic, with masked facies, left-sided tremor, and inability to rise from a chair or walk unassisted. Similar episodes, lasting 1 or 2 hr, occurred at irregular intervals each day, despite many revisions of her L-DOPA regimen.

She had to quit work and would not go out alone, for fear of becoming "stuck" on the street. At home, she compressed all of her activities into mobile periods, realizing that she could accomplish nothing while akinetic. Reactive depression became severe, especially as akinetic periods gradually occupied three-fourths of her waking hours rather than their original one-third.

Confronted with such a distressing pattern in many patients, we have tried to define its characteristics as well as those of the patients it affects. We have examined the patients' onset and development of parkinsonism, associated illnesses and medications, response to L-DOPA, and side effects from it. In addition, we have compared mobile and immobile periods among patients for time of day, duration, body part affected, relationship to medications, meals, activity, and associated symptoms. As an aid to these investigations, patients completed a diary grid sheet, as illustrated in Fig. 1. "On" or good periods were left blank, while "off" or bad periods were shaded in. Times of meals and medication were also listed.

This report offers such observations on 29 patients with definite "on-off" effect culled from approximately 300 patients with parkinsonism fol-

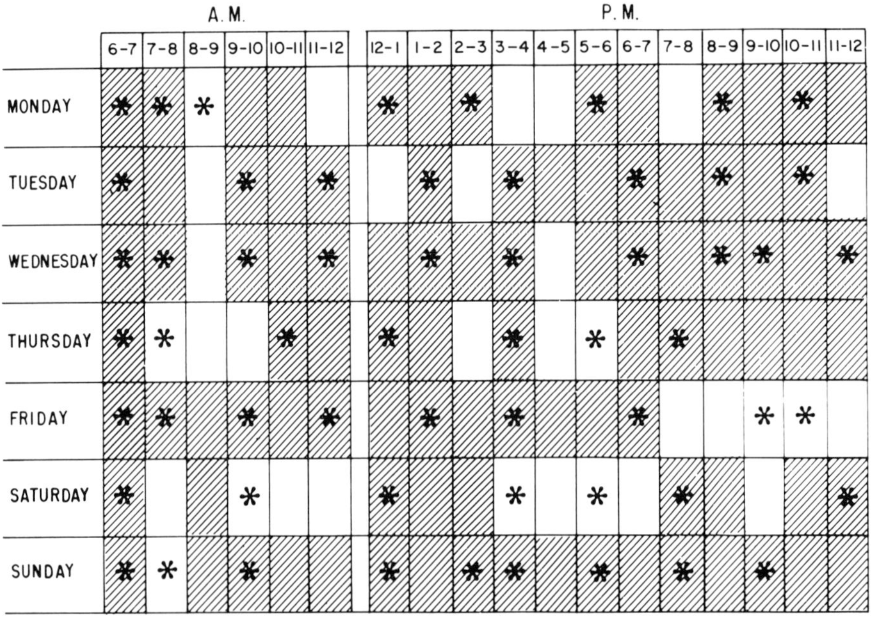

FIG. 1. Diary grid sheet completed by Mrs. B., showing the temporal pattern of clinical oscillations. "Off" periods (akinesia, tremor) are shaded, and "on" periods (mobile with dyskinesia) are left open. 500-mg doses of L-DOPA are indicated by asterisks. The "off" periods do not fall at any certain time, and they show no clear-cut relationship to time of L-DOPA dosage.

lowed at the New York Hospital–Cornell Medical Center. All but one of these patients have been seen at Cornell throughout their course of DOPA treatment, and 16 of them are from the group of 100 patients we have described several times (1, 2). This incidence of 16% in patients who started DOPA 4 years ago is the minimum, since we have found other patients with milder variations and we expect that more patients will develop oscillation in performance as time goes on.

CHARACTERISTICS OF THE "ON–OFF" EFFECT

Each patient complained of periodic reversion to untreated status for short times every day. This initial symptom was preceded by diffuse constant weakness in only five patients. Duration of L-DOPA therapy until an "on–off" effect was first noted averaged 28 months and ranged from 8 to 50 months (Table 1). Eighteen patients acquired the effect between 13 and 36 months after DOPA started, seven patients after 37 months or more, and four before 12 months of therapy. Severe oral facial or limb dyskinesia accompanied "on" or good periods in 20 of our 29 patients. Their hyperactive

TABLE 1. Duration of L-DOPA treatment prior to "on–off" effect

Months	<12	13–24	25–36	37+
Number of patients	4	7	11	7

motor status, flush or sweat, and rapid decline into an akinetic condition was dramatic. The end of an "off" period was often heralded by the onset of dyskinesia. In contrast, one woman had dyskinesia while "off," with bilateral akinesia and tremor, and a man became dyspneic with panting attributed to diaphragmatic dyskinesia and tremor as well. The seven remaining patients who did not have prominent dyskinesia were those whose "on–off" switches were the least marked.

The principal difficulty during "off" periods was poor gait in 16 patients, diffuse akinesia in 9, tremor in 6, and unintelligible speech in 1 (Table 2).

TABLE 2. Type and location of major motor disability during "off" periods

Type		Location	
Gait	16	Legs	15
Akinesia	9	Arms	1
Tremor	6	Voice	1
Speech	1	Lateralized	3
Dyspnea	1	Diffuse	9

Legs were the principal body part affected in 13 of 18 patients who could localize their defect. Seven patients had "off" periods mainly in the morning, seven in the afternoon, and five in the evening. Times were variable for the other patients. "Off" periods clustered about the time of the L-DOPA dose in four patients. They lasted anywhere from $\frac{1}{2}$ to 5 hr but were 1 to 2 hr long in most patients.

Four patients were consistently worse following meals. One of them, a physician, noticed that high-protein meals made him worse than low-protein meals, and another man had been taking DOPA with meals and a dietary supplement (Metrecal®) to minimize dyskinesia. In contrast, three patients found that DOPA's effects were enhanced after meals, perhaps because of faster gastric emptying (3).

Painful cramps in thighs or calves accompanied "off" periods in four patients, and were the chief complaint of two of them. An unreasoned sense of panic was felt by two women, and three other patients were more easily confused during "off" periods. Prominent flushing of face and chest was noticed by three patients, while four others had increased sweating before or during "off" periods.

CHARACTERISTICS OF THE PATIENTS

Is there a special group of patients who are more likely to develop the "on–off" effect? We compared data from 28 patients with "on–off" effect with information about 84 of the first 100 patients to start L-DOPA at Cornell who have not developed the effect (Table 3). "On–off" patients averaged 62 years of age, while others averaged 69 years. There were about two men to each woman in both groups. Parkinsonism had been present for an average of 12 years of both groups, but began at age 50 in "on–off" patients and at age 57 in others.

TABLE 3. Clinical characteristics: "on–off" patients versus remainder of the treated cases

	"On–off"	Others
Number of patients	28	84
Age	62	69
Sex	17/m 11/f	55/m 29/f
Age at onset of Parkinson's	50	57
Duration of Parkinson's	12 years	12 years
Severity when first seen		
Severe	4	31
Moderate	23	48
Mild	1	5

"On–off" patients had less severe Parkinson's disease than others. Only 4 of 28 were classified severe when first seen by us, compared with 31 of the other 84 original patients. Only 14% of the original patients being treated for 2 years remained 75% or more improved by L-DOPA, while 33% of "on–off" patients enjoyed 75% improvement at 2 years (Table 4).

TABLE 4. *Percentage improvement after 2 years of L-DOPA therapy (percent of patients)*

Percent improved	"On–off" (27 pts.)	Original except "on–off" (56 pts.)
75+	33	14
50–74	45	29
49–	22	57

All but one of the "on–off" patients had abnormal movements in response to L-DOPA. Three of them were among seven patients who demonstrated an enhanced response to low doses of L-DOPA after withdrawal from chronic therapy (4). Ten patients developed mental changes while taking L-DOPA, seven of whom were strikingly confused or demented. Twenty-one of 29 patients had GI symptoms, mainly nausea. Thus, "on–off" patients appear to be more susceptible than usual to L-DOPA's effects, both good and bad.

One possible factor separating "on–off" patients from others might be the etiology of their parkinsonism. However, only five patients had sudden onset of symptoms or onset under age 40, which might suggest postencephalitic disease, and only two had definite history of encephalitis. Eight patients had undergone stereotaxic surgery prior to L-DOPA treatment. No patient had significant gastric or small intestinal disease which might have altered DOPA's absorption from the GI tract. L-DOPA dose averaged 4.75 g/day in "on–off" and 4.5 g/day in other patients after 2 years of treatment. Sixteen of 29 patients were taking anticholinergic medication, 4 tricyclic antidepressants, and 1 each amantadine and methylphenidate. Plasma DOPA levels (Dr. H. Spiegel, Hoffman LaRoche) did not correlate with clinical status in 2 patients.

COURSE AND TREATMENT OF THE "ON–OFF" EFFECT

"Off" periods of poor motor performance were subtle at first and seemed to be corrected by either increasing the dose of L-DOPA or spreading it out over the day. In effect, the patients were riding the crest of a wave of DOPA effect, often requiring toleration of severe dyskinesia and more and more DOPA to avoid falling into akinesia. Inevitably, they did fall behind within

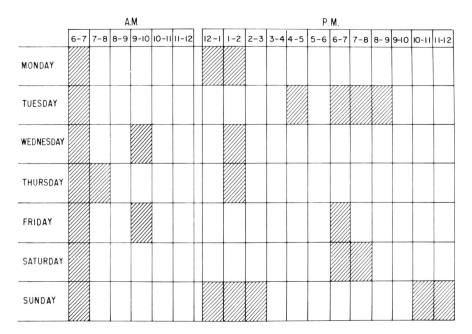

FIG. 2. Effect of a 7 g/day protein diet on Mrs. B's diary grid report. The "off" periods were greatly diminished, but dyskinesia became more prominent.

a few months, and then even hourly doses of DOPA were not sufficient to maintain good performance all day long. Lately, some of these patients have noticed an increasing percentage of the day occupied by poor function.

We have tried to correct this distressing development. We have administered peripheral DOPA decarboxylase inhibitors in order to bypass dose-limiting nausea, increase plasma levels of DOPA, and avoid rapid decreases in plasma level due to peripheral metabolism. Alpha-methyl-DOPA (5) was beneficial to three patients for more than a year, but lost its effect with most others. A double-blind trial of MK 486-DOPA in 24 patients resulted in 2 patients with marked benefit, 7 with mild improvement, and 3 who did not change on MK 486-DOPA, versus 1 with mild improvement and 11 the same or worse on placebo-DOPA. Limitation of dietary protein to 7 g/day for the patient described virtually eliminated her marked "on–off" effect (Fig. 2), although she was unresponsive to MK 486-DOPA, but failed to change another patient's course.

DISCUSSION

The "on–off" effect is a phenomenon of chronic L-DOPA therapy, and it seems to grow worse with time. The rapid changes in clinical status from hypermotility to akinesia bespeak a pharmacological rather than a structural change. This may be due to alteration of DOPA absorption from gut, DOPA transport across the blood–brain barrier, of central distribution or metabolism of DOPA, or of striatal dopaminergic receptor activity. Improvement of some patients by decarboxylase inhibitors and low-protein diet favors the peripheral postulates.

Barbeau (6) has described a similar group of patients with oscillation in clinical response to L-DOPA having akinesia alternating with dyskinesia. He postulates that diurnal variations in dopamine excretion, lowest in the afternoon, may correlate with clinical changes. However, the distribution of "off" periods throughout the day among our patients seems sufficiently random to exclude a straightforward diurnal phenomenon. Dr. Barbeau suggests that we may have to settle for lower therapeutic goals in order to avoid excessive L-DOPA doses which may adversely affect nondopaminergic systems in the brain. In this light, it has always been our therapeutic philosophy to achieve the highest DOPA dose possible, limited only by side effects or a perfect therapeutic response. Perhaps this accounts for the large number of patients we are seeing with oscillation in response to DOPA, although the dosage difference between "on–off" and other patients is not impressive.

Finally, Yamamura et al. (7) have recently described two siblings with juvenile parkinsonism and marked diurnal variation of motility without medication. This suggests that a primary central neurogenic factor may account for at least some instances of oscillation in parkinsonism response.

SUMMARY

Twenty-nine patients with Parkinson's disease taking L-DOPA who developed severe oscillations in response ("on-off effect") are described. Marked dyskinesia alternating with akinesia of the legs and gait abnormalities were common. The syndrome developed after 28 months of L-DOPA therapy in young, moderately affected patients who were more susceptible than most to good and bad effects of L-DOPA. Autonomic concomitants, leg cramps, and confusion accompanied "off" periods in some patients. Treatment with decarboxylase inhibitors and low-protein diet helped some patients, indicating that peripheral absorption or metabolism of L-DOPA may be important in the "on–off" phenomenon.

ACKNOWLEDGMENTS

This work was supported by the American Parkinson's Disease Association and grant RR–47, General Clinical Research Centers Program, National Institutes of Health.

REFERENCES

1. McDowell, F., Lee, J. E., Swift, T., Sweet, R., Ogsbury, J., and Kessler, J., *Ann. Int. Med.* 72, 29 (1970).
2. Lee, J. E., Sweet, R., and McDowell, F., *Ann. Int. Med.* 75, 703 (1971).
3. Bianchine, J., Calimlim, L., Morgan, J., Dujuvne, C., and Lasagna, L., *Ann. N.Y. Acad. Sci.* 179, 126 (1971).
4. Sweet, R., Lee, J., Spiegel, H., and McDowell, F., *Neurology* 22, 520 (1972).
5. Sweet, R., Lee, J., and McDowell, F., *Clin. Pharmacol. Therap.* 13, 23 (1972).
6. Barbeau, A., in: *Parkinson's Disease: Rigidity, Akinesia, Behavior,* Vol. 1, edited by J. Siegfried, Hans Huber Publishers, Bern, 1972, p. 152.
7. Yamamura, Y., Sobue, I., Ando, K., Iida, M., Yanagi, T., and Kono, C., *Neurology* 23, 239 (1973).

Advances in Neurology, Vol. 5
Raven Press, New York © 1974

Variations in the "On-Off" Phenomenon

Roger C. Duvoisin

Department of Neurology, Columbia University College of Physicians and Surgeons, New York, New York 10032

This report will be very brief; I shall merely present some speculations and ideas that represent my thinking on this problem for the past several years.

I like the term "on-off." It was suggested to us by some patients who used it themselves to describe the suddenness with which the DOPA response came on, as if someone had flicked a switch by the door, or the suddenness with which it disappeared. Also, the sense of being "on," or "turned on" in the popular meaning of the expression as used in the drug culture, is also, I think, reflective of the patient's subjective experience, and one the patients rather like, which often makes it difficult to reduce their dose.

All of us who have treated parkinsonian patients with DOPA for some time agree with the general description given by Dr. Sweet. I think the phenomenon is not related to the length of treatment with L-DOPA, because it can be seen within the first week and at times even on the first day of treatment when L-DOPA is given in combination with peripheral DOPA decarboxylase inhibitors. It is related to the severity of the disease before treatment. Dr. Sweet's expression "moderate severity" actually includes Stages 3, 4, and 5 of our classification of Parkinson's disease. The "on-off" phenomenon does not occur in the very mildly involved patients, but only in those patients who are severely enough involved to have some akinesia. The phenomenon becomes more severe as one progresses from Stage 2, through 3, and on through 4. In the very far advanced cases, corresponding to Stage 5, it is not so striking a phenomenon, but it still is present.

The patients who have been able to keep records of the hours that they are "on" versus the hours they are "off" have provided most of our information. The length and severity of the "off" periods become progressively greater month by month and year by year at about the same rate that I have come to expect progression of Parkinson's disease, prior to the advent of L-DOPA therapy. I believe it is an expression of the disease and an interaction between the disease state and treatment.

I would like to offer a speculation or two that have to my knowledge not yet been offered. We must remember that Parkinson's disease is a degenerative disease of the nervous system. With the progressive decline in the number of nerve cells in the substantia nigra, there is a progressive decline in the number of functional nigral neurons.

If, as the work of Katzman and others has suggested, there is a tremendous force toward collateral sprouting so that with progressive degeneration no synaptic sites are left unoccupied, and if the collateral sprouting is from adjacent dopaminergic neurons, we could see an enlargement of the field of supply of each nigral projection in the striatum, and that might be expected to cause a loss of the asynchrony necessary for smooth function. In a phenomenon analogous to that seen peripherally with motor neuron disease, we would get an increased synchrony of the DOPA effect analogous to the giant action potentials seen in amyotrophic lateral sclerosis in the muscle. This might account for the sharper rise and the sharper decline, as well as the shorter duration, of the DOPA response. In addition, we might anticipate that individually surviving and still functioning nigral neurons would have lost some of their capacity to store dopamine; consequently, the duration of the dopamine effect might also decline on that basis. These two speculations may be open to investigation in the near future by the techniques of Katzman and others.

It seems unlikely, therefore, that the "on-off" effect can be ascribed to abnormal metabolites, or will be readily susceptible to manipulation by pharmacologic means or by biochemical approaches. The DOPA decarboxylase inhibitors have been rather disappointing in their ability to improve the duration and length of the "on" periods.

Advances in Neurology, Vol. 5
Raven Press, New York © 1974

Plasma Levodopa and the "On-Off" Effect

D. B. Calne, L. E. Claveria, and J. G. Allen

*Department of Medicine (Neurology), Royal Postgraduate Medical School, London W12
OHS, England and Department of Biochemistry, Roche Products Ltd.,
Welwyn Garden City, Herts., England*

Over the last few years the terms "on-off" effect, oscillations in performance, and akinesia paradoxica have been coined to describe a new syndrome of transient motor deficit which has emerged in parkinsonian patients
receiving L-DOPA (1–7). The outstanding feature of this syndrome is hypokinesia. Spontaneous fluctuations in the severity of symptoms and signs,
including hypokinesia, have been recognized as a prominent feature of
parkinsonism long before the advent of L-DOPA, so there has been some
difficulty in deciding if the "on-off" effect really constitutes a new entity
related to L-DOPA therapy. Because of the severity, duration, and progressive problem in management posed by patients experiencing these phenomena while receiving L-DOPA therapy, most observers are convinced
that the "on-off" effect is something other than the transient spontaneous
exacerbation of parkinsonism well recognized before L-DOPA therapy.

Attempts to delineate the clinical features which characterize the "on-
off" effect have not, up to now, resulted in a single coherent description
which is universally accepted. There is general agreement that the dominant
feature of the "off" phase is hypokinesia, that the attacks start and stop with
dramatic abruptness over a few minutes, and that they generally last $\frac{1}{2}$ to
3 hr. Their duration is one factor discriminating between "on-off" effects
and spontaneous fluctuations seen in parkinsonian patients not receiving
L-DOPA, in whom transient clinical deterioration is commonly of shorter
duration, persisting for minutes rather than hours. Other components which
have been reported to accompany hypokinesia in the "on-off" attacks include hypertonia, hypotonia, tremor, dyskinesia, confusion, distress, and
flushing. Controversial reports have claimed that predisposing factors include such contradictory features as mild or severe parkinsonism, long or
short durations of L-DOPA therapy, high or low doses of L-DOPA. The
overall prevalence of "on-off" phenomena is approximately 10% in parkinsonian patients on routine L-DOPA therapy. As the pharmacological
mechanism of these episodic deteriorations of motor performance is not
known, no rational approach to their management is possible. Measures

which have been claimed to ameliorate these oscillations in performance include reduction of the total daily dosage of L-DOPA, more frequent administration of smaller doses of L-DOPA, temporary cessation of L-DOPA therapy, concomitant administration of extracerebral decarboxylase inhibitors, and limitation of dietary protein. None of these approaches to management has proved entirely satisfactory.

Barbeau (3) has recently presented observations indicating that "on-off" phenomena comprise four clinically distinguishable entities. He considered that some were related to an excessive intake of L-DOPA. In an attempt to obtain biochemical evidence which might be relevant to this claim, we have investigated the plasma concentrations of L-DOPA in a patient undergoing frequent oscillations in motor performance.

We studied a 67-year-old woman who had suffered from idiopathic parkinsonism for 14 years. She had moderate neurological disability and initially responded well to L-DOPA, taking 5 g per day for $2\frac{1}{2}$ years. She then began to experience episodes of severe dysphonia accompanied by confusion and a general deterioration in mobility. She was admitted to the hospital for observation. Her voice was recorded hourly on magnetic tape. Hourly blood samples were taken for estimation of L-DOPA as described by Reid et al. (8). The voice recordings were presented in a randomized order to two "blind" evaluators who graded the degree of dysphonia according to an arbitrary scoring protocol in which 0 represented normality and 4 indicated a severe reduction in the volume and quality of articulation such that the patient's voice hardly emerged over the background noise level of the recording. These quantitative assessments were then correlated with the plasma concentrations of L-DOPA, and it became evident that her deterioration in phonation coincided with the development of exceptionally high plasma levels, over 4 μg/ml. When the plasma concentration of L-DOPA returned to the more normal therapeutic range (approximately 1 to 2 μg/ml), her dysphonia improved. In addition to the high peak concentration of L-DOPA, it was notable that this patient absorbed the drug extremely rapidly, and the plasma half-life was longer (1.57 hr) than normal for a 1-g dose (1.08 hr). These findings are summarized in Fig. 1.

Changes were also observed in her confusion and facial hypokinesia which were evaluated according to an arbitrary clinical scoring protocol in which 0 represented normality and 4 indicated maximal deficit (9). Confusion and facial hypokinesia were both exacerbated when her plasma L-DOPA was high.

Although "on-off" reactions may well constitute a heterogenous group of phenomena, our observations indicate that some, at least, are manifestations of L-DOPA toxicity as suggested by Barbeau (3). Furthermore, it seems probable that unusual pharmacokinetics may be one contributing factor. These findings raise the question of how high doses of L-DOPA may exacerbate hypokinesia. Possible mechanisms include the formation

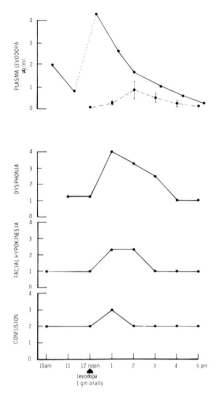

FIG. 1. Observations following an oral dose of 1.0 g L-DOPA between courses of breakfast at 8:00 A.M. and lunch at 12:00 noon. The dotted line indicates continuity of L-DOPA concentration in the blood: the rise must have followed the noon dose rather than preceded it. The broken line represents a normal range of plasma L-DOPA levels following 1 g orally, from (11). Simultaneous evaluations of dysphonia, facial hypokinesia, and confusion are shown to demonstrate their correlation with high plasma concentrations of L-DOPA.

of metabolites of L-DOPA which may be false dopaminergic transmitters, dopamine receptor blockers, inhibitors of L-DOPA transport systems, or inhibitors of cerebral DOPA decarboxylase (12). Alternatively, metabolites of L-DOPA may be leading to increased formation of acetylcholine (10). Further investigation of the concentrations of metabolites of L-DOPA in the plasma, urine, and cerebrospinal fluid may help to discriminate between some of these alternatives.

REFERENCES

1. Cotzias, G. C., Papavasiliou, P. S., and Gellene, R., *New Eng. J. Med.* 280, 337 (1969).
2. Barbeau, A., Gillo-Joffroy, L., and Mars, H., *Clin. Pharmacol. Ther.* 12, 353 (1971).
3. Barbeau, A., in: *Proceedings of the 4th International Symposium on Parkinson's Disease,* ed. by J. Siegfried, Huber, Bern (1972).
4. Markham, C. H., *Neurology* 22, 17 (1972).

5. McDowell, F., *Neurology* 22, 24 (1972).
6. Yahr, M. D., in: *Proceedings of the 4th International Symposium on Parkinson's Disease,* ed. by J. Siegfried, Huber, Bern (1972).
7. Damasio, A. R., Castro-Caldas, A., and Levy, A., in: *Advances in Neurology,* Vol. 3, ed. by D. B. Calne, Raven Press, New York (1973).
8. Reid, J. L., Calne, D. B., Vakil, S. D., Allen, J. G., and Davies, C. A., *J. Neurol. Sci.* 17, 45 (1972).
9. Calne, D. B., Reid, J. L., Vakil, S. D., Rao, S., Petrie, A., Pallis, C. A., Gawler, J., Thomas, P. K., and Hilson, A., *Brit. Med. J.* 3, 729 (1971).
10. Sethy, V. H., and Van Woert, M. H., *Neuropharmacology* 12, 27 (1973).
11. Dunner, D. L., Brodie, H. K. H., and Goodwin, F. K., *Clin. Pharmacol. Exp. Ther.* 12, 121 (1971).
12. Hornykiewicz, O., in: *Advances in Neurology,* Vol. 2, ed. by M. D. Yahr, Raven Press, New York (1973).

DISCUSSION

Dr. Cotzias: We can entertain some questions about the clinical description of the "on-off" phenomenon.

Dr. Goldberg: I will speculate some. We have heard the following: (1) that 3-methoxydopa blocks DOPA activity from Dr. Muenter; (2) that in the kidney 3-methoxydopamine is a dopamine antagonist; (3) that 3-methoxydopa accumulates; and (4) that 3-methoxydopamine does not block alpha or beta receptors.

Therefore, the clues lead me to think of 3-methoxydopa. If this were an important factor, you could still have flushing and tachycardia, and you would turn off the DOPA effect.

The treatment then would be: (1) stop the drug and see if 3-methoxydopa levels come down, not in the blood but in the tissues; and, (2) give an O-methyltransferase inhibitor, which may prevent the phenomenon.

Dr. Cotzias: Could you name such an inhibitor?

Dr. Goldberg: They are available but most of them are toxic. I think Dr. Brossi could come up with one.

Dr. Cotzias: I hoped you could name an inhibitor that is not a substrate which creates its own troubles.

Dr. Poirier: I would like to add a comment to Dr. Duvoisin's suggestion that there might be sprouting on the fibers after a cell is degenerated. I think, if I'm correct, this sprouting can take place from other incoming fibers and not necessarily from the dopaminergic. So you could expect sprouting from, for example, the thalamostriatal or cortical sites of fibers.

Concerning the "on-off" effect, especially dystonia, I would like to mention that we should not always believe that the effect occurs at the level of the striatum. When DOPA is given it is spread all over the brain, with dopamine, HVA, and abnormal metabolites throughout the brain. I would not be surprised to find out that dystonia is not due to an abnormal functioning at the level of the upper brainstem.

Dr. Roberts: I wonder if methylation is a problem, whether guanidoacetic acid might not trap some of the methyl groups and then cut down the phenomenon.

Dr. Cotzias: And this will form what compound?

Dr. Roberts: Creatine.

Dr. Yahr: I wouldn't want everybody to go away thinking that the methylated products are as pertinent to interfering with the DOPA response. If you give DOPA with a decarboxylase inhibitor, such as alpha-methyl-dopahydrazine, you increase the amount of methylated products in spinal fluid at least, and do not necessarily decrease the therapeutic response.

Advances in Neurology, Vol. 5
Raven Press, New York © 1974

The Clinical Physiology of Side Effects in Long-Term L-DOPA Therapy

André Barbeau

Department of Neurology, University of Montreal, and Department of Neurobiology, Clinical Research Institute of Montreal, Montreal 130, Quebec, Canada

INTRODUCTION

It has been repeatedly noted by many authors during the last few years that, after a certain time on high-dose-level L-DOPA therapy, there appears with progressively increasing frequency in some patients a variation in the level of performance during the day. These diurnal changes were first reported by Cotzias, Papavasiliou, and Gellene (1). Since then, different aspects of the oscillations have been described. In the present review we will attempt to summarize our own observations and to outline the avenues of possible fruitful physiological investigation.

Performance in the motor sphere may have many meanings depending on the initial motility of the subject, his achievement goals, and the method of measurement by the observer. For this study we utilized both subjective assessment by the patient of a comparison between his "best moments" and times when he was not well, or not "free," and objective measurements of performance on a standard series of simple tests (2). Using these criteria, we found that the majority of our patients who had been taking L-DOPA for a year or more (and as early as 6 months for those on L-DOPA plus Ro 4–4602 therapy) experienced a bimodal pattern of performance during the day, with good periods usually in the morning and early evening, and bad periods during which akinesia reappeared in the afternoon and late evening (3). Following Cotzias' lead, we modified drug regimens, protein content of diet, and other variables with some initial improvement, mainly in the less severe oscillations. But, as time passed, it became progressively more difficult to achieve any kind of satisfactory result as the variations became more pronounced (4). They were made worse by independent patterns of abnormal involuntary movements (A.I.M.), and there appeared, again with increasing frequency, a strange phenomenon marked by a rapid change-over from the "free" to the "rigid" (or "bad") conditions, or inversely. This "switch" effect has received the name "on-and-off phenomenon" because of its occasional very rapid unfolding (5). Some clinical characteristics of the patients during the "bad" periods made them different from the pre-DOPA experience and led us and others to use the term "akinesia paradoxica" (6, 7). Finally, as we will detail later, we became convinced that this process is progressive, leading eventually to a decompensation of the motor homeostatic mechanism and a state of dependence (6). For all these reasons, it became urgent to define clearly our terms before attempting some explanation of the underlying mechanism. The all-important question that must be answered, once the existence of these phenomena is acknowledged, is whether this is due to a side effect of long-term L-DOPA therapy, or to the natural progression of the underlying illness. Although at this stage our answers can only be partial, we will also attempt to face this problem.

DEFINITIONS

Akinesia

There is now overwhelming evidence that the only symptom clearly related to dopamine deficiency in the nigro-striatal system is akinesia (8–10). Rigidity and tremor may, secondarily, be modulated by the actual level of striatal dopamine, but are certainly more directly related to modifications in other systems using serotonin, acetylcholine, γ-aminobutyric acid (GABA), or other substances still unexplored as putative neurotransmitters. L-DOPA almost specifically corrects akinesia before it affects any other symptom. Therefore, if we say that akinesia reappears during some of the oscillations, we must clearly define this term to differentiate between it and other phenomena noted later. In another essay (6), we have analyzed in detail the phenomenon of akinesia, as we see it. According to that definition, akinesia is a defect in the "set" mechanism of motility (see infra) and includes the following components: (1) a defect in the initiation of movements, (2) a defect in kinetic melody, (3) a defect in the strategy of learning, and (4) a rapid fatiguability on repetitive tasks.

Motility

One of the most frequent causes of error in the clinical interpretation of our results has, we feel, been the misunderstanding of the concept of increased motility, which, of course, was the principal goal of our therapeutic approach. Indeed, too often we have equated decreased motility with akinesia. In previous studies (Fig. 1), we have outlined four main components of this process, all interrelated and all probably modulated by different monoamines: tone, rhythm, set, and drive (6, 11, 12). No useful movement can take place without an underlying pattern of correct tone in the appropriate sustaining muscles. The resting tone sufficient to maintain

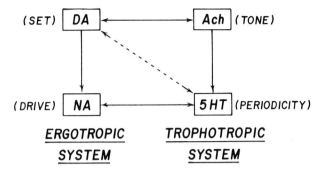

FIG. 1. Role of putative neurotransmitters in the various components of motility.

position at any given time is not enough; it must be supplemented by the preparedness of other muscle groups in anticipation of coming use, and following a preset pattern of movements. The evidence at hand implicates the gamma system in this process (13) and presupposes a central integration of the motor patterning and a timed signal system for the correct triggering of the operation. The sum total of these mechanisms we have called *set*. As demonstrated below, set is modulated by dopamine but, through a well-known reciprocal balance with acetylcholine (11), it also regulates individual muscle tone. Once the body has started its movement, it requires both a drive and a rhythm control mechanism to keep it going. The "drive," or motor, is an energy-spending system and utilizes the body's well-known ergotropic modulator: noradrenaline. Whenever rhythm is required, for example in walking, much of this energy can be conserved through the fine regulation imparted by serotoninergic systems, such as those in the brainstem, pineal, and hypothalamus (14, 15).

The two most important components of motility, as defined clinically, are "set" and "drive" (Fig. 2). Through a series of neuropharmacological experiments in our laboratory and elsewhere (16), it is now evident that a specific deficiency in dopamine will result in a state of "akinesia" in man and a variety of animals. In its more severe state, dopamine deficiency will cause progressively more important modifications in muscle tone, translated clinically into rigidity and occasionally catatonia. The use of L-DOPA, in animals as well as in man, almost always reverses the akinetic state. However, once akinesia is corrected, giving more L-DOPA will *not* result in increased motility, but in the appearance of a number of danger signals, such as abnormal involuntary movements of the facio-linguo-buccal type in man (4), or the "gnaw-compulsion" syndrome in rodents (17).

Similarly, it has now been clearly demonstrated that a specific depletion in noradrenaline (i.e., by blocking dopamine-β-hydroxylase and the reuptake process) will also result in reduced locomotion, occasionally in sedation. If the dopamine level is satisfactory (thus, if "set" is normal), specific cor-

ROLE OF CATECHOLAMINES IN MOTOR FUNCTION

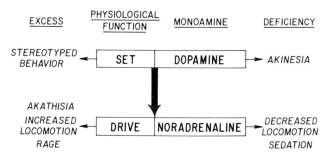

FIG. 2. The "set" and "drive" components of motility.

rection of this noradrenaline deficiency will permit resumption of normal motility. However, in the presence of a combined dopamine deficiency, no amount of noradrenaline will restore complete motility. On the other hand, overdose of noradrenaline with normal dopamine level will result in clinical akathisia ("need to move") and in overactivity of the animals, occasionally even in a rage reaction.

We emphasize again that once the "set" defect has been corrected by dopamine repletion, further motility is *not* obtained by giving more dopamine (a process which leads only to A.I.M.), but by supplying the proper amount of noradrenaline, or by specifically stimulating noradrenergic receptors (i.e., with Clonidine®). As we will attempt to demonstrate later, misunderstanding of this very principle is responsible for many of the long-term side effects noted under chronic L-DOPA therapy.

The "On-and-Off" Phenomenon

The initial response to L-DOPA therapy is usually one of remarkable increases in overall motility, with a reappearance of most previously lost associated movements. Unfortunately, this improvement does not usually continue for 1 or 2 years without the complications of abnormal involuntary movements or of the more obscure "on-and-off" phenomenon. The patient may be doing quite well when, without apparent reason, and not necessarily in association with a stressful situation, he suddenly feels very tired and, to the casual onlooker, rapidly returns to a state of akinesia, with expressionless or pained facies, stooped posture, and lack of motivation to move. This process is occasionally very rapid. I have seen it occur literally within a few seconds. This has prompted the comparison with an electrical "on-and-off" switch process. The akinetic state may last a few minutes or persist some hours. The return to normal (or at least the previous "well" state) may be equally rapid, but usually occurs more slowly, almost imperceptibly, often with the reappearance of dyskinesias. Indeed, the presence or absence of abnormal involuntary movements, and their time correlation to the recurring akinesia, is probably one of the important factors to be considered in the pathophysiology of the "on-and-off" phenomenon.

Whatever the speed of the switch process, the patient can often be observed to develop a strange pattern of behavior which is different from his pre-L-DOPA akinetic-rigid deportment. At first there are a number of autonomic manifestations: complete feeling of tiredness, profuse sweating or acute pallor, tachycardia and palpitations, dilated pupils, and occasional increases in blood pressure. The outward appearance of the patient is one of anxiety piercing an expressionless facial mask. This state will subside within 10 to 30 min, leaving a marked lassitude, some depressed or dejected feelings, and a complete lack of will to move. The patient wants to lie down and refuses to talk.

Later he will know that the episode is about to end and he will try, almost in a magical way, to hasten the moment by a series of preset, stereotyped behaviors which he has previously associated with success: gymnastic exercises, stamping of the foot, rotation of the head, wringing of the hands, and so on. These episodes may occur once or many times per day and are extremely distressing to both patient and family.

Akinesia Paradoxica

In addition to the above-noted phenomena, there also can occur some sudden "freezing" episodes during which the patient will be totally unable to move, or even to lift his feet from the ground, as if he were riveted to the floor. These episodes usually occur without prodromal symptoms, "in a clear blue sky" as it were. The opposite phenomenon has been well described. It is the classic story of the rigid, wheelchair-confined patient in a nursing home who, upon hearing the warning cry of "fire," will get up and run out of the house almost as rapidly as other, nonparkinsonian patients, only to "freeze" again on the lawn outside. This rare occurrence has received the name of "kinesia paradoxica." The phenomenon which we now describe, by association, could be called "akinesia paradoxica." It is not rare in patients on long-term L-DOPA therapy and need not be associated with stress or danger. Sometimes the sudden lack of proprioceptive and visual input, such as the crossing of a door threshold or a wide black band painted on the floor, or the simultaneous inpouring of too many sensory inputs (for example, in the middle of a busy street) will be sufficient to trigger the freezing. Examination of the patient at that time reveals the surprising finding of an almost total hypotonia along with the severely akinetic appearance. One can passively lift the legs, but the patient is absolutely unable to do so himself. He is literally "nailed to the ground." The first component of classical akinesia, the inability to initiate a movement, is present but accompanied by severe hypotonia and hyporeflexia instead of the usual rigidity and hyperreflexia seen before L-DOPA. We feel that this phenomenon deserves a special nosological place and, as such, a separate physiological explanation.

TYPES OF OSCILLATIONS IN PERFORMANCE

We have previously described in detail four types, or stages, in the diurnal oscillations seen in the performance of patients under chronic L-DOPA therapy (6). To permit a clearer understanding of our proposed explanation for these occurrences, we will again summarize our findings.

Type One (First-Stage) Oscillations

Type one (first-stage) oscillations (Fig. 3) are certainly the most frequently encountered of the variations in performance. The bimodal diurnal rhythm has been described before, with "good" periods in the morning and early evening and "bad" periods in the afternoon and late evening. The actual time course may, of course, be shifted one way or another by a few hours, but the bimodal pattern remains. There is no clear-cut correlation with time of ingestion of L-DOPA, but a heavy protein intake appears to

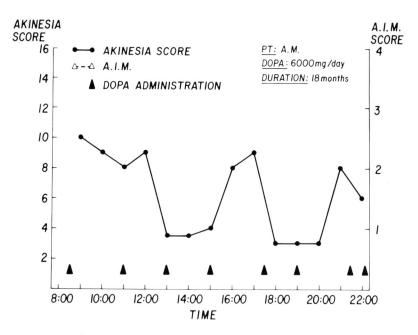

FIG. 3. Type one (first-stage) oscillations in performance.

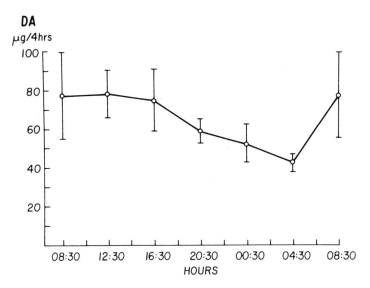

FIG. 4. Diurnal oscillations in the urinary excretion of dopamine in nine normal subjects (mean ± SEM). Subjects were studied under metabolic ward conditions on a constant diet and in the recumbent position.

increase the depth of the variations. Blood levels of DOPA sometimes tend to correlate with the same pattern, but unfortunately this is not a constant relationship. We have found a very similar rhythm in the diurnal urinary excretion of dopamine, with maximum activity in the morning and early afternoon, and a low in late afternoon and evening (Fig. 4 and Table 1). Since urinary excretion of dopamine can only reflect the general metabolism of this

TABLE 1. *Diurnal variations in catecholamines urinary excretion (nine normal subjects)**

Times	0830 1230	1230 1630	1030 2030	2030 0030	0030 0430	0430 0830
DA (μg/4 hr)	77.1 ± 22.8	78.1 ± 12.7	74.3 ± 15.8	58.8 ± 6.3	52.0 ± 10.4	42.8 ± 6.2
NA (μg/4 hr)	9.5 ± 2.6	8.4 ± 2.2	9.8 ± 1.9	7.5 ± 2.1	5.9 ± 1.7	6.7 ± 2.8
Volume (ml/4 hr)	693	1087	779	795	522	316
NA^+ mEq/4 hr	38.8	63.4	54.7	49.2	29.4	15
K^+ mEq/4 hr	16.5	25.7	13.9	8.9	7.1	8.3
Creatinine mg/4 hr	0.26	0.22	0.30	0.25	0.26	0.32

amine, we feel that this finding indicates that dopamine is not metabolized uniformly throughout the day, whether in the gastrointestinal tract, the brain, or the kidney. Thus, given a constant supply of L-DOPA, the oscillations in performance could reflect a temporary relative deficiency of dopamine at the effective sites. That this is probably the case is supported by the observation that type one oscillations can usually be influenced favorably by slight modifications in treatment schedules or diet. One other argument in favor of temporary deficiency is the complete absence of abnormal involuntary movements at this stage. Moreover, during these episodes there is a clear return to the previous akineto-rigid condition, albeit to a lesser degree than the pre-DOPA stage. Correlation with blood DOPA levels is usually good.

Most of the oscillations observed by Cotzias and during which his group *(This Volume)* have demonstrated changes in growth hormone discharges, with consequent releases of proteins and competition for transport mechanisms, appear to involve stage one, thus the phase of dopamine deficiency.

Type Two (Second-Stage) Oscillations

In type two (second-stage) oscillations (Fig. 5), the bimodal variations in performance become imperceptibly complemented by another, totally independent, diurnal pattern of facio-buccal, chorea-like, abnormal involuntary movements. These dyskinesias are at first clearly time related to the

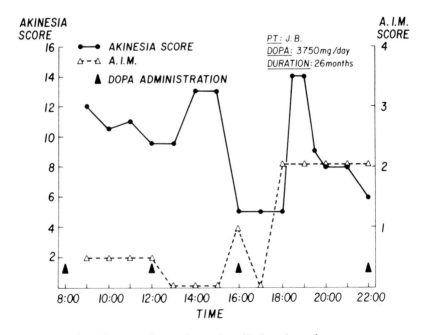

FIG. 5. Type two (second-stage) oscillations in performance.

ingestion of L-DOPA, appearing some $1\frac{1}{2}$ to 2 hr after almost each dose of the drug. A reduction in total dose will occasionally eliminate these movements, but usually at the expense of longer "bad" periods. Correction of the deficiency state thus becomes more of a problem, and simple schedule modifications usually do not suffice.

Type Three (Third-Stage) Oscillations

In type three (third-stage) oscillations (Fig. 6), the diurnal variations in performance noted in the first stage continue unabated, or even more pronounced. Now, however, the abnormal involuntary movements become more severe, usually prompting a reduction in dosage. Moreover, it appears that a pattern of relationship between the two previously independent oscillations is slowly being established. Sudden changes now occur. The "good" or "free" periods are usually preceded and occupied by the appearance of dyskinesias, which is sometimes severe. The patient is not annoyed by these movements, because he has come to realize that he is usually better when they occur and that he gradually, and occasionally rapidly, returns to the akinetic stage when they disappear. Examination during and immediately after the dyskinetic episodes reveals akinesia with hypotonia rather than rigidity. Only when the "bad" periods last more than a few hours is rigidity,

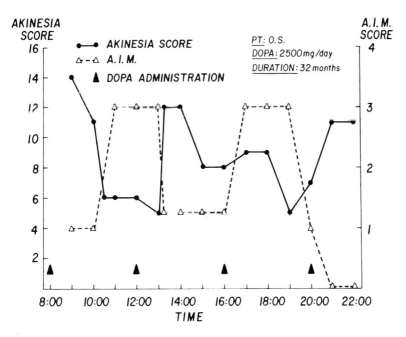

FIG. 6. Type three (third-stage) oscillations in performance.

as previously known, again noted. It is during stage three that the "on-and-off" phenomena previously described start to appear, as well as the sudden akinetic "crises" preceded or accompanied by a type of autonomic discharge. Because of all these side effects ("crises," dyskinesias, oscillations), the overall effectiveness of the L-DOPA therapy on motility appears diminished. However, it is our contention that this is not due to habituation, or loss of potency of L-DOPA, but to the positive addition of undesirable clinical features, probably because of overdosage. We shall return to this point later.

Type Four (Fourth-Stage) Oscillations

In type four (fourth-stage) oscillations (Fig. 7), the phenomena noted in stage three become the rule rather than the exception. The two previously independent oscillation patterns appear to merge completely. The patient is well only in the presence of severe dyskinesias. As soon as these disappear, he again becomes akinetic. The change from one state to the next is almost instantaneous and always reciprocal: presence of dyskinesias equals well-being; absence equals "bad" periods. During the latter, muscle tone is always diminished. Sudden freezing episodes occur frequently. We have reached a state of dependence on dyskinesias for satisfactory motility.

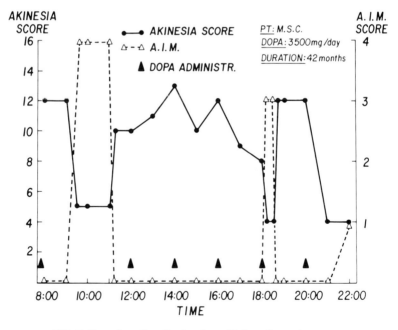

FIG. 7. Type four (fourth-stage) oscillations in performance.

One significant observation is regularly made by the patient himself: he will state, rather surprisingly to the unsuspecting physician, that the best moment of his day, except during severe dyskinesias, is *before* taking his first morning dose of L-DOPA! To us this means that both the dyskinesias and the *hypotonic* akinetic periods are *additive* phenomena. We are not dealing anymore with the simple deficiency akinesia of stage one. The only time when such a condition now exists is after the long nightly period of abstinence.

We realize, of course, that any clinical division of oscillations is by necessity schematic and incomplete. Others may add to or subtract from this working classification, or subdivide each stage into more facets. The important thing to remember is that we are observing a *continuum* of phenomena secondary to long-term L-DOPA usage. From a simple deficiency state, probably related to some intrinsic diurnal pattern of dopamine metabolism, the oscillations gradually become the result of superimposed "positive" symptoms such as the dyskinesias and the hypotonic "akinesia paradoxica." The end result in both cases is a *decrease* in motility. Because most of us had wrongly equated this decreased motility to a deficit in effective dopamine, our normal reaction was gradually to *increase* the total dose of L-DOPA, thus unwittingly ensuring the slow passage into the next phase, and further decreasing motility, while increasing dyskinesias and eventually reaching a state of homeostatic failure, or dependence on severe dyskinesias for any motility.

These were the clinical observations which we had made, and partially reported previously (6). It is obvious that once we became convinced of the existence of these phenomena, and mainly of the continuum, a number of important questions were raised.

PROGRESSION OF THE ILLNESS OR SIDE EFFECTS OF L-DOPA

The first and most important of these questions was to determine whether the progressive loss in motility observed in many, but not all, patients under high-level L-DOPA therapy was the result of progression of the disease, loss of efficacy of L-DOPA, or the presence of "positive" (added) side effects of the drug.

To answer this question, we devised the following experiment: our working hypothesis stated that if L-DOPA was causing both the dyskinesias and the late-stage oscillations in performance, a simple but slow reduction in dosage should result in a decreased incidence of both A.I.M. and oscillations (or at least a reduction in their severity) without loss of motor performance. If, on the other hand, these oscillations were due to progression of the illness or to loss of efficacy of the drug, including decreased responsiveness, then a reduction in dosage should make the patients worse.

We chose for this experiment 34 patients who had been on L-DOPA for a

TABLE 2. *Control group 1: Rapid reduction (N = 10 patients)*

Time (months)	L-DOPA dosage (g/day)	Patients with A.I.M.	Patients with oscillations							Performance weighed score (mean ± SE)
			No.	Severity						
				0	1	2	3	4		
0 (before)	4.4	10	10	0	1	3	3	3		25.8 ± 1.32
1	3.4	4	3	7	0	0	2	1		5.3 ± 1.09

minimum of 2 years (average dose equivalent to 4.2 g/day of L-DOPA at time of onset of experiment*). All of these patients manifested oscillations in performance *and* abnormal involuntary movements, thus none were in the simple, stage-one deficiency state. Over a period of 5 months, we voluntarily effected a very slow, gradual reduction in dosage equivalent to 1 g/day of L-DOPA per patient. This reduction was never more than 250 mg every 2 weeks, and often was of smaller magnitude. Over the next 5 months, the daily dosage of L-DOPA was again decreased slowly and gradually in this experimental group another 0.5 g/day on the average (usually 100 mg every month). The first control group consisted of 10 patients who had also been taking L-DOPA for 2 years (equivalent daily dose: 4.4 g of L-DOPA), all of whom manifested with dyskinesias and severe (stage two or above) oscillations in performance. In this group we effected a similar 1-g reduction over a period of only 1 month (250 mg/week). Finally, a second control group of 10 patients (average 4.1 g/day), all with A.I.M. and oscillations, was kept at a constant level for 10 months.

The results of this experiment are unequivocal. A rapid reduction by 1 g over a period of 1 month (control group 1) produced a definite worsening in all 10 patients, despite a lessening in the incidence of A.I.M. and abnormal oscillations (Table 2). Within 7 to 10 days, all patients had a return of their previous parkinsonian state and almost complete loss of the improvement thus far obtained with L-DOPA. This part of the experiment was therefore discontinued. In control group 2 (Table 3), where the dosage level of L-DOPA was kept at 4.1 g/day for 10 months without alteration, there was no improvement in the total incidence of A.I.M. or abnormal oscillations. In fact, there was a progressive further loss in the motor performance score of the order observed previously over a similar time period before investigating this phenomenon.

In the experimental group (Table 4), slow gradual reduction of the dose level produced only some transient loss of performance which never lasted

* For patients taking L-DOPA and Ro 4–4602 on a 4:1 ratio, the equivalence was calculated using a factor of 5 for conversion of the L-DOPA daily level.

TABLE 3. *Control group 2: No change in dosage (N = 10 patients)*

| Time (months) | L-DOPA dosage (g/day) | Patients with A.I.M. | Patients with oscillations | | | | | | Performance weighed score (mean ± SE) |
| | | | No. | Severity | | | | | |
				0	1	2	3	4	
0 (before)	4.1	10	10	0	2	2	2	4	23.6 ± 1.47
5	4.1	10	10	0	1	1	3	5	21.4 ± 1.28
10	4.1	10	10	0	0	2	2	6	18.2 ± 0.98

TABLE 4. *Experimental group: Slow reduction (N = 34 patients)*

| Time (months) | L-DOPA dosage (g/day) | Patients with A.I.M. | Patients with oscillations | | | | | | Performance weighed score (mean ± SE) |
| | | | No. | Severity | | | | | |
				0	1	2	3	4	
0 (before)	4.2	34	34	0	0	16	11	7	27.71 ± 1.59
5	3.2	4	19	10	6	10	8	1	26.56 ± 1.66
10	2.7	3	16	18	6	7	3	0	24.81 ± 2.50

more than 10 days. By the end of 5 months, only four of the original patients still manifested with dyskinesias, and only 19 still had significant oscillations. In all but one of the latter, there had been a reduction in the severity of the oscillations by at least one stage. Interestingly, this clear improvement in side effects was accomplished without any loss in motor performance, as measured objectively. Thus, in this group of patients, at least, it appears that we were administering *unnecessarily* nearly 1 g too much of L-DOPA per day to obtain similar performance results, at the expense of considerably more side effects. We therefore continued the experiment with a still further reduction equivalent to 0.5 g over the next 5 months. This resulted in little further change in the incidence of A.I.M. (Table 4), but in a significant reduction in the severity, if not the total incidence, of oscillations. Although the average motor performance score was not significantly decreased, it must be noted that in at least four cases there was a clinically significant loss (greater than 20% from baseline score). Thus, 30 of the original 34 patients still were performing at the same level 10 months later despite a daily reduction in dosage equivalent to 1.5 g of L-DOPA (average dose had now reached 2.7 g/day). This result was noted in addition to a very significant reduction in side effects. Only four patients seemed to have gone below a useful threshold.

What can we conclude from these experiments? It is obvious that many of the side effects noted during chronic L-DOPA therapy are not due only to progression of the illness, but are secondary to the wrong utilization of the drug. This was evident and well known with regard to the dyskinesias. We think that we have conclusively demonstrated that it applies equally well to the more severe oscillations in performance previously reported. Otherwise there is no way to explain their disappearance or decrease with a slow dosage reduction, *without* a simultaneous loss in motor performance. In fact, our second control group shows that such a loss is what should be expected over time when no dosage reduction is accomplished. Thus, our main conclusion is that the progressive loss in motor performance observed after long periods of continuous L-DOPA therapy is not due solely to progression of the illness (a factor that certainly plays a role), but that it is often the result of mismanagement. It is evident that in the great majority of our experimental group (30 of 34 patients), we were giving unnecessarily nearly 1.5 g of L-DOPA in excess of the minimum required to maintain performance at the level previously obtained during the first 2 years of therapy. No advantage was derived from this generosity. In fact, not only did we increase the cost to the patient of his treatment, but we were actually contributing to an evident decrease in motor performance and to abnormal involuntary movements, distressing at least to the observer.

Two restrictions must be placed on the above statement: first, it is clear that the reduction must be accomplished extremely slowly, especially when a high dose level had been maintained for a long time. This reduction must, in fact, be even slower than the gradual stepwise increase adopted earlier following Cotzias' suggestion. Second, it is also obvious that for each individual patient, there is a minimum (threshold) level below which one cannot further reduce the dosage without loss of performance. What this level is must still be found by trial and error, and it is too early to tell whether it is a constant or a variable reference point, even in an individual patient.

What we now seem to have demonstrated is that there are *two* dosage levels to strive for in the therapy of Parkinson's disease with L-DOPA: an *induction dosage* which may be quite high (4 to 6 g/day in our own experience) and *must* be reached slowly by stepwise increments. The end point here can be gauged according to the response of the patient in the motor sphere, but in no case should it exceed the minimum level at which dyskinesias are produced. In fact, we regard the appearance of abnormal involuntary movements as a danger signal! The second level is the *maintenance dosage,* which may be much lower and again must be reached, preferably voluntarily and not through the necessity of side effects, by an even slower gradual reduction. At the present time, the maintenance level in our experience appears to be between 2.5 and 3.5 g/day of L-DOPA. It will probably be lower as time goes on. This concept of two dose levels in the therapy of one disease, of course, is not new. It is well known for cortisone.

One further significant point in favor of the concept that the *severe* oscillations in performance are secondary to L-DOPA overdosage is the fact that in addition to a general decrease in their incidence, in every case we have observed a retrogression by at least one stage in their severity after a 10-month slow reduction in dosage.

Thus, L-DOPA does not lose efficacy with time, but when used in excess of a useful threshold, it can cause a reduction in motor performance, with or without a phenomenon of dependence on the presence of abnormal involuntary movements. Why is that? In the last part of this review we will attempt to answer this paradox.

THE PHYSIOLOGY OF LONG-TERM SIDE EFFECTS

The clue to the problem apparently lies in the observations previously referred to, indicating that in the more severe stages of oscillations we see a new form of akinesia, now accompanied by *hypotonia* rather than an increase in tone. This hypotonia may or may not be preceded by an autonomic discharge, and it does not last indefinitely, for it eventually disappears to flow into the more classical akineto-rigid state of dopamine deficiency, unless more DOPA has been given and A.I.M. reappear. We therefore postulate that it is a positive (additive) phenomenon and not the negative state of the usual form of dopamine-deficiency akinesia. Moreover, we think the above-noted clinical observations should help in orienting our further pathophysiological studies.

Many biochemical changes are known to take place in the brain after chronic L-DOPA overdosage. Figure 8 summarizes some possible events which may occur and may bear some relationship to the production of abnormal involuntary movements and the appearance of hypotonia with a reduction in motility or "drive," events which characterize the more severe stages of chronic L-DOPA overdosage. Each one of the modifications illustrated has been shown to occur in specific circumstances, but it is not yet known whether the full pattern can be found simultaneously, or which of the components is the most important:

(a) L-DOPA excess produces increases in brain dopamine concentration, in animals and in man (21). Even in Parkinson's disease, where dopamine concentrations are decreased, long-term treatment causes a return toward more normal levels of dopamine in the striatum (22). However, abnormal involuntary movements are usually not produced in humans given large doses of L-DOPA (up to 10 g/day) if they do not simultaneously have a dopamine deficiency. This has been shown in normal subjects (23) and in patients with amyotrophic lateral sclerosis (24). It thus appears that for dopamine — or its methylated derivatives (4, 12) — to produce abnormal

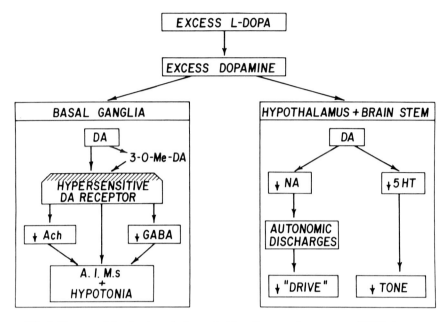

FIG. 8. The possible physiopathology of side effects on long-term L-DOPA therapy.

movements at the doses usually employed, it is necessary to have hypersensitive dopamine receptors in the striatum. Denervation hypersensitivity has been postulated in Parkinson's disease by Ungerstedt (25), and in Huntington's chorea by Klawans, Ilahi, and Ringel (26) and Barbeau (12). There is even evidence that after long-term usage of high doses of L-DOPA one can observe a further modification in receptor sensitivity. It has indeed been observed that in such cases it is often necessary to use smaller doses of L-DOPA to obtain equal results after a temporary cessation of the drug.

(b) Through mechanisms still unclear, hyperstimulation of dopamine receptors in the basal ganglia is accompanied by changes in the effective activation of the cholinoceptive and GABA-ergic receptors which modulate tone. We have previously shown that variations in dopamine concentrations result in changes in cholinergic activity (27). In Huntington's chorea, where hypersensitivity of dopamine receptors is also postulated (12, 26), secondary modifications in cholinergic receptor activity have been found (28, 29). Similarly, in that disease, where hypotonia and A.I.M. are the rule, decreases in GABA concentrations in the globus pallidus and putamen have now been reported (12, 30).

(c) Many authors (21, 31) have shown that high levels of dopamine can produce a decrease in brain serotonin concentrations and in the 5-HIAA levels in the cerebrospinal fluid (32) or urine (33). Ng, Chase, Colburn, and Kopin (34) have demonstrated that this phenomenon is the result of a displacement mechanism within nerve endings (or a false neurotransmitter effect). It is interesting that in Down's disease (mongolism), where blood serotonin levels are usually low, there is also a marked hypotonia which can be corrected by the use of the precursor 5-hydroxytryptophan (35). Thus, serotonin depletion, as a consequence of high L-DOPA levels, may be a further component of the induced hypotonia.

(d) A similar displacement (or "false transmitter") effect may contribute to the release of noradrenaline in the brainstem and hypothalamus, initially causing autonomic phenomena and later resulting in an effective noradrenergic deficiency. This deficiency is further reinforced by the feedback inhibition of dopamine synthesis caused by hyperstimulation of the dopamine receptors. Since noradrenaline is important in the "drive" (or "motor") component of movement, a decrease in motility is the paradoxical result of dopamine *excess*.

(e) Finally, we should attempt some explanation for the phenomenon of *dependence* on A.I.M. that we have described (stage four oscillations). However, at the present time there is very little experimental data to help us, except the recent demonstration that dopamine is probably involved in morphine and alcohol dependence and addiction (36–38). This subject should bear further extensive research.

CONCLUSIONS AND SUMMARY

In the present review we have been concerned with the long-term side effects of chronic high-dosage L-DOPA therapy, particularly abnormal involuntary movements (A.I.M.), oscillations in performance, and akinesia paradoxica. We have described four types of diurnal oscillations which are, in fact, four stages in a continuous process. The early (stage one) oscillations are the result of a variable deficiency in effective dopamine (secondary to an intrinsic circadian cycle of dopamine metabolism or to growth-hormone facilitated protein competition for transport sites). The more severe oscillations (stages two to four) are the result of additive phenomena due to L-DOPA overdosage. These phenomena involve the simultaneous production of abnormal involuntary movements and of a hypotonic akinesia. Clinical experiments designed to accomplish a slow, gradual reduction in L-DOPA dosage over a 10-month period conclusively demonstrate a marked reduction in the incidence and severity of these two side effects without loss of motor performance in almost all subjects. We conclude that in many patients manifesting A.I.M. and hypotonic akinesia, we were unnecessarily, and dangerously, giving between 1 and 1.5 g of L-DOPA *in excess* of the minimum requirements. From these observations, we propose two L-DOPA schedules in the therapy of Parkinson's disease: an *induction* dosage and a *maintenance* regimen. We further demonstrate that the progressive loss of motility observed on long-term treatment with L-DOPA is caused by our misunderstanding of the "set" and "drive" components of motility, resulting in overstimulation of dopamine receptors (with A.I.M. and hypotonia) and underfunctioning of noradrenergic "drive" mechanisms.

ACKNOWLEDGMENTS

The author would like to express his gratitude to his collaborators in these studies: Drs. M. I. Botez, M. Cousineau-Boyer, M. Boivin-Lesage; Misses D. Bédard, R. N., C. Larouche, R. N., and L. Paul. The present investigations were supported in part by grants from the Medical Research Council of Canada (MA-4938), the Department of National Health and Welfare of Canada (604-7-812), The United Parkinson Foundation, and the W. Garfield Weston Foundation.

REFERENCES

1. Cotzias, G. C., Papavasiliou, P. S., and Gellene, R., *New Engl. J. Med.* 280, 337 (1969).
2. Déry, J. P., De Groot, J. A., Laurin, C., and Barbeau, A., *Union Méd. Can.* 91, 842 (1962).
3. Barbeau, A., *Can. Med. Ass. J.* 101, 791 (1969).
4. Barbeau, A., Mars, H., and Gillo-Joffroy, L., in: *Recent Advances in Parkinson's Disease,* edited by F. H. McDowell and C. H. Markham, F. A. Davis, Philadelphia, 1971, *Contemporary Neurology,* Vol. 8, pp. 203–237.
5. McDowell, F. H., Lee, J. E., Swift, T., Sweet, R., Ogsbury, J. S., and Kessler, J. T., *Ann. Int. Med.* 72, 29 (1970).
6. Barbeau, A., in: *Parkinson's Disease: Rigidity, Akinesia, Behavior,* Vol. 1, edited by J. Siegfried, Hans Huber, Bern, 1972, pp. 151–174.
7. Boudin, G., Pépin, B., Guillard, A., Fabiani, J. M., and Haguenau, M., in: *Les mediateurs chimiques: leur rôle dans la physiopathologie de la motricité, de la vigilance et du comportement,* edited by P. Girard and R. Couteaux, Masson & Cie, Paris, 1972, pp. 79–97.
8. Hornykiewicz, O., *Pharmacol. Rev.* 18, 925 (1966).
9. Hornykiewicz, O., in: *Monoamines, noyaux gris centraux et syndrome de Parkinson,* edited by J. de Ajuriaguerra, Masson & Cie, Paris, 1971, pp. 143–157.
10. Barbeau, A., *Rev. Neurol.* 127, 253 (1972).
11. Barbeau, A., *Can. Med. Ass. J.* 87, 802 (1962).
12. Barbeau, A., in: *Advances in Neurology, Vol. 1: Huntington's Chorea, 1872–1972,* edited by A. Barbeau, T. N. Chase, and G. W. Paulson, Raven Press, New York, 1973, pp. 473–516.
13. Jung, R., and Hassler, R., in: *Handbook of Physiology,* edited by J. Field, American Physiological Society, New York, 1960, *Neurophysiology,* Vol. 2; ch. 35, pp. 863–927.
14. Jouvet, M., *Science* 163, 32 (1969).
15. Wurtman, R. J., Axelrod, J., and Kelly, D. E., *The Pineal,* Academic Press, New York, 1968, pp. 1–199.
16. Carlsson, A., *Pharmacol. Rev.* 11, 490 (1959).
17. Ernst, A. M., *Psychopharmacologia* 10, 316 (1967).
18. Wurtman, R. J., and Romero, J. A., *Neurology* 22(2), 72 (1972).
19. Barbeau, A., in: *Monoamines, noyaux gris centraux et syndrome de Parkinson,* edited by J. de Ajuriaguerra, Masson & Cie, Paris, 1971, pp. 385–402.
20. Barbeau, A., in: *Monographs in Human Genetics,* Vol. 6, edited by J. François, S. Karger, Basel, 1972, pp. 114–136.
21. Everett, G. M., and Borcherding, J. W., *Science* 168, 849 (1970).
22. Rinne, U. K., Sonninen, V., and Hÿppa, M., *Life Sci.* 10(I), 549 (1971).
23. Mena, I., Court, J., Fuenzalida, S., Papavasiliou, P. S., and Cotzias, G. C., *New Engl. J. Med.* 282, (1970).

24. Barbeau, A., *Can. Med. Ass. J.* 105, 450 (1971).
25. Ungerstedt, U., *Acta Physiol. Scand.* Suppl. 367, 69 (1971).
26. Klawans, H. L., Jr., Ilahi, M. M., and Ringel, S. P., *Confinia Neurol.* 33, 297 (1971).
27. Orzeck, A. and Barbeau, A., in: *L-DOPA and Parkinsonism,* edited by A. Barbeau and F. H. McDowell, F. A. Davis Co., Philadelphia, 1970, pp. 88–94.
28. Aquilonius, S. M., and Sjöström, R., *Life Sci.* 10, 405 (1971).
29. Klawans, H. L., Jr., and Rubovits, R., *Neurology* 22, 107 (1972).
30. Perry, T. L., Hansen, S., and Kloster, M., *New Engl. J. Med.* 288, 337 (1973).
31. Bartholini, G., Da Prada, M., and Pletscher, A., *J. Pharm. Pharmacol.* 20, 228 (1968).
32. Chase, T. N., *Neurology* 20(2), 36 (1970).
33. Barbeau, A., *La Revue du Praticien* 20, 5165 (1970).
34. Ng, K. Y., Chase, T. N., Colburn, R. N., and Kopin, I. J., *Science* 170, 76 (1970).
35. Bazelon, M., Paine, R. S., and Cowie, V. A., *Lancet* 1, 1130 (1967).
36. Blum, K., Merritt, J. H., Wallace, J. E., Owen, R., Hahn, J. W., and Geller, I., *Curr. Ther. Res.* 14, 324 (1972).
37. Sasame, H. A., Perez-Cruet, J., Di Chiara, G., Tagliamonte, A., Tagliamonte, P., and Gessa, G. L., *J. Neurochem.* 1953 (1972).
38. Sloan, J., Brooks, J., Eisenmann, A., and Martin, W., *Psychopharmacologia* 4, 261 (1963).

Advances in Neurology, Vol. 5
Raven Press, New York © 1974

The "On-Off" Effect

Arvid Carlsson

Department of Pharmacology, University of Göteborg, Göteborg, Sweden

For a better understanding of the "on-off" effect, the pharmacokinetic aspects appear to require more detailed studies. To what extent can rapid changes in the response to DOPA be correlated to variations in the plasma DOPA level? Relatively few correlative studies of this type appear to be available. It may be assumed, however, that the "on-off" effect can be explained in part, but not entirely, by such variations.

Another pharmacokinetic aspect deals with DOPA metabolites. The possibility that 3-O-methyldopa may antagonize the response to its parent compound DOPA has been brought up. I should like to add another possible mechanism. It is well known that catechols inhibit tyrosine hydroxylase, if present in sufficiently high concentration. After the administration of DOPA, catechol metabolites accumulate in the brain, e.g., dihydroxyphenylacetic acid (DOPAC). DOPAC may be expected to reach its peak concentration after its precursor dopamine. Thus the possibility exists that tyrosine hydroxylase remains inhibited during a phase of declining dopamine concentration. This inhibition might be of functional importance provided that dopamine synthesis from tyrosine still plays a significant role. Unfortunately, the investigation of this possible mechanism in the parkinsonian patient would probably prove very difficult.

Dr. Duvoisin pointed out that the natural time course of Parkinson's disease may be an important factor for understanding the "on-off" effect. From the theoretical point of view, this hypothesis is very attractive. The most significant factor in the development of Parkinson's disease might well be the number of available tyrosine hydroxylase molecules in the striatum. From our studies it appears that normally about one-third of these molecules are active, whereas the remaining two-thirds can be activated according to need. It seems possible, therefore, that about two-thirds of the nigrostriatal dopamine neurons can be lost without causing overt parkinsonian symptoms, possibly even more if we take into account the development of receptor supersensitivity. However, the minimum required number of neurons or enzyme molecules may not be constant but could depend on the demand put on the nigrostriatal dopamine system, e.g., by social stress as illustrated by Modigh's experiment referred to earlier.

Thus, at an early stage of Parkinson's disease there may still be a certain number of functioning nigrostriatal dopamine neurons, almost capable of coping with the situation at rest but overtly insufficient under less favorable, stressful conditions. If DOPA is administered at this stage, a good therapeutic response might be expected, for several reasons. Symptoms of overdosage at peak concentrations of DOPA should be infrequent, because excessive dopamine concentrations at receptor sites might be avoided by shutting off endogenous DOPA synthesis and by utilizing the reserve capacity of remaining storage sites. These stores would serve to prolong the responses to the individual doses.

At the other extreme we have the advanced stage of the disease, with but a few remaining striatal dopamine fibers. Now tyrosine hydroxylase activity and storage capacity are almost negligible. DOPA decarboxylase is likely to remain at a significant activity level for a long time and normally is present in considerable excess. At this stage the response to DOPA should be similar to that observed in the reserpine-treated animal, with great difficulty in finding the optimum dose level: either the dose is insufficient or it causes obvious overstimulation.

In conclusion, from a theoretical point of view, three different factors may be suggested as worthwhile investigating in the search for an explanation of the "on-off" effect: (1) rapid changes in the plasma (and brain) levels of DOPA and of metabolites possibly interfering with the response; (2) variations in the demands placed on the system under different conditions; and (3) decreased buffer capacity induced by the progressive loss of nigrostriatal dopamine neurons in the course of Parkinson's disease.

Advances in Neurology, Vol. 5
Raven Press, New York © 1974

Inhibition of DOPA Accumulation by Rat Brain at Critical L-DOPA Circulating Concentrations

W. D. Horst, G. Bautz, E. Renyi, and N. Spirt

Hoffmann-La Roche, Inc., Research Division, Nutley, New Jersey 07110

The clinical use of L-3,4-dihydroxyphenylalanine (L-DOPA) in the treatment of Parkinson's disease prompts a better understanding of the fate of this amino acid as it circulates through the brain.

We have previously shown that isolated perfused rat brains metabolize ^{14}C-L-DOPA in agreement with *in vivo* studies (1); therefore, the perfused rat brain appears to be an appropriate preparation with which to study the influence of circulating L-DOPA concentrations on its accumulation and decarboxylation in this tissue.

METHODS

Brains from male adult Royal Hart rats, anesthetized with urethane, were perfused through the internal carotid arteries according to Andjus (2), with the following modifications: the perfusion system was an open-ended type to avoid the recirculation of DOPA metabolites, and the pterygopalatine branch of the internal carotid artery was not occluded. The perfusion media were prepared with fluorocarbon in place of red blood cells as described by Sloviter (3). The brains were perfused at a constant rate of 1.6 ml/min. Brains were perfused for 2 min prior to the introduction of L-DOPA (Larodopa®). The L-DOPA perfusion lasted 15 min and was followed by a 2-min perfusion of L-DOPA-free media to eliminate DOPA from the vascular lumen. Brains were removed and homogenized in perchloric acid. DOPA, dopamine, and norepinephrine were separated through the use of alumina and dowex columns (4), then assayed fluorometrically (5, 6). In *in vivo* studies, rats or mice were sacrificed 30 min after the oral administration of L-DOPA (suspended in 5% gum acacia) and the brains removed.

RESULTS AND DISCUSSIONS

Figure 1 demonstrates the brain DOPA and dopamine concentrations following L-DOPA perfusions between 3 and 50 µg/ml of media. Brain

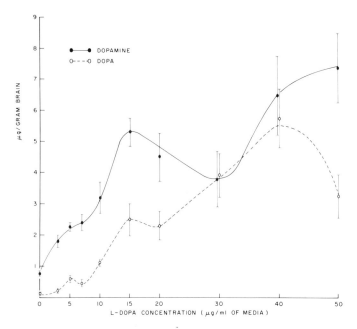

FIG. 1. The influence of L-DOPA concentrations on DOPA and dopamine accumulation by isolated perfused rat brains. Brains were perfused for 15 min with various doses of L-DOPA. Each point is the mean of six brains ± SEM.

norepinephrine levels were not influenced at all or only slightly elevated by DOPA perfusion and are not presented. Brain L-DOPA accumulation does not proceed in a regular or progressive manner with respect to increasing L-DOPA perfusion concentrations, but displays a series of plateaus and regressions. Tissue dopamine concentrations closely parallel tissue DOPA levels through the lower DOPA perfusion concentrations, but this relationship does not exist beyond 20 μg/ml of perfused L-DOPA.

The presence of DOPA decarboxylase in the walls of brain capillaries has been demonstrated by Bertler and others (7–9), and it was anticipated that the inhibition of this enzyme may aid in explaining the uneven accumulation of DOPA. In the following experiments, rats were pretreated with the decarboxylase inhibitor Ro 4–4602 [NI-(DL-seryl)-N^2-(2,3,4-trihydroxybenzyl)-hydrazine], 1 hr prior to the brain perfusion. The inhibitor (20 mg/kg) was given intraperitoneally, at a dose which has been shown to inhibit only peripheral decarboxylase (10, 11). Figure 2 demonstrates the accumulation of DOPA and dopamine in the presence of the inhibitor. Only at perfusion concentrations of 10 μg/ml or less did the inhibitor potentiate the accumulation of DOPA; at all other concentrations, pretreatment with Ro 4–4602 significantly decreased DOPA accumulation. Also, there is no

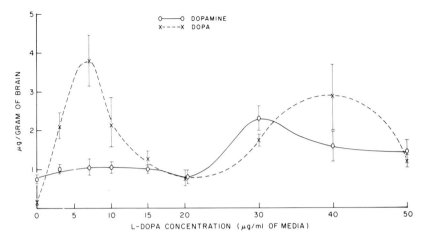

FIG. 2. Influence of peripheral decarboxylase inhibition on L-DOPA and dopamine accumulation by isolated perfused rat brains. The decarboxylase inhibitor Ro 4–4602 (20 mg/kg, i.p.) was administered 1 hr before the brains were isolated. Each point is the mean of six brains ± SEM.

significant accumulation of dopamine in the inhibited brains until an L-DOPA perfusion concentration of 30 μg/ml is employed. Perfused DOPA concentrations below 10 μg/ml caused a marked accumulation of DOPA but no increase in brain dopamine, suggesting that DOPA may be accumulated in peripheral sites within the brain from which it is not available for transport across the blood–brain barrier.

It is clear that a considerable portion of the brain dopamine increase following DOPA perfusion is due to the accumulation of dopamine in peripheral rather than central sites. This phenomenon has previously been described by de la Torre, Boggan, and Llovell (12). Presumably, this dopamine accumulation occurs within the walls of the brain capillaries or in areas of the brain outside the blood-brain barrier such as the median eminence or the area postrema.

Peripheral decarboxylase inhibition did not eliminate the regressions in brain DOPA and dopamine accumulation in the presence of increasing L-DOPA perfusion concentrations. To determine if this phenomenon occurs only in brain tissue, isolated rat hearts were also perfused with L-DOPA. Similar results were obtained in heart tissue as had been demonstrated in brains, although the fluctuations were not as great in heart tissue. In addition, rats were treated with various doses (250 to 1,000 mg/kg, p.o.) of L-DOPA, and the plasma DOPA levels were correlated with changes in heart and brain dopamine 30 min after the L-DOPA administration (Table 1). Even in the presence of increasing plasma DOPA levels, tissue dopamine concentrations decline and then recover, as was seen in the isolated tissue.

TABLE 1. *Correlation between plasma DOPA concentrations and dopamine levels in rat hearts and brains*

L-DOPA dose (mg/kg, p.o.)	Plasma (DOPA)	Brain (dopamine)	Heart (dopamine)
Control	1.25 ± 0.73	0.70 ± .03	0.10 ± 0.03
250	12.43 ± 2.74	1.30 ± .13	8.67 ± 2.31
500	15.00 ± 1.49	1.20 ± .08	7.59 ± 2.11
750	19.06 ± 1.45	1.07 ± .06	1.92 ± 0.21
1,000	24.78 ± 3.86	1.34 ± .13	9.38 ± 1.27

Each value is the mean of six values ± SEM expressed as micrograms per gram of tissue or milliliter of plasma. Rats were administered L-DOPA and sacrificed 30 min later.

Obviously, the oscillating accumulation of DOPA and dopamine in the presence of increasing circulating L-DOPA concentrations is not a function peculiar to isolated perfused brain tissue.

In contrast to rats, mice administered increasing doses (250 to 1,000 mg/kg, p.o.) of L-DOPA display continuously increasing brain concentrations of dopamine (Table 2).

The reason for these divergent oscillations remains unclear. We have unsuccessfully tried to eliminate them by inhibiting monoamine oxidase, catechol-O-methyl transferase, and DOPA decarboxylase, indicating that DOPA itself or a metabolite resulting from transaminase activity may be responsible. We have also monitored perfusion pressures in the presence of various DOPA concentrations. In isolated hearts there is a sharp increase in perfusion pressure which occurs at 20 μg/ml of DOPA and correlates well with the decline in heart DOPA and dopamine. Thus, the decline in tissue DOPA and dopamine accumulation may result from changes in the perfused vasculature which can then be overcome by increasing substrate

TABLE 2. *The influence of L-DOPA administration on mouse brain dopamine concentrations*

L-DOPA dose (mg/kg, p.o.)	Brain dopamine (μg/g)
Control	0.26 ± .03
250	0.79 ± .03
500	1.88 ± .20
750	2.90 ± .50
1,000	5.40 ± .29

Mice received L-DOPA and were sacrificed 30 min later. Each value is the mean ± SEM of six determinations.

concentrations. In perfused brain, however, we have not been able to demonstrate such changes in perfusion pressure, and so the significance of vascular changes with regard to DOPA and dopamine accumulation remains obscure.

Some parkinsonian patients undergoing L-DOPA therapy have been observed to exhibit pretherapy symptoms as L-DOPA doses were increased (13), while other patients whose symptoms are controlled with L-DOPA are known to revert, suddenly, to states of akinesia (14, 15). These temporary reverses in the efficacy of L-DOPA may be related to the inhibition of L-DOPA transport into the brain which occurs at critical circulating L-DOPA concentrations.

CONCLUSIONS

We have shown that in the presence of increasing L-DOPA perfusion concentrations, rat brain DOPA and dopamine accumulation does not proceed in a continuous elevation but progresses through a series of plateaus and regressions. This observation is not unique to isolated brains but occurs in heart tissue and *in vivo* as well. The reduction of DOPA and dopamine accumulation at critical L-DOPA circulating concentrations may be related to the "on-off" phenomenon observed in parkinsonian patients treated with L-DOPA.

REFERENCES

1. Horst, W. D., and Jester, J., *Life Sci.* (Part I) 10, 685 (1971).
2. Andjus, R. K., Suhara, K., and Sloviter, H. A., *J. Appl. Physiol.* 22, 1033 (1967).
3. Sloviter, H. A., and Kamimoto, T., *Nature* 216, 458 (1967).
4. Horst, W. D., and Jester, J., *Biochem. Pharmacol.* 20, 2633 (1971).
5. Laverty, R., and Taylor, K. M., *Anal. Biochem.* 22, 269 (1968).
6. Laverty, R., and Sharman, D. F., *Brit. J. Pharmacol.* 24, 538 (1965).
7. Bertler, A., Falck, B., Owman, C., and Rosengrenn, E., *Pharmacol. Rev.* 18, 369 (1966).
8. Owman, C., and Rosengren, E., *J. Neurochem.* 14, 547 (1967).
9. Constantinidis, J., De La Torre, J. C., Tissot, R., and Geissbuhler, F., *Experientia* 24, 130 (1969).
10. Bartholini, G., Bates, H. M., Burkard, W. P., and Pletscher, A., *Nature* 215, 852 (1967).
11. De La Torre, J. C., *J. Neurol. Sci.* 12, 77 (1971).
12. De La Torre, J. C., Boggan, W. O., and Llovell, R. A., *J. Pharm. Pharmacol.* 24, 481 (1972).
13. Cotzias, G. C., Papavasiliou, P. S., and Gellene, R., *New Engl. J. Med.* 280, 337 (1969).
14. Barbeau, A., *Lancet* I, 395 (1971).
15. Sroka, H., Eichhorn, F., Rutengerg, A., Radwan, H., and Bornstein, B., *J. Neurol. Sci.* 17, 61 (1972).

DISCUSSION

Dr. Muenter: I think there is not as much mystique to the "on-off" effect as we may sometimes be inclined to believe.

During the past 3 years we have studied the individual response curves of numerous patients after the morning dose of L-DOPA, measuring clinical aspects of Parkinson's disease as well as concentrations of DOPA, 3-O-methyldopa, and homovanillic acid in plasma at intervals of 45 minutes to 1 hour over a period of 4 to 5 hours. We find that some patients show what we have called "short-duration improvement" — that is, a dramatic reversal of clinical disability after the individual dose that usually reaches its peak within 1 to 2 hours after the dose and subsides within 3 to 4 hours after the dose. This short-duration improvement is invariably accompanied by a simultaneous increase and then decrease in the concentration of DOPA in plasma. Patients with this type of response curve will at times refer to the onset of short-duration improvement as being "turned on" and to the often rather abrupt disappearance of short-duration improvement as being "turned off."

Attempts to correlate short-duration improvement, or the "on-off" effect, with the total daily dose of L-DOPA is not very useful, for the following reason. A patient who is taking 4 grams of L-DOPA daily as four 1.0-gram doses may demonstrate the short-duration improvement after each dose. However, if the total daily dose of 4 grams is given as eight 500-milligram doses, the short-duration improvement will either be markedly attenuated or disappear completely. For this reason it is the individual single dose of L-DOPA rather than the total daily dose that is meaningful in regard to short-duration improvement.

Another important point is that short-duration improvement shows a statistically highly significant correlation ($p < 0.01$) with the clinical severity of the disease prior to treatment with L-DOPA: the more severe the disease, the more likely it is that the patient will experience short-duration improvement. This observation corroborates the earlier remarks of Dr. Carlsson and suggests that the progressive loss of nigrostriatal neurons is the structural event that results in short-duration improvement in response to L-DOPA. It is of interest that some of the true therapeutic failures of L-DOPA tend to occur in patients with severe clinical disability (more advanced than that observed in patients who still show the short-duration improvement). One may speculate whether this ultimate lack of response to L-DOPA is related to the anatomic loss of most or all of the nigrostriatal neurons.

Dr. Fahn: I am impressed with Dr. Muenter's points. I think there are maybe two types of "on-off" effects. One is the acute, suddenly appearing "off" effect, and then later, after a period of time, coming back "on" again. Another one is a slower one and does correlate with plasma levels. This is the type where the patient says, "My DOPA lasts only about 3 hours; then it wears off and I slow down again." He takes the next dose and gets back "on" again. This type I think does correlate with plasma DOPA levels. The other one is more mysterious, and I think it's the one most of us are talking about.

Dr. Cotzias: Dr. Papavasiliou will probably corroborate your statements by showing that the first variety responds to diet whereas the other one does not.

Dr. Mones: I want to make two comments. First, there is another aspect of the oscillation the patients have. Some patients oscillate by days; that is, the patients have good days and bad days, with no obvious reason for the variation. Secondly, if the "on-off" effect is due only to the fact that there are very few nigral neurons left, then you must explain why it seems to take so long for the "on-off" effect to appear after the patient starts to take L-DOPA; it seems to take 6 months or so. There should be some patients who are started with L-DOPA who have just a few neurons left and develop the "on-off" effect quickly.

Dr. Boshes: Intermittency of function is inherent to the disease. You have only to do a graphic recording of speech and of motion (patient walking) to see the extra pauses. When a patient comes into your waiting room and you ask him into your consultation room, as he comes through the doorway he freezes, probably just from adding in that extra stimulus. The "on-off" is absolutely inherent to the disease, and I think you're seeing an exaggeration of it.

If a patient is resting quietly, he will have no tremor, and at the same time the electroencephalogram will contain little alpha. If you call to the patient at that moment, he will not start to have tremor, but the electroencephalogram becomes desynchronized and the tremor starts after 100 to 150 milliseconds. This, I think, is what Dr. Barbeau pointed out in his diagram. There are multiple neurochemical intermediators and we are dealing with a very complex system.

If a patient has had a thalamotomy with the tremor erased in the right hand, and he is asked to write with his left hand, the initial tremor immediately returns, showing that it is possible neurochemically to wire around the defect to produce the intermittency of response.

Dr. Yahr: I think the time sequence of developing "on-off" is more apparent than real. True, it takes time during which the individual has been treated with DOPA, and the delay may be a year or so. But if you use DOPA plus a decarboxylase inhibitor, the "on-off" effects can be seen at an earlier date. It may be the amount of pharmacological activity delivered to the damaged striatum rather than the time interlude itself.

Dr. Sandler: There seem to be as many explanations for the "on-off" phenomenon as there are participants here, so I shall add my own. I look on it as sort of a special case of the pyridoxal phosphate phenomenon which itself is a false transmitter competing with other transmitters in the brain. Thus one would guess that dietary aldehydes may simulate the way that pyridoxal combines with dopamine, and that dietary aldehydes may combine with dopamine to form false transmitters to compete with whatever is the transmitter in the central nervous system. This would explain the dietary overtones and undertones, at least in this situation.

Dr. Krnjević: I wonder whether some of these very striking changes in function may be a reflection of large or appreciable variations of cerebral blood flow. This could obviously be reflected, especially in tissue which is presumably working at its limit. Even a small change in oxygenation can make a rather striking difference in function. A very simple and obvious test for this would be administration of small amounts of CO_2 to increase the local PCO_2, which would increase cerebral blood flow remarkably.

Dr. Roberts: In view of Dr. Barbeau's very interesting suggestion about the balance between dopamine and norepinephrine, I wonder if methylation might become a rate-limiting step as DOPA will drain off methyl groups. Is there any relationship to food intake and, particularly, to the choline and methionine content? Does supplementation with methionine and choline have any effect?

Dr. Yahr: I wish I had a positive answer. We have tried methionine and it does not push the reaction that way.

Dr. Barbeau: I just want to confirm what Dr. Yahr said. I do not think the progression of disease can be the only explanation, or the loss of cells, because with Ro 4–4602 we get the "on-off" reactions much earlier, but not necessarily in the more severely involved patients.

I want to answer the remark by Dr. Boshes that the "on-off" response is inherent to the disease. It is true that oscillations and freezing are inherent to the disease, but what we are seeing in the severe oscillations is freezing with hypotonia and not the freezing that we observed before, which is the main point of difference between the two. You cannot explain this away as being just the result of the disease continuing.

Dr. McGeer: Dr. Cotzias, I'm surprised that people haven't looked more into the therapeutic possibilities of altering GABA levels in brain in the treatment of Parkinson's disease. By giving loads of DOPA to patients, possibly there is competition for pyridoxal phosphate in the conversion of DOPA to dopamine and glutamic acid to GABA. At least in the substantia nigra we're fairly certain that GABA acts in an antagonistic way to dopamine. It seems as though the descending gabaminergic tract has its synapses on the dendrites of dopaminergic cells. It may be that you're just on a threshold, and that a load of DOPA has a dramatic effect on the levels of GABA in brain. I mention this to encourage people to look into the therapeutic possibilities of agents which raise or lower the levels of GABA.

Dr. Cotzias: We have tried gamma-hydroxybutyric acid and it was totally worthless in our hands.

Dr. McGeer: Well, gamma-hydroxybutyric acid may or may not change GABA levels in brain but it does change dopamine.

Dr. Poirier: I fully agree with the suggestion of Dr. Carlsson that we must know more about the pharmacological kinetics of the metabolism of dopamine. He has given us a very nice example with which to attack this.

I add that we have some information along this same line of one of his suggestions. We have given DOPA chronically to cats for several weeks by mouth, and this leads to a reduction in the activity of tyrosine hydroxylase in the brain.

Advances in Neurology, Vol. 5
Raven Press, New York © 1974

Short- and Long-Term Approaches to the "On-Off" Phenomenon

Paul S. Papavasiliou, George C. Cotzias, and Ismael Mena

Medical Research Center, Brookhaven National Laboratory, Upton, New York 11973

INTRODUCTION

Although the long-term therapeutic effects of L-DOPA are fairly constant in some parkinsonian patients, late in the treatment others develop diurnal oscillations of the control of parkinsonism (the so-called "on-off" phenomenon) with or without the emergence of dyskinesia (1). The "on-off" phenomenon may also be defined as sudden or gradual episodic reemergence of the parkinsonian symptoms which had been brought under control earlier with L-DOPA. It has varied in severity and in frequency from one patient to the next. In some patients it was managed by changing doses and schedules but in others it has persisted unaltered for a long time. It has occasionally progressed to become an incapacitating, difficult problem. A common reason for the incapacitation is that the coexistence of dyskinesia precludes the administration of L-DOPA in doses sufficient for full and constant control of the symptoms of parkinsonism.

We present a short-term and a long-term approach to this problem. The short-term approach, involving the use of apomorphine, has been effective in all patients studied. The long-term approach, involving the use of a metabolic inhibitor and protein restriction, has been effective in most participating patients and might therefore qualify for the management of the "on-off" phenomenon.

BACKGROUND

We were impressed by patients' reports emphasizing temporary loss of the therapeutic effects of L-DOPA following a high-protein meal. We thought that this might be due (a) to impeded reactivity of the brain (namely, something similar to a postprandial somnolence); (b) to oscillations in the catabolism of L-DOPA in peripheral tissues; or (c) to competition between the neutral amino acid L-DOPA and equivalent alimentary amino acids on their way to the brain.

It must be emphasized that although a number of patients have developed the "on-off" phenomenon without any other accompanying limitation to therapy, perhaps an even larger number developed it as a consequence of manipulating the doses of L-DOPA to avoid some complication, such as the development of involuntary, adventitious, intermittent, dyskinetic movements. Trying to avoid dyskinesia by diminishing the L-DOPA dose which has caused it has often initiated episodes of the "on-off" phenomenon or has aggravated them when already present. Control of the "on-off" phenomenon also implies, therefore, some concomitant control of dyskinesia.

That the reactivity of the brain to dopaminergic stimulation was not impeded during this phenomenon was shown by using single and multiple injections of apomorphine detailed below. We induced alterations in the catabolism of aromatic amino acids, including that of L-DOPA, by inhibiting their peripheral decarboxylation with the L-aromatic amino acid decarboxylase inhibitor α-methyldopa hydrazine (MK-486) (1, 2). Since combined therapy by itself resulted in some improvement in the diurnal stability of the symptomatic control, we thought that full stabilization of the neurological status might be accomplished by also diminishing the intake of amino acids which are substrates for the aromatic amino acid decarboxylase, in addition to inhibiting decarboxylation. We therefore tested the effects of various protein intakes on the stability of the symptomatic control produced with L-DOPA given either alone or with MK-486.

Reports that L-DOPA releases growth hormone in man (3, 4) led us to studies (5) in which administration of growth hormone in mice promoted, potentiated, and prolonged the cerebral effects of L-DOPA. These will be discussed by Dr. Ismael Mena together with the long-term release of growth hormone in parkinsonian patients under treatment with L-DOPA, elsewhere in this volume.

INJECTED APOMORPHINE AND THE "ON AND OFF" PHENOMENON

The effects of injected apomorphine (1.5 to 3.0 mg, s.c.) on this phenomenon in parkinsonian patients were evaluated in double-blind tests by scoring 24 items on a 0 to 4 scale for 2 hr (6, 7). Patients were given either single or multiple injections (six times a day for 2 to 43 days) which alleviated whatever major symptom of Parkinsonism might have emerged during steady treatment with L-DOPA. In nine patients with parkinsonism receiving L-DOPA alone or with MK-486, apomorphine was given during episodic but predictable periods of reemerging tremor, rigidity, or akinesia. In five patients with reemerging tremor and rigidity, apomorphine abolished both symptoms, while in four patients who had predominantly reemerging akinesia, this drug induced improvement varying from 25% in one patient to 50 or 100% in the others. These same effects were always induced in three patients when apomorphine was injected by the nurses when needed.

These findings were interpreted as indicating that the central neurons remained responsive to dopaminergic stimulation during these episodes. This raised the question of whether serial injections might not totally prevent their diurnal reemergence. Injections of apomorphine were therefore given six times a day in three patients at 2- to 3-hr intervals, with reproducible but temporary improvement of the reemerging symptoms. By contrast, placebo injected in patients off or on L-DOPA diminished their scores by a maximum of 15%.

In the absence of L-DOPA, apomorphine reduced tremor and rigidity, but not akinesia. The control of akinesia during coadministration of L-DOPA (7) suggested that the two drugs acted synergistically (8).

Apomorphine injected during the temporary decline or disappearance of L-DOPA-induced symptomatic control has invariably aborted this phenomenon if given in sufficient doses. This restitution of control has, however, also induced preexisting involuntary movements. As explained by Dr. Cotzias elsewhere in this volume, this dyskinesia-producing effect of apomorphine was totally reversed when sufficient amounts of the drug were given during episodes of DOPA-induced dyskinesia instead of during the temporary loss of symptomatic control.

The side effects of apomorphine preceded the antiparkinsonian effects and were less pronounced in L-DOPA-treated patients. They included nausea, salivation, occasional vomiting, orthostatic hypotension, pallor, weakness, sweating, and dizziness. The emetic effects became progressively less, but signs of addiction or withdrawal were not found (7).

LONG-TERM APPROACH TO THE "ON-OFF" PHENOMENON

Administration of MK-486

Early in these studies, the oscillations in the diurnal control of parkinsonism raised the question of their reflecting intermittent metabolic changes in the peripheral catabolism of L-DOPA. It seemed, therefore, that the inhibition of the catabolism of L-DOPA exclusively in peripheral tissues might provide a more steady therapeutic control of parkinsonism. Preliminary but encouraging results were obtained with D,L-α-methyldopa hydrazine (MK-485), as reported earlier (1, 2).

In subsequent studies, 18 patients with parkinsonism, showing episodic reemergence of tremor, rigidity, and bradykinesia as the predominant manifestations while on L-DOPA alone, received the L-isomer of the inhibitor (MK-486), which reduced the requirements of L-DOPA about 75%. While this combination resulted in satisfactory to excellent stability of control in 12 patients with mild to moderate intermittency of their symptoms, in six patients with severe intermittency, only mild improvement of the "on-off" phenomenon was induced in spite of several changes of the daily doses, of the schedules, and of the ratios of L-DOPA to MK-486.

By contrast to these six difficult cases, others benefited from readjustments of the daily dose, including administration of a larger number of doses than the six times a day originally prescribed.

Dietary Approach to the "On and Off" Phenomenon

Some patients reported that a meal rich in protein aggravated their symptoms temporarily. This, coupled with the fact that the peripheral inhibitor tended to stabilize the patients' performance, suggested that investigations of the effects of protein intake might result in a better control of this phenomenon.

Nine inpatients, whose diurnal control ranged from stability to nearly total, unpredictable instability, were studied on a metabolic ward. They had been receiving L-DOPA or L-DOPA plus MK-486 for the last 2 to 7 years and represented advanced cases of parkinsonism.

In the first period of the study, L-DOPA (1.8 to 8.0 g/day) was administered alone in six doses per day. In the second period, the patients were given MK-486 (25 mg, six times daily) plus L-DOPA (0.45 to 2.2 g/day). Each period lasted for 5 weeks, during which the following diets were given: (a) standard house diet containing 1 g protein/kg per day divided into three meals for 10 days; (b) 1 g protein/kg per day given in eight isocaloric meals; (c) 10 g protein per day in three meals with equal distribution of fat, protein, and carbohydrate, for 4 days; (d) 2 g protein/kg per day divided in three meals with the same protein, fat, and carbohydrate content for 4 days; (e) 0.5 g protein/kg per day in eight meals for 6 days. The isocaloric feature of the meals was incorporated because of the patients' reports that their performance was not altered by bulky meals but only by high-protein intakes. The neurological symptoms of each patient were scored twice a day before and during all phases of the dietary studies, and ergometric measurements were made six times a day with an automated ergometer. During the first period of this study, while L-DOPA was administered without the inhibitor and while the diet was varied, we observed some stabilization of the neurological state in the six patients who had the "on-off" phenomenon but no particular benefit in the three patients with relatively steady performance. Meals with high-protein content tended to diminish the therapeutic effects of L-DOPA, whereas low-protein diets potentiated and stabilized the therapeutic effects (Table 1). From these observations it appeared that the "on and off" phenomenon presented by six of these patients might have been due to the competition between L-DOPA and alimentary amino acids on their way to the brain, as postulated under Background. This explanation proved less than sufficient.

The second period consisted of diminishing the dose of L-DOPA by co-

TABLE 1. *Mean ± SE of the neurological scores obtained in six patients under the dietary regimens indicated*

Daily protein intake	L-DOPA		p <	L-DOPA + MK-486		p <
	8 a.m.	3 p.m.		8 a.m.	3 p.m.	
1 g/kg body wt	26 ± 2	40 ± 3	0.001	21 ± 2	24 ± 4	0.6
1 g/kg body wt 8 meals	25 ± 3	38 ± 2	0.002	26 ± 3	19 ± 2	0.08
10 g	25 ± 3	24 ± 4	0.9	16 ± 1	18 ± 2	0.4
2 g/kg body wt	26 ± 3	54 ± 3	0.0001	31 ± 4	39 ± 5	0.3
0.5 g/kg body wt 8 meals	20 ± 2	34 ± 6	0.02	18 ± 1	21 ± 2	0.3

administering MK-486 while the intake of the alimentary amino acids was varied by varying the protein intake as described above. If the transport of L-DOPA was diminished during the increased protein intake, this competition should become more pronounced when the L-DOPA dose was decreased by the inhibitor, thus aggravating the "on-off" phenomenon. When the episodes of diurnal intermittency (the number of decreases of work output and the number of increases of the disability scores by more than 50%) were counted in five patients over a period of 4 days (Fig. 1), it was found that MK-486, which had diminished the requirements for L-DOPA, had also induced greater stability in the symptomatic control when given to patients receiving 0.5 g protein/kg of body weight per day. In three additional patients with parkinsonism tested on standard as well as low-protein diets (0.5 g/kg per day) while receiving combinations of L-DOPA plus MK-486 for several months, potentiation of the pharmacological effect and greater stability of symptomatic control were found with the lower protein intake. In a group of three patients, who exhibited frequent and severe "on-off" phenomenon, the frequency of L-DOPA administration was varied from 3 to 15 times a day. It was observed that the higher the number of daily doses, the larger was the total tolerated daily dose, the better the diurnal stability, and the fewer the side effects. These experiences indicated that some patients require more frequent dosage schedules than the original six times a day recommended by us (1).

It should be reemphasized that in some of the patients, the temporary, diurnal, intermittent disappearance of L-DOPA-dependent symptomatic control had been brought about while diminishing the doses of L-DOPA in order to diminish L-DOPA-dependent dyskinesias. The combined dietary-pharmacological regimen which diminished the "on-off" phenomenon appears to have also increased our capability to manage the excessive in-

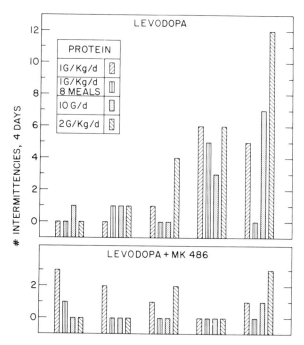

FIG. 1. The number of "intermittencies" recorded over a 4-day period by ergometry in eight patients while receiving the diets indicated. Note that MK-486 diminished the "intermittencies" despite having markedly diminished the dose of L-DOPA.

voluntary movements in several of these patients. Some of them have been on this combined regimen for several months with satisfactory results and without neurological or nutritional complications.

DISCUSSION

The "on-off" phenomenon was observed originally during our early studies (1, 2) and was reported to emerge either as an isolated phenomenon or as a consequence of diminishing the dose of L-DOPA, after drug-dependent dyskinesia. This latter consideration suggested that the lower doses of L-DOPA were incapable of saturating the brain constantly, rather than that the brain itself had become intermittently refractory to the drug. This conclusion has been confirmed by the short-term abortion of this phenomenon with injected apomorphine. This, in turn, argued in favor of either irregular transport of the drug or of its interception on the way to the brain. This latter hypothesis appears confirmed by the step-wise diminution of the "on-off" phenomenon in several of our patients, achieved first by coadministering the DOPA decarboxylase inhibitor MK-486 (2), and now by imposing, in addition, dietary protein restrictions.

Our early hypothesis that L-DOPA was being competed against by alimentary amino acids for transport into the brain was proven to be insufficient as an explanation by the experiments reported here. In fact, we cannot yet formulate a new hypothesis to account for the effectiveness of the combined dietary-pharmacological regimen presented here, since we do not yet fully comprehend the mechanisms of action either of L-DOPA, of the DOPA decarboxylase inhibitor, or of our dietary maneuvers. This ignorance, however, does not preclude the use of this experimental regimen, provided that both its safety and its effectiveness are confirmed on a long-term basis. Regarding the safety of administering 0.5 g protein/kg of body weight per day to mature or elderly patients, this protein intake slightly exceeds the minimum intake formulated for the child-bearing age by the World Health Organization (10). Similarly, there is thus far neither theoretical nor experimental evidence that such a dietary regimen is incompatible with L-DOPA or MK-486, assuming that the requirements for vitamins and minerals are met. Still, we must emphasize the experimental nature of this regimen.

In addition to having diminished the "on-off" phenomenon, this combined regimen seems to have increased both the milligram potency of L-DOPA and the margin between induction of therapeutic effects versus side effects such as dyskinesia. These conclusions are, however, based on a small number of carefully studied patients and can be confirmed or negated only by equally meticulous studies conducted elsewhere.

CONCLUSION

A short-term reversal of the "on-off" phenomenon was imposed by injections of apomorphine (1 to 3 mg, s.c.). Although this reversal by apomorphine was effective in all patients studied, it was not fully satisfactory because it was often accompanied by reemergence of preexisting dyskinesia. By contrast, the long-term combined dietary-pharmacological regimen described here (which was not effective in all patients) appeared devoid of this drawback and is therefore worthy of careful confirmation.

ACKNOWLEDGMENTS

This work was supported by the U.S. Atomic Energy Commission, The National Institutes of Health (grant NS 09492–03), the Charles E. Merrill Trust, and Mrs. Katherine Rodgers Denckla.

REFERENCES

1. Cotzias, G. C., Papavasiliou, P. S., and Gellene, R., *New Engl. J. Med.* 280, 337 (1969).
2. Papavasiliou, P. S., Cotzias, G. C., Düby, S. E., Steck, A. J., Fehling, C., and Bell, M. A., *New Engl. J. Med.* 286, 8 (1972).
3. Boyd, A. E., Lebovitz, H. E., and Pfeiffer, J. B., *New Engl. J. Med.* 283, 1425 (1970).

4. Boyd, A. E., Lebovitz, H. E., and Feldman, J. M., *J. Clin. Endocr.* 33 (5), 829 (1971).
5. Cotzias, G. C., Tang, L. C., and Mena, I., in: *Neuroscience Research,* Vol. 6, I. J. Kopin and S. Ehrenpreis, Eds., Academic Press, New York *(in press)*.
6. Cotzias, G. C., Papavasiliou, P. S., Fehling, C., Kaufman, B., and Mena, I., *New Engl. J. Med.* 282, 31 (1970).
7. Düby, S. E., Cotzias, G. C., Papavasiliou, P. S., and Lawrence, W. H., *Arch. Neurol.* 27, 474 (1972).
8. Cotzias, G. C., in: *The Harvey Lectures,* Academic Press, New York and London *(in press)*.
9. Mena, I., Cotzias, G. C., Bell, M. A., and Potter, D. W., *Neurology (submitted for publication)*.
10. *Protein Requirements,* Report of a Joint FAO/WHO Expert Group. Wld. Hlth Org. techn. Rep. Ser. 301, 5 (1965).

Advances in Neurology, Vol. 5
Raven Press, New York © 1974

The "On-Off" Side Effect of L-DOPA

Charles H. Markham

Department of Neurology, UCLA School of Medicine, Los Angeles, California 90024

The "on-off" effect is one of the more troublesome problems in long-term L-DOPA therapy of Parkinson's disease. It may be defined as sudden fluctuations in parkinsonian symptoms, particularly akinesia and rigidity, sometimes interdigitated with L-DOPA-induced choreoathetosis, in individuals with Parkinson's disease who are on long-term L-DOPA therapy.

Since the question has been raised (1) that the method of administration of L-DOPA may be a factor in the production of the "on-off" effect, let me briefly review our present and past techniques. We (2, 3) start giving 500 mg L-DOPA daily for 4 to 7 days, increase it to 1.0 g per day for the second 4 to 7 days, and increase it in similar steps until the patient reaches a level of 3.0 g per day. The dosage is then increased over 2 to 3 months to a point of maximum benefit for symptoms, until significant side effects occur, or until a level of 8.0 g per day is reached. The daily dosage is divided into four to six allotments. If nausea or vomiting occurs early in the institution of therapy, the increases are spaced farther apart. In a few patients we achieved maximal dosage in several weeks; none of these developed the "on-off" effect.

The incidence of the "on-off" effect, as determined in an initial series of 100 patients followed for 5 years, plus another 81 followed for 1 to 3 years, is 11% (10 and 9 patients, respectively). All of these patients developed indications of it in the first 3 years of therapy, most by 2 years, and none earlier than 9 months.

The "on-off" patients may be characterized as follows. The great majority (17/19) were males, as compared to a 2-to-1 predominance of males in our main series (3). Their average age at the time of L-DOPA therapy was 54, whereas it was 62 in our total group. They were in Stages II, III, and IV of Parkinson's disease and this was not different from the entire series. All had moderate to marked initial improvement from L-DOPA. The average optimum dose of L-DOPA at 1 year was 5.3 g daily for the patients with the "on-off" effect, and 4.3 g daily in the total group. All had intact or nearly intact mentation. At least 2/3 of the group could be described by several of the following terms: tense, anxious, compulsive, rigid, chronic worrier, overly sensitive. These qualities were present before the "on-off" effect occurred and were prominent even compared to the total parkinsonian group.

Some 89% (17/19) of our patients with the "on-off" effect had some choreoathetosis in the first year of treatment before the "on-off" effect began. Yet very few of our total group of patients who had choreoathetosis early went on to develop the "on-off" effect. Thus, in our initial series evaluated at 30 months, 22% (20/91) had had choreoathetosis as a management problem in the previous year. In the first year the figure was 39% (38/97). Further, we had the suspicion that we could have induced choreoathetosis in most of our patients if we had pushed the dosage far enough. All this indicates that choreoathetosis early in treatment is a frequent occurrence and is an even more frequent precursor to a later "on-off" effect.

When we first began to hear from our patients about the symptoms we now call the "on-off" effect, we recorded the patients' descriptions, saw a fragment of the phenomenon in the out-patient clinic, or occasionally observed the patient in the hospital. It became clear there were too many variables to recall so we devised the table shown in Fig. 1 for the patient, family member, or nurse to fill in. The other figures in this chapter were derived from such weekly tabulations.

The development of the "on-off" effect typically began as a complaint of suddenly being unable to move. One nearly symptom-free patient occasionally found himself 'frozen' in a chair. He had no idea when he sat down whether he would be able to rise quickly to his feet, as had been his wont in the previous year on L-DOPA, or whether he would be 'stuck' for 10 to 20 min. Some patients seemed to have an akinetic episode every few days in the morning (see Fig. 2); others would have episodes in the afternoons or randomly throughout the day. Most episodes would occur 2 or 3 hr after some dosage of L-DOPA.

About the same time, or somewhat later, most patients found that the effects of the usual dose of L-DOPA did not last as long. They would experience a mild return of tremor or akinesia 2 or 3 hr after a dose of L-DOPA. As the doses were spaced closer together and increased, the choreoathetosis side effect either appeared or got worse. At first these tended to occur 1 to 2 hr after a given dosage of L-DOPA, at a time when there was maximal benefit for the Parkinson's disease (see Fig. 3). However, one man repeatedly had choreoathetosis develop when the parkinsonian symptoms were reappearing 3 or 4 hr after a given dose. We confirmed this pattern during a period of hospitalization.

Still later, as the doses of L-DOPA were lowered and/or administered closer together, a few patients had a continuous but variable degree of both parkinsonian symptoms and choreoathetosis (see Fig. 4). Most ended up with isolated episodes of akinesia and/or choreoathetosis (see Fig. 2). Of the 19 patients, 14 had choreoathetosis as a significant aspect of the "on-off" effect.

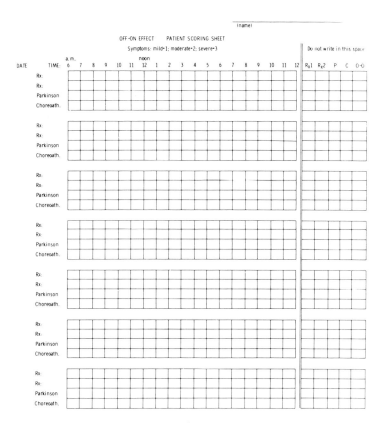

FIG. 1. Daily tabulation of drugs, parkinsonian symptoms, and L-DOPA-induced choreo-athetosis, to be kept by the patient or his family.

We have now observed the "on-off" effect in these 19 patients for 1 to 4 years. All still have it. All had a period of worsening but, as we adjusted the treatment (see below), most improved somewhat and then reached a state of equilibrium. In this state eight have continued to work or are living a near-normal retirement; the remainder are more incapacitated.

Environmental or psychological factors are very important in the precipitation of a bout of the "on-off" effect. Most of our patients have found that anxiety or emotional stress will precipitate akinesia, or tremor, or perhaps surprisingly a severe episode of choreoathetosis. We see these reactions in parkinsonian patients who are not suffering from the usual repetitive "on-off" effect, so anxiety should not be considered a specific precipitant to the "on-off" phenomenon.

Several of our patients have found that heavy exercise will precipitate a bout of choreoathetosis; one man has given up chopping wood and has bought a power saw for this reason.

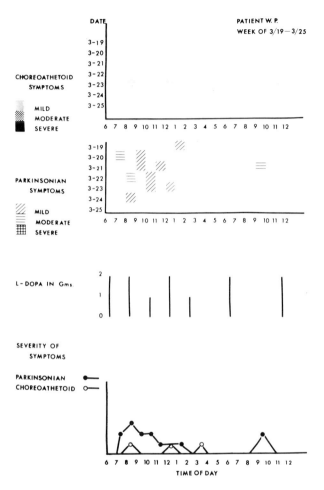

FIG. 2. To show daily occurrences of choreoathetosis (top graph), parkinsonian symptoms (second graph), dosages of L-DOPA (third graph), and a weekly summation (bottom graph) of choreoathetosis (open circles) and parkinsonian symptoms (closed circles). The weekly summation represents a combination of frequency and severity. After 3 years on L-DOPA, this patient developed intermittent akinesia and then intermittent choreoathetosis when L-DOPA was increased.

Another precipitant to a bout of akinesia is a large meal, particularly one high in protein (4). Two patients avoided eating for this reason and lost much weight.

From the treatment standpoint, initially we altered the dose of L-DOPA and gave the other drugs below on the basis of a verbal history. It became clear there was much variability in taking the medicine at the time prescribed and in reporting the physical symptoms. Many patients did not know and could not be easily taught to distinguish between what was tremor and

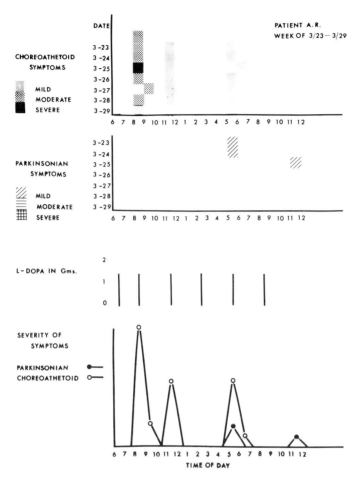

FIG. 3. After 2 years on L-DOPA, patient A.R. developed bouts of akinesia throughout the day. Increasing the L-DOPA caused the situation shown: akinesia on a few afternoons, and a daily severe episode of choreoathetosis.

akinesia and what was choreoathetosis; it often required several visits to clarify this difference. Once this was accomplished, however, we found the data forms (see Fig. 1) filled in by the patients to be of enormous help both in determining what was happening and in knowing what to tell the patient he should do next.

If the principal element in the "on-off" state was recurrent akinesia, closer spacing of the doses of L-DOPA usually helped. If there was a reasonably predictable time at which the akinesia occurred, increasing the amount of the preceding dose helped. The administration of one or even two doses

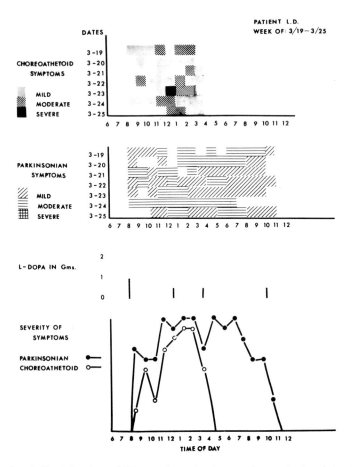

FIG. 4. Patient L. D. at the time of this graph was having nearly constant and simultaneous parkinsonian symptoms and choreoathetosis, after having had a more typical off-on effect earlier.

in the middle of the night reduced early morning akinesia. In four cases, eating smaller, more frequent meals seemed to help.

If bouts of choreoathetosis constituted the main difficulty, lowering the dose or taking the dose with larger meals sometimes helped. Avoiding heavy physical work or trying to avoid situations of emotional tension proved helpful in certain patients.

We have tried a number of drugs without applying strict controls. Medicines such as diazepam (Valium ®), chlordiazepoxide HCl (Librium ®), and meprobamate helped to a modest degree in certain patients, probably through their tranquilizing effect. Certain other drugs occasionally helped, possibly by a more direct action on the monoamines. Desipramine (Pertofrane®) and protriptyline (Vivactil®), whose principal action is thought to be increasing brain norepinephrine synthesis (5) without altering dopamine synthesis, seemed to produce a reduction in both akinetic and choreoathetoid episodes. Imipramine (Tofranil®) and amitriptyline (Elavil®) have also helped. The phenothiazines (we have used largely Compazine ®), whose main action appears to be that of blocking catecholamine action at the postsynaptic receptor site, may also help. The smoothing action of these drugs with such different actions on dopamine may be secondary to mood-altering characteristics from action on other monoamines elsewhere in the brain.

Six of our patients have insisted they have had fewer akinetic episodes while taking DOPA decarboxylase inhibitors (three were on MK-486 and three on Ro 4-4602). On the other hand, two users have not had their on-off state improved. In no instance was the L-DOPA-induced choreoathetosis improved. Papavasiliou et al. (7) have reported similar results.

We have not tried it, but fusaric acid, an inhibitor of dopamine-beta-hydroxylase, has been reported (8) to improve L-DOPA-induced choreoathetosis and might alter that aspect of the "on-off" effect. A catechol-O-methyltransferase (COMT) inhibitor, N-butylgallate, has also been reported (9) to reduce choreoathetoid movements induced by L-DOPA, but we have not used this.

Certain drugs clearly have not helped the "on-off" effect but these conclusions are based on trials of only a few patients each: these include dextro-amphetamines, methamphetamine, and monoamine oxidase inhibitors.

We have one patient whose "on-off" problem was helped by stereotaxic surgery. Prior to surgery he had predominantly left-sided parkinsonian rigidity plus akinesia. Response to L-DOPA became episodic and about the same time he began to have severe intermittent choreoathetosis. A stereotaxic thalamic ventralis lateralis lesion markedly improved the contralateral rigidity, and allowed a marked reduction in the dosage of L-DOPA. He now takes 2 g of L-DOPA a day and has a modest degree of akinesia and choreoathetosis which generally occur together.

Finally, the "on-off" effect may be benefited by stopping the L-DOPA completely for several days and then starting it again at a lower dosage. Since there is a marked worsening of the Parkinson's disease when L-DOPA is stopped, it serves to warn the patient and doctor that at least some L-DOPA will be indicated.

DISCUSSION

There appear to be two key parts to the "on-off" effect. One is that L-DOPA becomes less effective in bringing about remission of parkinsonian symptoms; the already brief duration of action of a given dose becomes still less. Also, there is greater variation in reaction from one dose to the next. The causes for variation in response earlier in L-DOPA therapy (such as stress, anxiety, physical effort, and food intake) become more powerful. And stress and anxiety are notorious for enhancing parkinsonian symptoms regardless of therapy or lack of it. These factors suggest to us that the "on-off" effect, which affects about 11% of our patients, represents simply an exaggeration of already precariously rapid degradation of exogenous L-DOPA.

The other major component of the "on-off" effect is the choreoathetosis. The close temporal linking of the choreoathetoid with the parkinsonian portions of the "on-off" effect supports our earlier view (3) that these two phenomena are associated with a common mechanism, the utilization of dopamine. Further, almost 90% of our patients who later developed the "on-off" effect had choreoathetosis during the induction phase of L-DOPA or in the first year of therapy. Goldstein and his colleagues (10) showed that L-DOPA given in combination with a DOPA decarboxylase inhibitor suppressed parkinsonian-like tremor secondary to ventromedial midbrain lesions and evoked complex repetitive movements in monkeys, which may be the animal counterpart of human choreoathetosis.

In the human, the usual variety of L-DOPA-induced choreoathetosis occurs, with few exceptions, in those individuals with Parkinson's disease (11, 12). It may be due to denervation sensitivity secondary to a portion of striatal neurons losing their nigrostriatal dopamine terminations (13), or it could be due to flooding the striatum with too much dopamine, causing otherwise normal dopamine receptors to become hyperpolarized (the inverse of the chronic depolarization produced by too much acetylcholine at the neuromuscular junction). Excess DOPA could be decarboxylated in the remaining nigrostriatal terminations or possibly in noradrenergic or serotoninergic terminations (14, 15). Or, a deficiency of methyl donors might lead to the dopamine being retained for too long in the striatum (16). When proof does come, we suspect it will show that both the L-DOPA-induced improvement in the parkinsonian symptoms and the L-DOPA-induced choreoathetosis are due to action at the dopamine receptors.

Let us assume the main cause of the "on-off" effect is the major variation in the delivery of dopamine to its receptor sites in the striatum. A part may well be due to alterations in decarboxylation in the brain of L-DOPA, possibly in nondopaminergic neurons containing L-aromatic amine decarboxylase and under strong influences of the limbic brain. But at least as strong a case can be made for a disturbance outside the CNS. Since 98 to 99% of L-DOPA is metabolized peripherally, including the brain capillary endothelium (17), a slight fluctuation could cause significant changes on the small fraction of intact L-DOPA destined for the brain. Delayed gastric emptying or the very presence of an intact stomach may reduce the amount of L-DOPA (18, 19) available for absorption, presumably in the jejunum (20). The L-DOPA is apparently metabolized in the gastrointestinal wall and in the first pass through the liver such that even at peak levels relatively little is found in the central circulation (21–23). In the plasma some L-DOPA is free, some is bound to protein, and some is in red blood cells; the total amount in blood is highly variable (21, 24). Any minor variation in these processes could alter either in amount or in time the L-DOPA available to the central nervous system. If non-brain transamination or decarboxylation of L-DOPA were to occur slightly more rapidly in a small proportion of humans with Parkinson's disease, perhaps the "on-off" effect might result. However, the "on-off" effect is clearly not a pure enhancement of peripheral DOPA decarboxylase; otherwise the DOPA decarboxylase inhibitors would more completely correct the condition.

Emotions play a major role in the "on-off" effect. The patient who is in a chronic anxiety state or who is a compulsive worrier seems more likely to develop the "on-off" effect, and a given bout of either akinesia or choreoathetosis is frequently triggered by an emotional upset. One may speculate that such stress could either work its effect peripherally by, for example, increased catabolism of amino acids, or centrally by increased limbic system demands on a precariously functioning striatum. The ultimate explanation of the "on-off" effect will have to include its exaggeration by certain emotional states.

There are a number of testable situations implicit in the above comments that could lead to significant improvement in the treatment of the "on-off" effect (and probably other aspects of Parkinson's disease as well). For example, holding the blood (or spinal fluid) levels of L-DOPA constant by prolonged and controlled intravenous administration of this drug in patients with the "on-off" effect should clarify its central or peripheral origin. Secondly, methods of selectively enhancing transport across the blood-brain barrier such as making DOPA (or dopamine) transiently lipophilic (25) might point the way both to the cause of present side effects and to better methods of treatment. Until then, however, we are limited to present clinical measures which may have a smoothing effect on the enormous swings of intracranial and extracranial L-DOPA.

REFERENCES

1. Barbeau, A., in: *Parkinson's Disease, Vol. 1*, p. 152. Hans Huber, Bern (1972).
2. Treciokas, L. J., Ansel, R. D., and Markham, C. H., *Calif. Med.* 114, 7 (1971).
3. Markham, C. H., *Neurology* 22, 17 (1972).
4. Mena, I., and Cotzias, G., *Fed. Proc. Abst.* 32(3), #346 (1973).
5. Neff, N. H., and Costa, E., in: *Antidepressant Drugs*, p. 28. Exerpta Medica Foundation, Amsterdam (1967).
6. Andén, N.-E., Carlsson, A., and Häggendal, J., *Ann. Rev. Pharmacol.* 9, 119 (1969).
7. Papavasiliou, P. S., Cotzias, G. C., Düby, S. E., Steck, A. J., Fehling, C., and Bell, M. A., *New Eng. J. Med.* 286, 8 (1972).
8. Mena, I., Court, J., and Cotzias, G. C., *JAMA* 218, 1829 (1971).
9. Ericsson, A. D., *J. Neurol. Sci.* 14, 193 (1971).
10. Goldstein, M., Battista, A. F., Ohmoto, T., Anagnoste, B., and Fuxe, K., *Science* 179, 816 (1973).

11. Barbeau, A., *Canad. Med. Assoc. J.* 101, 791 (1969).
12. Ansel, R. D., and Markham, C. H., in: *L-DOPA and Parkinsonism*, p. 69. F. A. Davis Co., Philadelphia (1970).
13. Ungerstedt, U., *Acta Physiol. Scand.* Suppl. 367, 69 (1971).
14. Butcher, L. L., Engel, J., and Fuxe, K., *J. Pharm. Pharmacol.* 22, 313 (1970).
15. Everett, G. M., and Borcherding, J. W., *Science* 168, 849 (1970).
16. Wurtman, R. J., Rose, C. M., Matthysse, S., Stephenson, J., and Baldessarini, R., *Science* 169, 395 (1970).
17. Bertler, A., Falck, B., Owman, C., and Rosengrenn, E., *Pharmacol. Rev.* 18, 369 (1966).
18. Rivera-Calimlim, L., Dujovne, C. A., Morgan, J. P., Lasagna, L., and Bianchine, J. R., *Europ. J. Clin. Invest.* 1, 313 (1971).
19. Fermaglich, J., and O'Doherty, D. S., *Dis. Nerv. Sys.* 33, 624 (1972).
20. Milne, M. D., *Clin. Pharmacol. Ther.* 9, 484 (1968).
21. Abrams, W. B., Coutinho, C. B., Leon, A. S., and Spiegel, H. E., *JAMA* 218, 1912 (1971).
22. Peaston, M. J. T., Bianchine, J. R., and Hersey, M., referred to in Abrams et al. (21).
23. Tissot, R., Bartholini, G., and Pletscher, A., *Arch. Neurol.* 20, 187 (1969).
24. Hinterberger, H., *Biochem. Med.* 5, 412 (1971).
25. Creveling, C. R., Daly, J. W., Tokuyama, T., and Witkop, B., *Experientia* 25, 26 (1969).

Advances in Neurology, Vol. 5
Raven Press, New York © 1974

Variations in the "On-Off" Effect

Melvin D. Yahr

*Department of Neurology, Columbia University College of Physicians and Surgeons,
New York, New York 10032*

Variability in intensity of symptoms and inconsistent responses to therapeutic agents are not an uncommon phenomena in parkinsonism. Indeed, there are few disorders of the central nervous system as capricious in this regard as this particular symptom-complex. We are all familiar with the patient whose examination varies with the hour of the day, the environment in which it is carried out, and a host of other factors including some undoubtedly motivational in origin. The striking episodes of voluntary motor responses — the so-called "paradoxical akinesia" — are examples par excellence of the unpredictable nature of this disorder. However, there is something unique and different about the so-called "on-off" reaction, a phenomenon which has made its appearance since the introduction of levodopa in the treatment of parkinsonism.

Characteristically, patients suffering from this reaction experience periods in which a complex form of the akinetic-rigid state occurs with a complete lack of movement, akin to that seen in an advanced stage of parkinsonism. Seemingly it comes on precipitously, without apparent causation, and may or may not bear a relationship to the ingestion of a scheduled dose of L-DOPA. After a variable period of time, its resolution occurs in as unpredictable a manner as its onset. Although usually the "on-off" reaction makes its appearance after an extended period of use of L-DOPA, this relationship to the duration of the treatment program may be more apparent than real. Indeed, since the combined use of L-DOPA with a peripheral decarboxylase inhibitor has been introduced, its occurrence has been noted at an earlier date following initiation of treatment. Perhaps of greater importance than the temporal relationship to treatment is the predilection for this reaction to occur in patients who have experienced an initial beneficial response, sustained this effect for a period of time, and then developed induced involuntary movements. This has suggested to us an alteration in the pharmacodynamics of L-DOPA interacting with some feature of the parkinsonian process. In analyzing a group of such patients we have to date been unable to identify clinical characteristics of their parkinsonian process which correlates with this reaction. Admittedly, this is a limited preliminary survey and a more comprehensive study including the many heterogeneous factors operating in this disorder may well reveal predictive factors. At any rate, it would appear at this time that the "on-off" effect is linked to the "DOPA effect" in the nervous system in a way that is far from clear. It is even less clear as to what can be done for its alleviation until more information regarding its underlying mechanism becomes available.

Early on, when we first encountered this phenomenon we were impressed by patient reports indicating an alteration in their response to L-DOPA. The phrases consistently used were "some doses of L-DOPA are not as effective as others" or "the effect of a dose does not last as long as it did before." In view of this, we undertook monitoring blood levels over an interval of time which covered periods in which the "on-off" effect occurred. Although there are obvious limitations to such studies and, indeed, blood levels are markedly variable from one patient to the next, there are instances, in contrast to Dr. Calne's report, in which an intimate relationship with the therapeutic response can be seen. Such an instance is indicated in Fig. 1. This patient was experiencing numerous "off" periods throughout the day. Over a 6-hr interval his parkinsonian state and blood levels of DOPA were recorded hourly. During the "off" periods, exceedingly low levels of plasma DOPA were found. However, when an "on" period is recorded a rise above

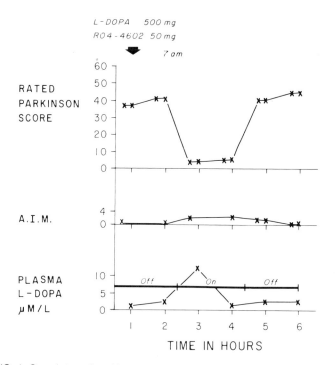

FIG. 1. Correlates of parkinsonian status with plasma levels of L-DOPA.

5 micromoles per liter is recorded. In fact, a blood level of such an amount or higher was required for this patient to maintain his functional capacity. Unfortunately, such a sustained blood level of DOPA could not be maintained without the concomitant occurrence of a disabling degree of involuntary movements.

I do not mean for a moment to suggest that this is the situation in all instances, nor that blood levels necessarily reflect what is occurring in the brain. However, it does raise the possibility that following the administration of a substantial amount of an aromatic amino acid such as DOPA, alterations in its transport, storage, or metabolism may well develop with resultant unpredictable adverse central nervous system reactions.

Concerning our present approach to dealing with the "on-off" effect, one can do little more than indulge in a number of therapeutic maneuvers. These are summarized in Table 1. In actuality they are, in the main, attempts to individualize the treatment program for a given patient. They can be applied seriatim in the order given or in any sequence one wishes, for indeed no consistent responses have been found. At best what one hopes for is to reduce the severity of this disturbing reaction to a minimum without compromising the beneficial effects of L-DOPA.

TABLE 1. *Therapeutic measures in the treatment of "on-off" reaction*

1. Maintain established L-DOPA dosage—alter dosing schedule using multiple small doses.
2. Increase daily L-DOPA dosage—with or without change in dosing schedule.
3. Reduce daily L-DOPA dosage—with or without change in dosing schedule.
4. Temporary discontinuation of L-DOPA—reinstitute L-DOPA starting with lower dosage and gradually increase.
5. Addition of ancillary anti-parkinsonian agents.
6. Replacement of L-DOPA by L-DOPA plus peripheral decarboxylase inhibitors.
7. Dietary modification—restriction of protein intake/multiple small meals.

DISCUSSION

Dr. Cotzias: This reminds me of the early days when we were trying to find one dose of levodopa to fit all patients, although we knew that no two patients with parkinsonism look or are similar. It seems to me that we are still looking for one treatment of the phenomenon.

Dr. Roberts: Diet seems to have some effect. I wonder whether attention has been paid to the microorganisms in the gut, and whether there have been experiments where the gut has been sterilized to see if this would affect the responses for a period.

Dr. Markham: We tried to do this, without any significant effect, in several patients with the "on-off" effect.

Dr. Cotzias: Dr. Markham, can you give us a schedule concerning the use of tranquilizers?

Dr. Markham: I've had the largest experience with Compazine. If I were going to use a tranquilizer I would prefer to use Elavil or Vivactil.

Dr. Klawans: I wouldn't want to correlate Elavil or Vivactil with Compazine or Thorazine in parkinsonian patients. I think the actions of the drugs are entirely different.

Dr. Markham: Although these drugs do indeed have very different actions on a biochemical level, either the Thorazine type of drug or the tricyclic drugs may have a smoothing effect on some of these "on-off" phenomena, and will allow a slight reduction in the amount of L-DOPA needed.

Dr. Klawans: Our experience in patients who have gotten even small to medium doses of tranquilizers, although not specifically for the "on-off" effect, is that this decreased the efficacy of L-DOPA and increased the daily requirement, not decreased it. I would like to know of others' experiences with tranquilizers.

Dr. Barbeau: I would tend to lean toward what Dr. Klawans just said. Personally, my experience with the phenothiazines has not been good, and certainly not useful in the "on-off" phenomenon.

Dr. Cotzias: We have had in-between experiences and therefore anything hopeful might be interesting.

Dr. Coleman: In view of the fact that some patients seem to profit from a low protein diet, I would like to suggest the 24-hour urine specimen for uric acid be done on patients who have the "on-off" effect and compare these values with those patients on L-DOPA who are not having the "on-off" effect. It is now known that there is a subgroup of humans who have abnormal, increased purine synthesis. These patients tend to have four sets of phenomena, including psychiatric disease. I think it would be interesting to compare purine synthesis in the patients who have the problem with those who do not.

Dr. Cotzias: That is an interesting point. Dr. Chase?

Dr. Chase: We have been interested in the possibility that the "on-off" effect was either peripherally mediated (having something to do with bio-availability of L-DOPA to the central nervous system) or a central nervous system effect perhaps related to the receptors. One way of studying this is to maintain constant plasma L-DOPA levels in patients who have severe "on-off" effects. We found we can turn off the "on-off" effect by maintaining a constant level. I think this supports the concept that this is simply a problem of supplying a constant dose of L-DOPA to the central nervous system. As a practical matter, one might get around this problem by using a sustained-release form of L-DOPA. We have tried those which are available thus far, and in our experience they are really not sustained-release L-DOPAs and they have not been very successful.

Dr. Cotzias: May I bring the discussion back to the dialogue between Dr. Carlsson and Dr. Duvoisin?

Dr. Duvoisin: I'm going to take advantage and just ask a question. Is it possible that some of the DOPA analogues that Dr. Brossi discussed before would have high protein binding and therefore provide a more sustained blood level? I doubt whether the various animal models which have been used to test the potential anti-parkinsonian benefit of these compounds would have taken that aspect into consideration. My own experience with the various neuroleptic agents, and this includes reserpine, is that in the end all you are doing is the same thing as adjusting the DOPA dose and it makes the therapy more complicated. I admit that there are occasional patients who somehow are benefited by a very small dose of a neuroleptic agent.

There is one agent that we've stumbled on recently and haven't studied too extensively: cyproheptadine, otherwise known as Periactin, which is marketed as a serotonin antagonist. This will reduce the DOPA effect but not very strongly. It may reduce some of the DOPA side effects, notably dyskinesias and thermal paresthesia, and might be more useful than the others mentioned.

Dr. O'Reilly: I offer one therapeutic suggestion I have not heard so far: this is that we reduce the number of patients per neurologist. This is not facetious really because the "on-off" effect, when it's severe, is a cause of great anxiety to the patient and to the physician, and it is more difficult to deal with when you have a lot of patients.

In my own experience, adjusting the dosage and slowly reducing the total dose is sufficient, without any other manipulations.

The question I have is this: Is it possible that you might do better with the addition of amantadine? There are one or two patients who, when I added amantadine to their regimen, seemed to have a smoother therapeutic benefit from L-DOPA. It is possible you might do well to add amantadine at a time when you reduce the total daily dose.

Dr. Sibley: It seems to me that to understand the "on-off" effect one must understand the prolonged "on" effect that many patients have on DOPA. In my experience patients who have experienced a great therapeutic benefit from DOPA can usually discontinue the drug for a day or two with impunity. Why is this? Is there DOPA storage in the surviving nigral neurons?

Dr. Cotzias: I can only agree with you. Dr. Yahr?

Dr. Yahr: I agree that this may happen for a period of two or three days with DOPA, but the same thing happens with trihexyphenidyl. I wonder whether those neurons that have been turned "on" are capable of going on and working and producing some of the transmitters that subserve their function. This is a phenomenon we see after you discontinue treatment with any of the anti-parkinsonian drugs.

Dr. Cotzias: But I think with DOPA it's a little more pronounced.

Dr. Yahr: In some patients it is more pronounced, and in others it is not. I have also seen precipitous turn-offs by stopping their other drugs.

Dr. Katzman: I just wanted to comment about the possible competition of amino acids for DOPA uptake in the brain. The blood-brain barrier to DOPA really consists of two steps. The first is the transport of DOPA as an amino acid across the capillary endothelium; competition, I believe, would occur whether or not you gave DOPA decarboxylase inhibitors or other amino acids. Therefore, the dietary effect on this action would be pronounced whether or not you gave DOPA decarboxylase inhibitors.

The other part of the blood-brain barrier is the decarboxylation that takes place in the rat capillary endothelium, but which may be less important in primate capillary endothelium. And I think the decarboxylase inhibitors are probably acting on other structures peripherally rather than on the brain capillaries in man.

I have one question. Nobody has yet commented on Dr. Brossi's statement that there is one-tenth of 1% 6-hydroxydopamine in commercial DOPA preparations. This means that a patient receiving $4\frac{1}{2}$ grams of DOPA per day is receiving 4.5 micrograms of 6-hydroxydopamine a day. I do not know if it gets across the gut, but if some of it did, it might deplete the amount of sites for storing dopamine in the periphery of the body.

Dr. Alvord: All that I've heard in this session, and I apologize to Dr. Cotzias for not knowing anything at all about the "on-off" effect, suggests that this is a very heterogeneous population of patients you're dealing with, just as heterogeneous as those we see at autopsy.

My hypothesis is that, as suggested with the uric acid problem, there is a subgroup of parkinsonians who are particularly susceptible to this "on-off" effect. I wonder if there is agreement on the general incidence of this at about 10 to 20%? If so, and if they're generally the younger patients who are less severely involved, this would fit with the group that has neither Lewy bodies nor Alzheimer tangles.

And so my question would be whether any of your patients had the misfortune to die but the good fortune to be autopsied.

Dr. Cotzias: Since there would be as many answers as there are investigators, I propose that they get to you in private.

Dr. Stern: First, the definition of a severe "on-off" effect is not that easy.

Dr. Sweet has very stringent criteria for the "on-off" effect; based on these, only five of our 80 patients would be included.

Second, I'd like to state that we all have diurnal variations. And the parkinsonians have them as well.

Third, the proximity of the toxic effect to the optimal effect (by toxic effect I mean dyskinesia development) can very easily be managed by taking the patient off L-DOPA. When we take patients off L-DOPA, they usually do better than before, after they are reinstituted on L-DOPA.

And finally, categorically as a clinician, I would like to state that our data so far reveal that there has been no really significant reduction of the effectiveness of L-DOPA in the treatment of Parkinson's disease.

Dr. Cotzias: That's good news in this dismal atmosphere.

Dr. Klawans: We've heard about the diurnal variation of parkinsonism which, of course, occurs in patients who are not on L-DOPA. Are there any data on the use of a very remarkably reduced protein diet and diurnal variations in parkinsonian patients who are not on L-DOPA?

Dr. Papavasiliou: The effectiveness of the diet in this population while off DOPA therapy is not as pronounced as while on therapy.

Advances in Neurology, Vol. 5
Raven Press, New York © 1974

Dopaminergic Involvement in Hypothalamic Function: Extrahypothalamic and Hypothalamic Control. A Neuroanatomical Analysis

Kjell Fuxe, Menek Goldstein, Tomas Hökfelt,
Gösta Jonsson, and Peter Lidbrink

Department of Histology, Karolinska Institutet, 104 01 Stockholm, Sweden, and Department of Psychiatry, New York Medical Center, New York, New York 10016

It is well known that there exist ascending dopamine (DA) pathways from the mesencephalon to the neostriatum and parts of the limbic forebrain (1–4). A short intrahypothalamic tubero-infundibular DA system has also been described (see reviews 5 and 6). With the help of immunohistochemical studies on DOPA decarboxylase (DDC) (7), new types of pharmacological models (8), and ontogenetic studies (9 and 10), it has been possible to obtain evidence for the existence of new types of DA systems in the limbic system and in the neocortex. New types of small neurons containing a monoamine-like transmitter, possibly DA, may also exist in the preoptic area and within the hypothalamus. These results support the view of Thierry, Stinus, Blanc, and Glowinski (11), who, on the basis of biochemical evidence, have postulated the existence of neuronal DA stores in the cerebral cortex.

In this article the DA pathways in the brain will be described in detail, including particularly a description of previously unknown systems of DA terminals and cell bodies. The various types of DA systems will be discussed in relation to their possible influence on hypothalamic function. In this discussion the neuronal circuits between the limbic forebrain and the basal ganglia on the one hand and the preoptic area and the hypothalamus on the other hand will be considered.

NIGRO-NEOSTRIATAL DA PATHWAY

This pathway originates from the substantia nigra (Fig. 1) (group A9 according to ref. 5) and from adjacent ventrolateral mesencephalic reticular formation (group A8). The DA fibers aggregate in the medial part of the substantia nigra and ascend in the area ventralis tegmenti and the dorsolateral hypothalamic area. Then they pass laterally into the lenticular part of

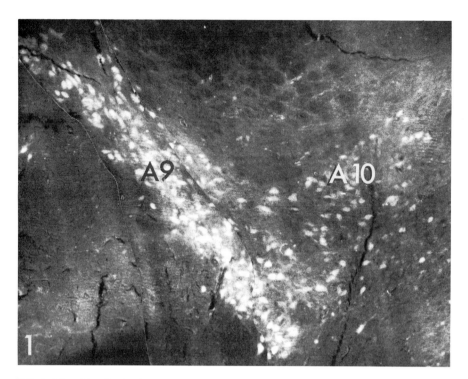

FIG. 1. DA cell bodies in the substantia nigra (group A9) and in the paranigral area (group A10). Group A9 is localized in the left part of the picture. Treatment with Ro 4–4602 (50 mg/kg, i.p.) 30 min before L-DOPA (200 mg/kg, i.p.). The animals were killed 1 hr after the DOPA injection. All animals were pretreated with reserpine (10 mg/kg, 24 hr before killing). A marked increase in fluorescence intensity is observed in group A9, which has become strongly fluorescent. The increases in group A10, on the other hand, are only weak to moderate. (From ref. 8.) ×125.

the internal capsule and reach the neostriatum via the fibrae capsulae internae. A very dense plexus of very fine terminals is formed in the neostriatum (Fig. 2). The highest density of nerve terminals is found in the caput and the lowest density in the cauda of the neostriatum. In ontogenetic studies (9, 10) and studies using the tyrosine hydroxylase inhibitor α-methyltyrosine, evidence has been obtained that two "types" of DA terminals may exist in the neostriatum. Thus, in the postnatal rat, strongly fluorescent islands of terminals can be observed scattered over the neostriatum (Fig. 3), whereas the rest of the striatum has a very weak fluorescence. Strong fluorescence is also observed at this stage of the development on the border between the striatum and the cerebral cortex. Since these islands have also been observed in adult animals following tyrosine hydroxylase inhibition, these islands probably not only represent a developmental phenomenon but also are present in the adult stage. The fact that these islands are unmasked

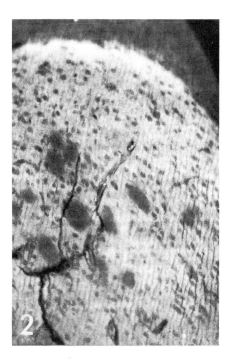

FIG. 2. Nucleus caudatus of normal rat. A strong diffuse DA fluorescence is present in the neuropile due to the presence of a densely packed plexus of DA nerve terminals. ×160.

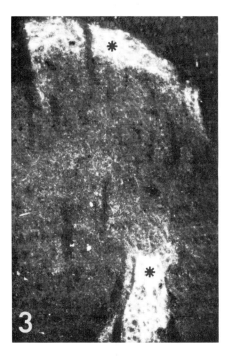

FIG. 3. Neostriatum of a postnatal rat (7 days old). A strongly fluorescent island of DA terminals is observed to the right in the picture (∗), whereas the rest of the neostriatum has a relatively low density of weakly fluorescent terminals. A strong fluorescence is also observed in DA terminals on the border (∗) between the cortex cerebri and the neostriatum (top of the picture). (From ref. 9.) ×120.

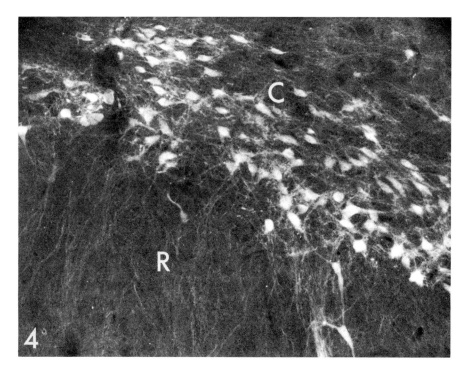

FIG. 4. DOPA decarboxylase immunofluorescence in DA cell bodies in the zona compacta (C) of the substantia nigra. Specific DDC immunofluorescence is observed both in the cell bodies and the processes of the cells. R = zona reticulata. (From ref. 7.) ×160.

following tyrosine hydroxylase inhibition may suggest that they have a lower turnover of DA than the other terminals in the striatum. Studies on the striatum using the Vibratome ® technique (see ref. 7) or infusion of saline have also suggested that the DA present in the terminals of the islands may be more strongly bound to the DA granules than the DA in the other neostriatal terminals. It is at the present time unknown whether or not the DA terminals of these islands stem from a particular part of the substantia nigra or from some other area of the mesencephalon or the hypothalamus.

Fluorescence histochemical studies after DOPA administration in combination with a decarboxylase inhibitor (Ro 4–4602 or MK-486) have revealed that the substantia nigra is heterogenous (Fig. 1) (8, 12). Thus, the DA cell bodies in the lateral caudal part of the substantia nigra, including those in the zona reticulata, show a much stronger increase in fluorescence after DOPA injection than those in the rostro-medial part of the area. In view of the fact that the dorsolateral part of the neostriatum shows a greater increase in fluorescence intensity after DOPA than does the medio-caudal part of the striatum, it might be proper to subdivide the nigro-striatal DA

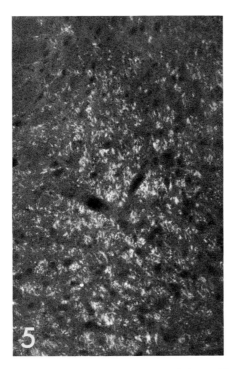

FIG. 5. DDC immunofluorescence in nigro-neostriatal DA fibers. The DA fibers exhibit a strong specific immunofluorescence and are observed to pass through the capsula interna. (From ref. 7.) ×160.

pathway into a medial and a lateral DA pathway. Such a subdivision has in fact been suggested by Poirier et al. (13; see also 12).

By immunofluorescence studies using antibodies against DDC (7), it has now also become possible to map out the nigro-striatal DA pathway. The results confirm in principle the findings made with the Falck-Hillarp technique demonstrating catecholamine (CA) fluorescence. However, the immunofluorescence technique has the advantage that the DA pathway itself also becomes strongly fluorescent, and thus the DA fibers can be mapped out in detail in the intact brain.* The distribution of DDC immunofluorescence-positive cells in the substantia nigra is practically identical with that for nerve cells demonstrating specific DA fluorescence. All the DA cell bodies and their dendrites and axons were observed to exhibit a strong fluorescence localized to the cytoplasm (Fig. 4). Thus, the processes of the

---

*Strong DDC immunofluorescence is, for example, observed in the DA fibers as they traverse the globus pallidus, explaining Hornykiewicz's findings (41) of high homovanillic acid levels in the globus pallidus.

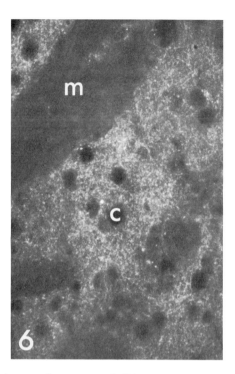

FIG. 6. Specific DDC immunofluorescence in DA nerve terminals of the neostriatum. The individual DA terminals are observed as moderately fluorescent dots. A somewhat higher density of DDC-positive terminals are observed in the middle part of the picture (c). This island may correspond to the fluorescent islands found with the Falck-Hillarp technique (see Fig. 3). m = fibrae capsulae internae. (From ref. 7.) ×400.

cells can be much better visualized with this immunofluorescence technique than after the Falck-Hillarp technique (Fig. 5). In the neostriatum, the individual DA terminals having a moderate fluorescence intensity (Fig. 6) could be observed more easily than is the case with the routine Falck-Hillarp technique for demonstrating DA stores, probably because of diffusion problems. Therefore, with DDC antibodies it was possible to study the density of the DA terminals in various regions of the brain. A higher density was found in the caput than in the cauda, in agreement with the fluorescence histochemical studies according to Falck-Hillarp. It should be underlined that it was possible to observe islands of strongly fluorescent terminals, the terminals of which were more closely packed than those in the surrounding areas (Fig. 6). These islands may correspond to the CA-fluorescent islands found in ontogenetic studies and in the adult brain after tyrosine hydroxylase inhibition.

POSSIBLE RELATION TO THE HYPOTHALAMUS

From the presently available neuroanatomical evidence (see 14), it seems clear that changes in DA receptor activity in the striatum can only indirectly influence hypothalamic activity. Thus, it should be emphasized that the existence of pallido-hypothalamic fibers is questionable. However, information of changes in the striatum can probably reach the hypothalamus via the globus pallidus and the medial thalamic nuclei. The latter probably send fibers down into the lateral hypothalamus. Another indirect route could be by changing activity in ascending reticular pathways, since the globus pallidus sends fibers down into the reticular formation with or without relaying through the nucleus ruber.

THE MESO-LIMBIC DA PATHWAY

The meso-limbic DA pathway innervates several areas of the limbic forebrain, and most of the axons originate from the large DA cell group surrounding the interpeduncular nucleus medial to the substantia nigra (2–4). The DA pathway to the limbic forebrain seems to ascend immediately ventromedial to the nigro-striatal DA pathway. All known DA terminal systems in the limbic forebrain are localized to the subcortical areas. DA terminals have been described in the following areas: nucleus accumbens, all layers of the tuberculum olfactorium, nucleus amygdaloideus centralis, dorsolateral part of the nucleus interstitialis striae terminalis, areas in the nucleus of the diagonal band (15–17).

Recently, a new pharmacological model has been discovered which will allow selective demonstration of DA neurons in the brain (8). This model is based on the fact that following DOPA treatment in combination with a peripheral decarboxylase inhibitor to reserpine-pretreated rats, selective accumulation of CA occurs in the DA nerve terminals. In agreement with previous studies, accumulation of CA was observed in the areas described above, whereas known 5-hydroxytryptamine (5-HT) and noradrenaline (NA) nerve terminals remain nonfluorescent. In addition, appearance of strong CA fluorescence was also observed in CA nerve terminals in the lateral septal nucleus (Fig. 7). The results suggest that these terminals represent DA nerve terminals, and therefore a DA system may exist that innervates the septal area. These very fine terminals appear to establish very fine axo-somatic and axo-dendritic contacts with cells in the lateral septal nucleus.

The mechanism for this selective accumulation of CA in the DA terminals may be a reserpine-resistant binding of CA to the DA granules (see 18), a binding which does not appear to exist to the same extent in NA terminals. In agreement with this view, it has been found in *in vitro* experiments that high concentrations of NA will accumulate in the DA nerve terminals

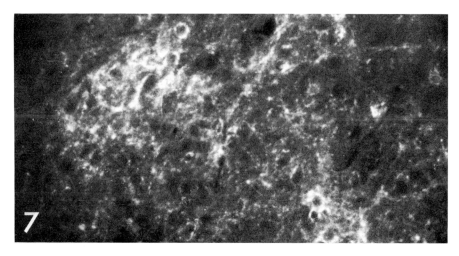

FIG. 7. Nucleus septalis lateralis of a rat treated with reserpine, Ro 4–4602, and DOPA as described in text to Fig. 1. A strong CA fluorescence has appeared in a plexus of CA terminals in this nucleus. These terminals may represent a previously undiscovered system of DA nerve terminals making, for example, close axo-somatic contacts with some of the nerve cells. (From ref. 8.) ×330.

following reserpine treatment (Fig. 8), but not in the NA and 5-HT nerve terminals (8). In view of the high background fluorescence that occurs in the cortical areas after DOPA treatment, and also in view of possibilities for diffusion during the Falck-Hillarp procedure, the *in vitro* experiments have been performed especially to map the possible DA terminals in the cortical areas as suggested by Thierry et al. (11). It was found that a varying percentage of the CA terminals in different parts of the cortex cerebri

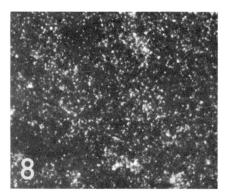

FIG. 8. Smear of a slice of the neostriatum after incubation for 30 min with a high concentration of NA (10^{-5} M). The rat was pretreated with reserpine (10 mg/kg, 24 hr before killing). A large number of strongly fluorescent dots are observed due to the accumulation of CA in these terminals. (From ref. 8.) ×300.

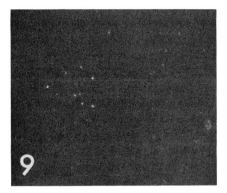

FIG. 9. Smear of a slice from the cortex cerebri which has been incubated with a high concentration of NA (10^{-5} M). The rat was pretreated with reserpine (10 mg/kg, 24 hr before killing). Only a small minority of the CA nerve terminals in the cerebral cortex have been able to accumulate CA and show a strong fluorescence. These terminals which exhibit a reserpine-resistant binding of CA may represent a previously unknown system of DA terminals in the cerebral cortex. They have a clear-cut regional distribution. (From ref. 8.) ×300.

(Fig. 9) show a reserpine-resistant binding of CA. These terminals were particularly frequent, for example, in the dorsal and anterior part of the frontal and cingular cortex (8), whereas very few were observed in the occipital cortex. Terminals accumulating CA following reserpine treatment were also found in the hippocampal formation. There may therefore exist a cortical DA innervation which has a regional distribution. *In vivo* experiments using the Vibratome ® technique to avoid diffusion combined with the reserpine–Ro 4–4602-DOPA model (Hökfelt, Ljungdahl, and Fuxe, *unpublished data*) have also suggested the existence of reserpine resistant accumulations of CA in nerve terminals in the rostro-medial part of the cortex cerebri, especially in the gyrus cinguli. The origin of the DA innervation in the limbic and frontal/ cortex is unknown. The findings of Thierry et al. (11) suggest that the cell bodies are not localized to the mesencephalic DA cell groups. One possibility is that they may originate from DA cell groups in the hypothalamic areas such as the group A13 lying dorsomedial and dorsal to the nucleus dorsomedialis hypothalami (see 6, 15, 19, 20). It seems possible that the large group A10 can be divided into several subgroups which may supply the axons to the various areas of the subcortical limbic system described above. However, no experimental data are yet available to support this view.

In view of the above, there is good evidence for the existence of considerable DA innervation of various parts of the limbic forebrain. It is well known that the limbic forebrain has rich connections with the hypothalamus, and it is thus quite conceivable that this dopaminergic input into the limbic system could have a considerable influence on hypothalamic function, such as the control of the activity in the peptidergic neurons governing the activity of the anterior pituitary.

Information of changes in DA receptor activity in the nucleus accumbens and in the tuberculum olfactorium can probably reach the hypothalamus via the medial forebrain bundle. It may also be pointed out that the tuberculum olfactorium is a secondary relay in the olfactory pathway, and thus the DA synapses here can modify the olfactory input into the hypothalamus. The neuroendocrine function of the nucleus accumbens is as yet unknown.

The amygdala has rich connections with the hypothalamus via the striae terminalis and the ventral amygdala-hypothalamic pathway. The activity of these pathways can be influenced by the DA terminals in the central amygdaloid nucleus, and furthermore, the striae terminalis innervates its red nucleus, which is also partly innervated by DA nerve terminals. After relaying in this nucleus, the fibers probably continue to the hypothalamus, and thus we have here an additional dopaminergic influence which can modify the input into the hypothalamus from the amygdala.

The septal area also send fibers into the hypothalamus, mainly via the medial forebrain bundle, and here again a dopaminergic influence exists in the lateral septal nucleus which can modify this input. By way of the fornix, the hippocampal formation governs activity in the hypothalamus. It is also known that the gyrus cinguli connects with the hippocampal formation via the area entorhinalis, which also may be dopaminergically innervated (8). Thus, the dopaminergic innervation of the gyrus fornicatus and the hippocampal formation can influence hypothalamic function by changing the activity in the fornix system.

On the basis of the available neuroanatomical evidence on the connections between the limbic system and hypothalamus and on the distribution of DA terminals within the limbic forebrain, it seems likely that there exists an extrahypothalamic dopaminergic control of hypothalamic function, for example, of its neuroendocrine control mechanisms.

THE TUBERO-INFUNDIBULAR DA NEURONS

The tubero-infundibular DA neuron system originates mainly from the nucleus arcuatus and the ventral part of the anterior periventricular hypothalamic nucleus and innervates the external layer of the median eminence (5, 6, 21–25). Recently, it has been demonstrated that the rostral part of the nucleus arcuatus is concerned mainly with the dopaminergic innervation of the intermediate lobe and the neural lobe of the pituitary gland (26). A number of CA-containing nerve cells probably containing DA are also found in the most rostral periventricular hypothalamic area (8, 20, 25, 27, 28). Björklund and Nobin (20) have named this group A14. A few cell bodies have also been described in the retro-chiasmatic area (20, 25). The innervation areas of these DA nerve cells are unknown, but it cannot be excluded that some of them participate in the innervation of the external layer of the median eminence.

The plexus of DA nerve terminals in the external layer of the median eminence is particularly dense in the lateral part of the median eminence. In ultrastructural analysis using potassium permanganate as a fixative, it has been possible to study quantitatively the CA nerve endings in this area. It was shown (29) that about 33% of all nerve endings in this area belong to monoamine neurons. This is the highest density of the monoamine terminals so far found in the brain. In the neostriatum, the density varies between 10 and 15% (18). The plexus of DA terminals is less dense in the medial area, where the DA boutons, for example, surround the capillary loops. With the help of pharmacological analysis using α-methyl-DOPA-hydrazine and treatment with dopamine-β-hydroxylase (DBH) inhibitors, it has been shown that the internal layer of the median eminence contains primarily NA nerve terminals (16, 17).

Recent studies on the use of antibodies against DBH are also in agreement with this view, since the plexus of DBH-containing nerve terminals in the internal layer is practically identical to that found with the Falck-Hillarp technique (7). In addition, the immunofluorescence studies on DBH have revealed the existence of a small percentage of DBH-containing terminals in the most lateral part of the external layer immediately adjacent to the primary capillary plexus. These terminals have previously been overlooked, mainly because of technical problems associated with the Falck-Hillarp technique when attempting to differentiate between DA and NA. These NA terminals, which have not previously been described may, in view of their location, have an important functional role in the control of the release of the hormones from the peptidergic neurons. It should be emphasized, however, that of course the DA nerve terminals are in a vast majority among the CA terminals in the external layer and play the major role in the control of release of the releasing and inhibitory factors from the peptidergic neurons.

The functional role of the DA terminals in the median eminence has been studied extensively by our own group (see reviews 5-7). The findings suggest that the tubero-infundibular DA neurons participate in the control of gonadotropin secretion by inhibiting luteinizing hormone releasing factor (LRF); follicle stimulating hormone releasing factor (FRF) secretion and by enhancing prolactin inhibitory factor (PIF) secretion. The evidence is based on results from amine turnover studies on the system in various endocrine states and after injection of various types of hormones as well as studies on the effect of monoaminergic drugs on the ovulation process in adult and immature rats following injection with pregnant mare serum. It may be pointed out that new types of DA receptor-stimulating agents such as ET-495 (30, 31) and ergot alkaloids (e.g., ergocornine) (32) have been found to cause a blockade of ovulation. The mechanism for these effects on the secretion of the factors involved in the control of gonadotropin secretion could be by an axo-axonic interaction at the level of the median eminence (33). Thus, the DA release could act to enhance the secretion of PIF and to inhibit the secretion of LRF. The functional role of the NA terminals in the internal layer and in the external layer is so far unknown.

OTHER DA CELL GROUPS IN THE HYPOTHALAMUS

A densely packed nerve cell group of CA cell bodies (A13) is localized in the dorsal hypothalamic area dorsal to the nucleus dorsomedialis hypothalami. Caudally, these cells are found to lie surrounding the medial and ventral surface of the tractus mamillo-thalamicus. Another CA cell group is also found in the dorsocaudal hypothalamic area partly within the nucleus posterior hypothalami at the border between mes- and diencephalon (A11) (6, 15, 19, 20, 28, 34). The innervation areas of these CA nerve cells are as yet unknown. They do not appear to participate in the innervation of the external layer of the median eminence, since in hypothalamic islands no decrease in the fluorescence intensity is observed in the external layer of the median eminence, in spite of the fact that groups A13 and A11 are not included in the islands. It can be speculated that these cell groups are involved in the innervation of the limbic forebrain and the neocortex. The evidence for their dopaminergic nature is based on findings from studies using DOPA, from microspectrofluorometric analysis, and from immunohistochemical studies on DOPA decarboxylase. Thus, in the same way as the DA cell bodies in the mesencephalon, they show considerable increases in fluorescence in response to DOPA after decarboxylase inhibition and they have a relatively high DOPA decarboxylase immunofluorescence.

DOPA-POSITIVE CELL GROUPS IN THE HYPOTHALAMUS AND IN THE PREOPTIC AREA

These nerve cells cannot be shown to exhibit any endogenous specific CA fluorescence using the Falck-Hillarp technique for demonstration of CA. However, they become markedly to strongly fluorescent following treatment with DOPA in combination with a peripheral decarboxylase inhibitor with or without reserpine pretreatment (8, 28). The DOPA-positive cells are found in the area surrounding the nucleus suprachiasmaticus within the nucleus periventricularis preopticus (Fig. 10) and in the nucleus preopticus lateralis down to the retrochiasmatic area. Other DOPA-positive cells are found within the area of the nucleus dorsomedialis hypothalami, within the perifornical area, and within the tubero-mamillary nucleus dorsal to the premamillary area (see 8).

All these nerve cells contain relatively high amounts of DOPA decarboxylase immunofluorescence (see 7), and they also have the ability to accumu-

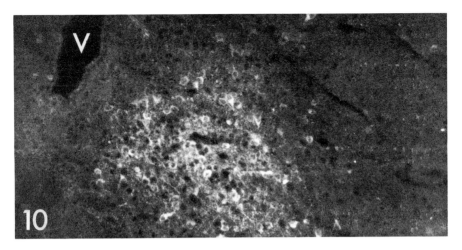

FIG. 10. Periventricular preoptic area. Moderate to strong specific DDC immunofluorescence is observed in small rounded nerve cells lying dorsally and also rostrally and
laterally to the nucleus suprachiasmaticus and also within the adjacent medial preoptic
nucleus. The dots in the background among the nerve cells probably represent the axons
from this densely packed DDC-positive nerve cell group. These nerve cells show no endogenous CA fluorescence and may represent nerve cells utilizing a monoamine-like
transmitter substance, possibly DA. V = third ventricle. (From ref. 8.) ×160.

late exogenous CA (see 6, 35). The axons of these nerve cells have been
found to have a weak to moderate DDC immunofluorescence. The transmitter of these nerve cells is unknown, but the findings suggest that it may
be a monoamine-like transmitter and possibly DA itself. It is interesting
that certain endocrine cell systems that produce peptide hormones also have
the ability to take up exogenous DOPA or amines, although they do not contain an endogenous amine which can be visualized with the Falck-Hillarp
technique (see, e.g., 36–39). It may therefore be speculated that the DOPA-
positive cells may contain an amine and/or a peptide hormone.

In view of the location of these DOPA-positive nerve cells, for instance,
in the medial preoptic region close to the suprachiasmatic nucleus, they may
play a considerable role in the control of, for instance, gonadotropin secretion, since the preoptic-tubero tracts governing the peak secretion of LRF
probably originate from the preoptic area (see 40).

CONCLUSIONS

The present review article favors the idea that the DA neurons in the
brain may have a wider distribution than has previously been believed. DA
terminals probably exist in the septal region as well as in various parts of the
cortex cerebri including the hippocampal formation. Particularly, a dopa-

minergic mechanism controlling activity in the limbic cortex must be postulated. The present morphological findings therefore support the view of Thierry et al. (11) that cortical DA neuronal stores exist. However, the regional distribution of the DA nerve terminals in the cortical areas must be emphasized. Furthermore, it should be pointed out that the dopaminergic innervation of the neostriatum and the limbic forebrain is heterogenous. Thus, in addition to the diffuse DA innervation in both areas, there are strongly fluorescent islands of DA terminals which seem to have a low DA turnover and a different degree of binding of DA to the amine granules. It is postulated that not only can the tubero-infundibular DA neurons participate in the control of neuroendocrine function, but also that the DA nerve terminals in the septal area, in the nucleus accumbens, in the tuberculum olfactorium, and in the limbic cortex could represent an important extrahypothalamic dopaminergic control of neuroendocrine events in the hypothalamus. The existence of other DA cell groups in the hypothalamus besides the well-known A12 group in the arcuate nucleus is described (see 20). They are found mainly in the dorsal and dorsocaudal hypothalamic areas. Their innervation areas are unknown, but it is speculated that they could contribute to the innervation of the cortical areas. Finally, there exist in various parts of the hypothalamus, and especially in the periventricular medial preoptic area, relatively large numbers of DOPA-positive cells which contain DOPA decarboxylase and are capable of accumulating exogenous amines. These small nerve cells may act with monoamine-like transmitters, and by way of their location it is postulated that they could have important neuroendocrine functions. It cannot be excluded that they might represent new types of DA neurons with very low endogenous amine fluorescence in their cell bodies.

The idea is favored, however, that the tubero-infundibular DA neurons still represent the major mechanism by which DA influences neuroendocrine functions.

ACKNOWLEDGMENTS

This work has been supported by grants (B73-04X-715-08A, B73-04X-2887-04C, B73-04X-2295-06B) from the Swedish Medical Research Council, Svenska Lifförsäkringsbolags nämnd för medicinsk forskning and Population Council (M 73. 73).

We thank Mrs. K. Andreasson, Mrs. M. Baidins, Mrs. A. Eliasson, and Miss B. Hagman for excellent technical assistance.

REFERENCES

1. Andén, N.-E., Carlsson, A., Dahlström, A., Fuxe, K., Hillarp, N.-Å., and Larsson, K., Life Sci. 3, 523 (1964).
2. Andén, N.-E., Dahlström, A., Fuxe, K., Larsson, K., Olson, L., and Ungerstedt, U., Acta Physiol. Scand. 67, 313 (1966).

3. Fuxe, K., Hökfelt, T., Jonsson, G., and Ungerstedt, U., in: *Contemporary Research in Neuroanatomy*, p. 275, Springer, New York (1970).
4. Ungerstedt, U., *Acta Physiol. Scand.* Suppl. 367, 1 (1971).
5. Fuxe, K., and Hökfelt, T., in: *Frontiers in Neuroendocrinology*, Ganong, W. and Martin, L. eds., p. 47, Oxford University Press, New York (1969).
6. Hökfelt, T., and Fuxe, K., in: *Median Eminence: Structure and Function*, p. 181, Karger, Basel (1972).
7. Hökfelt, T., Fuxe, K., and Goldstein, M., *Brain Res.* 62, 461 (1973).
8. Lidbrink, P., Jonsson, G., and Fuxe, K., *Brain Res. (in press)*.
9. Olson, L., Seiger, A., and Fuxe, K., *Brain Res.* 44, 283 (1972).
10. Tennyson, V. M., Barrett, R. E., Cohen, G., Côté, L., Heikkila, R., and Mytilineou, C., *Brain Res.* 46, 251 (1972).
11. Thierry, A. M., Stinus, L., Blanc, G., and Glowinski, J., *Brain Res.* 50, 230 (1973).
12. Butcher, L. L., Engel, J., and Fuxe, K., *J. Pharm. Pharmacol.* 22, 313 (1970).
13. Poirier, L. J., Bouvier, G., Bedard, P., Boucher, R., La Rochelle, L., Olivier, A., and Singh, P., *Rev. Neurol. (Paris)* 120, 15 (1969).
14. Nauta, W. J. H., and Haymaker, W., in: *The Hypothalamus*, p. 136, Charles C. Thomas, Springfield, Ill. (1969).
15. Fuxe, K., *Z. Zellforsch.* 65, 573 (1965).
16. Carlsson, A., Dahlström, A., Fuxe, K., and Hillarp, N.-Å., *Acta Pharmacol. et Toxicol.* 22, 270 (1965).
17. Corrodi, H., Fuxe, K., Hamberger, B., and Ljungdahl, Å., *Europ. J. Pharmacol.* 12, 145 (1970).
18. Hökfelt, T., *Z. Zellforsch.* 91, 1 (1968).
19. Fuxe, K., Hökfelt, T., and Nilsson, O., *Neuroendocrinology* 5, 107 (1969).
20. Björklund, A., and Nobin, A., *Brain Res.* 51, 193 (1973).
21. Carlsson, A., Falck, B., and Hillarp, N.-Å., *Acta Physiol. Scand.* 56, Suppl. 196, 1 (1962).
22. Fuxe, K., *Acta Physiol. Scand.* 58, 383 (1963).
23. Fuxe, K., *Z. Zellforsch.* 61, 710 (1964).
24. Fuxe, K., and Hökfelt, T., *Acta Physiol. Scand.* 66, 243 (1966).
25. Lichtensteiger, W., and Langemann, H., *J. Pharmacol. Exp. Ther.* 151, 400 (1966).
26. Björklund, A., Moore, R. Y., Nobin, A., and Stenevi, U., *Brain Res.* 51, 171 (1973).
27. Lichtensteiger, W., *Brain Res.* 4, 52 (1967).
28. Butcher, L. L., Engel, J., and Fuxe, K., *Brain Res.* 41, 387 (1972).
29. Ajika, K., and Hökfelt, T., *Brain Res. (in press)*.
30. Corrodi, H., Fuxe, K., and Ungerstedt, U., *J. Pharm. Pharmacol.* 23, 989 (1971).
31. Corrodi, H., Farnebo, L.-O., Fuxe, K., Hamberger, B., and Ungerstedt, U., *Europ. J. Pharmacol.* 20, 195 (1972).
32. Corrodi, H., Fuxe, K., Hökfelt, T., Lidbrink, P., and Ungerstedt, U., *J. Pharm. Pharmacol. (in press)*.
33. Schneider, H. P. G., and McCann, S. M., *Endocrinology* 85, 121 (1969).
34. Jonsson, G., Fuxe, K., and Hökfelt, T., *Brain Res.* 40, 271 (1972).
35. Fuxe, K., and Ungerstedt, U., *Europ. J. Pharmacol.* 4, 135 (1968).
36. Falck, B., and Owman, Ch., *Adv. Pharmacol.* 6A, 211 (1968).
37. Tjälve, H., *Acta Physiol. Scand.* Suppl. 360, 1 (1971).
38. Ericson, L. E., M. D. Thesis, University of Göteborg (1972).
39. Sundler, F., M. D. Thesis, University of Lund (1973).
40. Wurtman, R. J., *Neurosci. Res. Program Bull.* 9, 172 (1971).
41. Bernheimer, H., and Hornykiewicz, O., *Klin. Wschr.* 43, 711 (1965).

Advances in Neurology, Vol. 5
Raven Press, New York © 1974

Behavioral, Physiological, and Neurochemical Changes after 6-Hydroxydopamine-Induced Degeneration of the Nigro-Striatal Dopamine Neurons

Urban Ungerstedt, Tomas Ljungberg, and Göran Steg*

*Department of Histology, Karolinska Institutet, Stockholm, Sweden, and *Department of Neurology, Sahlgrenska Sjukhuset, Göteborg, Sweden*

It is well established that a degeneration of the nigro-striatal dopamine (DA) neuron system is the single most important lesion in the etiology of Parkinson's disease (1). The strategy in the creation of a model syndrome has therefore been the production of DA denervations in experimental animals (2). The following is an account of such experiments on rats using a highly specific chemical degeneration technique.

THE 6-HYDROXYDOPAMINE DEGENERATION TECHNIQUE

Intraventricular and intracerebral injections of 6-hydroxydopamine (6-OH-DA) cause a highly specific degeneration of noradrenaline (NA) and DA neurons (3–5). Intraventricular injections tend to cause a widespread, nonlocalized degeneration of catecholamine neurons, while stereotaxically localized, intracerebral injections of 6-OH-DA make possible lesions aimed for certain well-defined pathways (6, 7). The specificity of the 6-OH-DA-induced degeneration is in all probability dependent on the selective uptake of 6-OH-DA into catecholamine-containing neurons, which are killed by the subsequent intraneuronal oxidation of 6-OH-DA (8). However, the specificity of the 6-OH-DA-induced degeneration is clearly dose dependent, and too large a concentration will cause nonspecific damage of cerebral tissue (6). This has recently been pointed out by Poirier, who produced large, nonselective lesions in rats with a concentration of 10 μg of 6-OH-DA per μl of the injection fluid. At a concentration of 2 μg/μl, however, the lesion is remarkably specific, and in a recent series of electron-microscopically investigated 6-OH-DA lesions, *nonspecific lesions* larger than 0.2 mm were produced in only 2 of 18 animals (9). As a comparison, the *specific lesion* of

DA cell bodies in the substantia nigra had a diameter of about 2 mm. Stereotaxic injection of 6-OH-DA into the substantia nigra of rats may thus serve to produce an experimentally useful model syndrome for Parkinson's disease.

The ascending NA pathways in the rat pass close to the substantia nigra. A 6-OH-DA lesion, therefore, will unavoidably cause some destruction of NA axons. In order to account for the functional effects of such a lesion, the substantia nigra-lesioned animals are always compared to animals lesioned farther caudally in the brain, thus involving only ascending NA axons without affecting the DA neurons. It should be pointed out that a partial destruction of the NA pathways, such as that resulting from a degeneration of the NA cell bodies in the locus ceruleus, often occurs as well in the parkinsonian patient.

SYMPTOMATOLOGY

The bilaterally DA-denervated rat (but not the NA-denervated rat) shows a range of well-defined behavioral symptoms that are closely related to the clinical syndrome. The animal is severely akinetic. The akinesia is relieved only for short periods of time when the animal is activated by, for example, handling. There is an obvious rigidity which, however, does not seem to be as profound as that seen in humans. The rigidity is confined mostly to the hindlegs, which are held widely separated from the body. There is also a pronounced crouched back posture, possibly a sign of tonic changes in the back muscles, and the animal "tiptoes" in a characteristic manner. There are often signs of a fine tremor. The frequency is considerably faster (20 per second) than that seen in human parkinsonism. At present it is difficult to say if this indicates a different mechanism or if it is a characteristic feature of the rat species. It is not as pronounced in the rat symptomatology as in the human. Finally, the rat shows a serious adipsia and aphagia, which lead to death unless the animal is supported by careful tube feeding. The symptom is not one of food aversion, but rather an inability to initiate food seeking and ingestion. This symptom may seem unrelated to Parkinson's disease, in contrast to the previously mentioned symptoms. However, the DA-denervated rat should probably be compared to the most serious cases of Parkinson's disease, where the patient needs help with the ingestion of food and water.

FUNCTIONAL BASIS FOR THE SYMPTOMS

In order to understand the functional background of the symptoms described above, we have attempted a neurological, electrophysiological, and pharmacological analysis of the DA-denervated animals. The neurological deficits become particularly evident in the unilaterally denervated animal

(10). When sensory stimuli (auditory, visual, olfactory, and tactile) are applied to the side of the body ipsilateral to the lesion, the animal shows a normal orienting reaction to the stimulus, while there is no such reaction when the stimuli are applied to the side contralateral to the lesion. This "sensory neglect" of olfactory, visual, and auditory stimuli shows a slow recovery over a period of 2 weeks, while there seems to be no recovery of the ability to orient toward tactile stimuli. The fact that the animal is able to orient toward certain kinds of sensory stimuli while not toward others shows that there is a true sensory neglect and not simply a motor impairment. The nature of this deficit is not clear, but preliminary EEG studies show that sensory stimuli induce cortical activation, while there is no behavioral reaction. This may indicate that there is a deficit in the final sensory-motor integration rather than a block of the afferent sensory signals. Such a deficit may well arise from a disturbance of striatal activity, in view of its anatomical position as part of a cortico-striato-thalamo-cortical loop, as well as the known sensory convergence on the striatal cells (Krautheimer and Abbe Ferrard 19). These observations may contribute to an understanding of the akinesia, the difficulties in initiating movement, and thus the adipsic and aphagic state of the bilaterally DA-denervated rat.

In order to find a functional correlation to the rigidity following degeneration of the nigro-striatal DA system, we have studied the changes occurring in efferent stretch reflex mechanisms and the effect of drugs that reduce rigidity in the animals. Bilaterally 6-OH-DA-denervated rats were studied in a spinal preparation under superficial anesthesia (for details of the preparation, see ref. 11). The left dorsal and ventral roots of the segment innervating the calf muscles were cut distally. The dorsal root was electrically stimulated with single pulses, and recordings were made from two pairs of recording electrodes attached to thin filaments of the divided ventral root. This arrangement makes it possible to identify the fast α and the slow γ action potentials. Animals with bilateral 6-OH-DA lesions have considerably higher α efferent responses than normal animals, without a corresponding increase of γ responses. Intravenous injection of L-DOPA and apomorphine lowers the ratio between α and γ potentials; that is, it brings it back toward normal values. In Fig. 1 these results are compared to the results obtained by Arvidsson et al. (11) on reserpinized animals. The 6-OH-DA-denervated rat approaches the reflex pattern of the reserpinized animal. However, in the 6-OH-DA rat, L-DOPA in a dose of 10 mg/kg eliminates rigidity and induces changes in α and γ responses to dorsal root stimulation, whereas in the reserpinized, unlesioned animal, 100 mg/kg of L-DOPA is required to induce corresponding changes. This is probably due to the fact that the long-standing denervation has induced a stronger receptor supersensitivity than the reserpine treatment.

In the rigid 6-OH-DA rat, there is a spontaneous activity in both α and γ efferents. After L-DOPA injection (10 mg/kg), the rigidity and the tonic

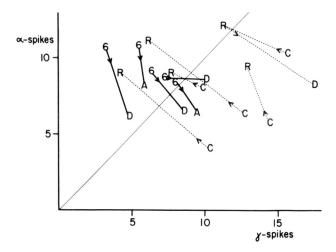

FIG. 1. The effect on the number of α and γ spikes appearing in the ventral root filament reflex response to dorsal root stimulation of apomorphine and L-DOPA. The number of γ spikes is plotted on the abscissa and the number of α spikes on the ordinate. The broken lines show the α and γ responses in the normal unoperated rat (C) and the changes induced by reserpine, 6 to 7 mg/kg, i.v. (R), and in one rat after later injection of L-DOPA, 100 mg/kg, i.v. (D). The continuous lines show 6-OH-DA-lesioned rats (6), and the effects of L-DOPA, 10 mg/kg, i.v. (D) and apomorphine, 0.25 mg/kg (A). Each point represents the mean values of 5 to 10 reflex exposures. Arrows indicate the time order of events.

α discharge ceases and the γ efferent activity increases. During L-DOPA as well as apomorphine, there occur sudden bursts of α efferent activity simultaneously with contractions of the intact innervated muscles. It is intriguing to speculate that these contractions are comparable to dystonic movements in the L-DOPA-treated parkinsonian patient. The rigidity of the bilaterally 6-OH-DA-lesioned rats is easily evident in the EMG as a tonic reflex response to muscle extension and as a tonic motor unit discharge at rest. After the administration of L-DOPA or apomorphine, spontaneous tonic motor unit discharges cannot be obtained, and the tonic EMG response to muscle extension is decreased or abolished. However, the bursts of α efferent activity are accompanied by spontaneous phasic bursts of EMG and the appearance of an initial phasic component in the response to muscle stretch.

The electromyographic demonstration of the rigidity pattern of the bilaterally 6-OH-DA-lesioned rat completes the picture of the akinetic-rigid model syndrome and stresses its parallelism with the human parkinsonian syndrome. The high α and comparatively low γ efferent activity level revealed both in spontaneous and reflex discharge in the 6-OH-DA rat, which is reversed to lower α and higher γ discharge rates by L-DOPA and apomorphine, supports the concept that the nigral dopamine lesion shifts the balance between the α and γ routes of efferent muscle control toward a dominance for the α route. The phasic stretch reflex pattern in the electromyogram and the bursts of phasic α activity in the ventral root filament may be related to the hyperkinetic behavior induced by apomorphine and L-DOPA.

Apart from changes in "sensory-motor integration" and spinal reflexes, there are important neurochemical changes in the denervated striatum. These become obvious if the bilaterally DA-denervated animal is treated with a drug that affects DA neurotransmission. Amphetamine, which is known to release DA (12), induces hyperactivity in the normal animal. However, after bilateral removal of the nigro-striatal DA system, the animal shows no reaction to amphetamine (13). Conversely, apomorphine, which is known to stimulate DA receptors, induces a strong hyperactivity in doses that do not affect a normal animal. Previous studies on unilaterally DA-denervated animals (14) have shown that this overstimulation is due to a postsynaptic supersensitivity that develops after the DA denervation. Similarly, L-DOPA induces a strong hyperactivity in doses that do not affect a normal animal. This effect may be prevented by pretreatment with a DOPA-decarboxylase inhibitor (Ro 4–4602), indicating that DOPA needs to be converted to DA in order to exert its effect. The degeneration-induced supersensitivity of the DA receptors is in all probability the underlying functional change that makes possible the substitution therapy with DOPA in Parkinson's disease.

SUBSTITUTION EXPERIMENTS

The above has been an attempt to demonstrate the behavioral deficits following a bilateral degeneration of the nigro-striatal DA system and to analyze some of the underlying neurological, electrophysiological, and neurochemical changes. However, animal models may also be used to detect and evaluate the therapeutic response to certain drugs. In a recent article we have outlined a series of behavioral test situations used to study various aspects of the therapeutic response to a drug (7). However, we feel that there is a distinction to be made between behavioral tests based on, for example, a hyperactive response following DA receptor stimulation and a test revealing substitution back to "normal behavior," which undoubtedly is a better representation of the clinically useful response. We have recently tried to create test situations where a substitution back to normal levels of behavioral activity may be detected.

In order to test for normal ability to coordinate movements, we have used an ordinary treadmill, where the animal is forced to move in pace with the moving surface in order not to bump into the wall at the rear of the moving band. In this situation, apomorphine or DOPA brings back motor coordination at doses too low to induce hypermotility, sniffing, or gnawing; that is, it restores normal abilities without inducing a behavioral excitation that may well correspond to the human hyperkinesias seen after DOPA.

In order to test the possibility of restoring more complicated learned behavior, rats were trained to run a maze for a water reward. This behavior involves both the spatial task of finding the way through the maze and the subsequent drinking of water. Fully trained animals lost their ability to run the maze after a bilateral DA denervation. However, substitution with low doses of apomorphine brought back both the ability to run the maze and to drink water; that is, the animal temporarily recovered from the akinesia as well as the adipsia.

In conclusion, there is an intriguing similarity between the symptoms following a bilateral 6-OH-DA-induced degeneration of the nigro-striatal DA system and the clinical picture of Parkinson's disease. The model makes possible an analysis of the physiological and neurochemical bases for the disease as well as a behavioral quantification of the therapeutic properties of various drugs.

REFERENCES

1. Hornykiewicz, O., *Pharmacol. Rev.* 18, 925 (1966).
2. Sourkes, T. L., Poirier, L. J., and Singh, P., in: *Third Symposium on Parkinson's Disease,* E. & S. Livingstone, Ltd., Edinburgh and London, 1969, p. 54.
3. Ungerstedt, U., *Europ. J. Pharmacol.* 5, 107 (1968).
4. Bloom, F. E., Algeri, S., Groppetti, A., Revuelta, A., and Costa, E., *Science* 166, 1284 (1969).
5. Uretsky, N. J., and Iversen, L. L., *Nature* 221, 557 (1969).
6. Ungerstedt, U., in: *6-Hydroxydopamine and Catecholamine Neurons,* Malmfors, S. E. and Thoenen, H. eds., North-Holland Publishing Company, New York, 1971, p. 101.
7. Ungerstedt, U., Avemo, A., Avemo, E., Ljungberg, T., and Ranje, C., in: *Symposium on the Treatment of Parkinsonism,* Raven Press, New York, 1973.
8. Jonsson, G., and Sachs, C., *Europ. J. Pharmacol.* 9, 141 (1970).
9. Hökfelt, T., and Ungerstedt, U., *Brain Res. (in press).*
10. Ljungberg, T., and Ungerstedt, U., *Brain Res. (in press).*
11. Arvidsson, I., Roos, B.-E., and Steg, G., *Acta Physiol. Scand.* 67, 398 (1966).
12. Carlsson, A., Fuxe, K., Hamberger, B., and Lindqvist, M., *Acta Physiol. Scand.* 67, 481 (1966).
13. Ungerstedt, U., *Acta Physiol. Scand.* 82, 69 (1971).
14. Ungerstedt, U., in: *Monoamines and the Central Grey Nuclei,* Proceedings of the IV Bel-Air Symposium, Genève and Paris, 1971, p. 165.

Advances in Neurology, Vol. 5
Raven Press, New York © 1974

A New Experimental Model of Hypokinesia

Gerard P. Smith and Robert C. Young

Department of Psychiatry, Cornell University Medical College, and Edward W. Bourne Behavioral Research Laboratory, New York Hospital, Westchester Division, White Plains, New York 10605

Hypokinesia, a hallmark of Parkinson's disease, is a failure of motor performance under some stimulus conditions. The failure of motor performance under some stimulus conditions, but not others, is difficult to understand. The defect is primarily in the initiation of movement. The power of some stimulus conditions to reveal the defect suggests a disorder of sensory-motor integration.

Experimental models of hypokinesia have been produced by lesions in a variety of subcortical sites, including the hypothalamus (1). Since all of these animal models show a deficit in motility under all stimulus conditions tested, the animal models do not mimic the human defect.

As part of our study of the behavioral functions of central catecholamine neurons in rats (2, 3), we have observed a defect in the initiation of motor performance after intrahypothalamic microinjections of 6-hydroxydopamine (6-OHDA). The motor defect occurred in only three stimulus conditions. Because microinjections of 6-OHDA produced a relatively selective loss of catecholamine neurons and because the failure to initiate motility was restricted to certain stimulus conditions, we believe this preparation will be a useful animal model for the experimental analysis of the hypokinesia of Parkinson's disease.

MATERIALS AND METHODS

The technique of Ungerstedt (4) was used to microinject 6-OHDA into the anterolateral hypothalamus just above the caudal edge of the optic chiasm in male rats weighing 200 to 400 g. The stereotactic coordinates for the anterolateral injection site were A 7.0, RL 2.0 and 8.0 down from the dura (all distances are in millimeters according to the atlas of De Groot, ref. 5). All injections were bilateral. Each injection consisted of 4 μl of distilled water containing 6-OHDA (6.5 μg base/μl) and ascorbic acid (0.4 μg/μl). Isovolumetric injections of ascorbic acid (0.4 μg/μl) in distilled water were made to control for nonspecific damage produced by the penetration of the cannula and injection of fluid.

Ungerstedt previously reported small areas of nonspecific damage (greatest diameter was approximately 0.3 mm) revealed by light microscopy using this microinjection technique in rats (4). Review of our material is consistent with Ungerstedt's results. It is important to note, however, that Poirier, Langelier, Roberge, Boucher, and Kitsikis (6) reported more extensive damage after midbrain injections of 6-OHDA in cats and after intraventricular injections in rats. Reasons for the difference in the extent of nonspecific damage have not been determined, but the variability of damage makes histological control essential. (See the chapter by Ungerstedt in this volume).

RESULTS

The first demonstration of hypokinesia after anterolateral hypothalamic injections of 6-OHDA was the observation that rats failed to move in an open field, but moved normally in their home cages. After vehicle injections at the same site, rats moved normally in both the open field and their home cages. Results of a representative pair of rats appear in Fig. 1.

Note that after 6-OHDA, the home-cage activity of Rat PC 35 measured by interruption of a photocell beam was low on the first postinjection day. Home-cage activity returned to normal by the third postinjection day and remained normal thereafter. Despite normal motility in the home cage, Rat PC 35 failed to move in the open field on days 3, 5, and 7. Since the dissociation between motility in the open field and motility in the home cage was not produced by the vehicle injection in the same site in Rat PC 34, the failure to move in the open field was specifically linked to 6-OHDA and not to nonspecific damage by microinjection. The defect of motility in the open field was also apparent in rats tested 30 days after anterolateral hypothalamic injections of 6-OHDA, so that the defect was not related to recovery processes during the immediate postinjection period.

The second demonstration of hypokinesia in rats after anterolateral hypothalamic microinjections of 6-OHDA was discovered by our colleague Sechzer while the rats were being handled for routine weighing. She noted that 6-OHDA-injected rats did not extend their forelegs when they hung over a table top. Formal neurological testing revealed that these rats had a selective loss of visual placing, that is, they failed to extend and place their forelimbs on any nearby solid object when they hung in the air with their limbs free. Vibrissae placing, chin placing, tactile placing, righting responses, and hopping reactions were all intact (7). This emphasizes the critical nature of the stimulus conditions in this form of hypokinesia. Visual placing was lost immediately after microinjection of 6-OHDA, and it did not recover spontaneously in rats examined for up to 6 months. Vehicle microinjections

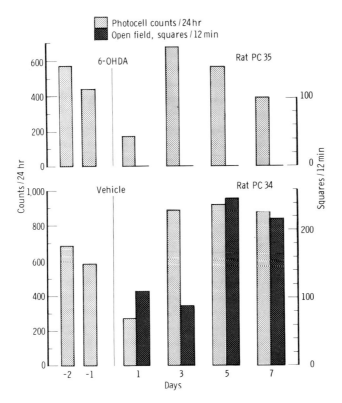

FIG. 1. Activity of two rats in their home cages was measured by interruption of a photocell beam across the middle of the plastic cages. Home-cage activity (counts/24 hr) is displayed for 2 days immediately before and 4 days after bilateral microinjection of 6-OHDA or vehicle into the anterolateral hypothalamus. On the four postoperative days displayed, the rats were removed from their home cage for two 6-min trials in the open field. The open field was an enclosed rectangle (76 cm × 93 cm) with a floor divided into 8-cm squares. Motility in the open field is presented as squares traversed in 12 min. The major result was that microinjection of 6-OHDA in Rat PC 35 produced a selective deficit in open-field motility, but vehicle injection in Rat PC 34 did not.

did not abolish visual placing, so this defect in motor performance was also a specific effect of 6-OHDA.

The third demonstration of hypokinesia in the 6-OHDA rats occurred during an attempt to train rats in a one-way active avoidance test (8). Training was done in a Plexiglas chamber (Grayson Stadler model 1111; internal dimensions were 30.5 cm long, 30.5 cm wide, and 15.3 cm high). The chamber was divided into two compartments of equal size by a partition which had a sliding door (14.0 cm long) at one end. The safe compartment (right side) had a smooth vinyl floor laid over the shock bars. The shock compartment (left side) had a floor of stainless steel bars (0.25 cm in diameter) that were separated by 1 cm. Current was supplied to the floor bars of the shock compartment by activating a constant-current shock generator equipped with a shock scrambler (Grayson Stadler model 700 GS). White noise entered both compartments from a speaker fixed to the roof of the test chamber.

Avoidance training of each rat began with the foot-shock current equal to the rat's jump threshold. Jump threshold was the minimal current at which a rat consistently lifted its rear paws off the shock bars. A trial began when the sliding door in one end of the partition was removed. If the rat crossed from the safe compartment to the shock compartment within 5 sec, this movement (approximately two rat body lengths) was considered an *avoidance* response. If the rat did not cross within 5 sec, foot shocks (1 Hz, 1 sec duration) were delivered through the shock bars for 10 sec. If the rat crossed during the train of shocks, this movement was considered an *escape* response. If the rat did not move out of the shock compartment during the 10-sec train of shocks, the rat was coaxed by hand into the safe compartment. The rat was left in the safe compartment until just before the next trial began. The intertrial interval was about 30 sec. Training was continued for 70 trials or until the rat reached the behavioral criterion of nine consecutive avoidance responses.

Although all 12 rats injected in the anterolateral hypothalamic sites with 6-OHDA moved into the safe compartment after receiving foot shock (escape responses), 9 of the 12 rats did not make the *same* movement in response to the removal of one end of the partition (avoidance response). Vehicle-injected rats acquired the avoidance response readily and achieved the behavioral criterion (Table 1).

The failure of 6-OHDA rats to move in response to the complex cue of removing the partition was not altered by increasing the shock current or by the acute administration of L-DOPA. This defect in motility persisted as late as 198 days postinjection.

TABLE 1

Treatment	n	Avoidance responses (median percent)	Number of rats achieving behavioral criterion
6-OHDA	12	0	2 (17%)
Vehicle	8	55	8 (100%)

Number of avoidance responses is presented as median percent of total trials. Nine of 12 rats injected with 6-OHDA did not make avoidance responses. One 6-OHDA rat made 2 avoidances. Two other rats made 20 and 32 avoidances, and both achieved the behavioral criterion of 9 consecutive avoidance responses. All eight vehicle-injected rats achieved criterion. Percent avoidance responses of vehicle-injected rats ranged from 28 to 68%.

DISCUSSION

After anterolateral hypothalamic injections of 6-OHDA, rats fail to move in an open field, to place visually, and to acquire an active avoidance response. The failure to move is the failure of certain stimulus conditions to control central motor mechanisms. Under our conditions, remote stimuli which are sensed by distance receptors fail to control movement; proximate stimuli of touch and foot shock retain their usual effectiveness. Since there is no histologic evidence that the 6-OHDA injections damaged the distance receptors directly, the defect is central and may be tentatively considered perceptual.

The failure to move is not the result of inability of the motor system to produce the movement. The evidence for this is that other stimulus conditions (e.g., touching vibrissae to a table edge or delivering foot shock in the avoidance training chamber) elicit motor responses (vibrissae placing and escape responses, respectively) which look very similar to the motor responses that fail to appear in visual placing and avoidance training.

This experimental hypokinesia is related to the catecholaminergic damage produced by 6-OHDA, because vehicle injections did not produce hypokinesia. Anterolateral hypothalamic 6-OHDA injections significantly reduced hypothalamic and forebrain concentrations of norepinephrine and dopamine, but did not decrease the concentration of dopamine in the caudate nucleus (3). Thus, our experimental hypokinesia was related to catecholaminergic damage in the hypothalamus, limbic system, or cerebral cortex, but not to damage of the nigro-striatal pathway.

We believe the hypokinesia produced by anterolateral hypothalamic injections of 6-OHDA has several characteristics which make it an attractive model of the hypokinesia of Parkinson's disease: (a) it is easily produced; (b) the failure to move occurs only under certain stimulus conditions; (c) the hypokinesia is tentatively considered the result of a perceptual defect; two recent studies have found a significant defect in perceptual organization in a series of Parkinsonian patients (9, 10); and (d) it is the result of catecholaminergic damage in the hypothalamus; hypothalamic catecholamines are also abnormally low in Parkinson's disease (11).

Like all models, this one will be judged by the experiments it provokes.

ACKNOWLEDGMENTS

The research was supported by U.S. Public Health Service grant NS 08402. G.P.S. is a Research Career Development Awardee 7-K04-NS38601.

REFERENCES

1. Poirier, L. J., in: *Recent Advances in Parkinson's Disease,* F. A. Davis Co., Philadelphia, 1971, p. 102.

2. Smith, G. P., Strohmayer, A. J., and Reis, D. J., *Nature New Biol.* 235, 27 (1972).
3. Smith, G. P., in: *The Neuropsychology of Thirst,* H. V. Winston and Sons, Washington, D.C. *(in press).*
4. Ungerstedt, U., in: *6-Hydroxydopamine and Catecholamine Neurons,* American Elsevier Publishing Co., New York, 1971, p. 101.
5. De Groot, J., *Trans. Roy. Netherl. Acad. Sci.* 52, 1 (1959).
6. Poirier, L. J., Langelier, P., Roberge, A., Boucher, R., and Kitsikis, A., *J. Neurol. Sci.* 16, 401 (1972).
7. Sechzer, J. A., Ervin, G. N., and Smith, G. P., *Anat. Rec.* 175, 439 (1973).
8. Levin, B. E., and Smith, G. P., *Neurology* 22, 433 (1972).
9. Meier, M. J., and Martin, W. E., *JAMA* 213, 465 (1970).
10. Loranger, A. W., Goodell, H., McDowell, F. H., Lee, J. E., and Sweet, R. D., *Brain,* 95, 405 (1972).
11. Bernheimer, H., Birkmayer, W., and Hornykiewicz, O., *Klin. Wschr.* 41, 465 (1963).

DISCUSSION

Dr. Duvoisin: I've begun working, using Dr. Ungerstedt's technique, on the analogies with clinical Parkinson's disease that one can see in the mouse. These are really quite extraordinary, and I'd like to mention just one.

The rotating rat has its analogy in the patient. Many patients with Parkinson's disease have a scoliosis, which is almost invariably contralateral. This scoliosis is reduced by DOPA and may even be reversed, although at doses that give severe dyskinesia. Thus, the model is almost exactly analogous to that shown in the rat.

Dr. Boshes: The sensory defect phenomenon is seen best after thalamotomy, because the contralateral limb, although nontremorous, is completely neglected, both in man and in monkey, unless the opposite limb is immobilized. Fred Mettler showed that monkeys will not use the contralateral hand after such an operation unless the other limb is tied down, and I have shown the same thing in humans.

The syndrome is augmented when you injure the rubro-thalamic pathway by doing a ventrolateral nucleus thalamotomy.

Dr. Barbeau: In my laboratory a few years ago Dr. Joubert showed a very clear baresthesia loss in parkinsonian patients, especially the akinetic patients.

Dr. Cotzias: Any further correlations from what you heard from the previous speakers with regard to clinical syndrome?

Dr. Poirier: In the studies where we used 6-hydroxydopamine, both in the rat and the cat, we made our observations after several days when the morphological changes had had a chance to take place. I would like to show you the effect of an injection of 6-hydroxydopamine in the cat. The cat brain is eight to ten times larger than the rat brain, and we give an amount proportional to that usually given to rats for such experiments. This was injected in the frontal horn of the several cats. The destruction followed the dynamics of the cerebrospinal fluid; the right frontal lobe was destroyed, along with the foramen of Monroe, the hypothalamus, the aqueduct, and the fourth ventricle. Everywhere the destruction followed the gravitational flow. The ependyma is completely destroyed, leaving debris, phagocytosis, sick cells, and a glial reaction.

Dr. McGeer: I'm sure what Dr. Poirier says may be correct, under certain conditions. But I'd like to describe some experiments done by Dr. Mailer in our laboratory. We put 3 milligrams of 6-hydroxydopamine locally into the substantia nigra, as Dr. Ungerstedt does, and then looked for degeneration by the Fink-Heimer technique. We saw degeneration confined to the established tracts for dopaminergic neurons. It was most exclusively confined to the neostriatum, but in some cases there was cell damage in the midbrain. You may also see degeneration in the olfactory tubule and the nucleus accumbens. But, had there been nonspecific degeneration in the substantia nigra, then there would have been heavy degeneration in the thalamus, because the principal pathway from the substantia nigra, pars reticulata, is to VL of the thalamus. There was no degeneration at all there except very small amounts which we also saw with control injections.

So I think this establishes that Dr. Ungerstedt's method does give selective degeneration of dopaminergic neurons, which is important for his animal model.

When you put 6-hydroxydopamine into the substantia nigra and produce this selective degeneration, there still seem to be preserved some nigrostriatal tracts. In other words, we do not believe that all of the tracts running from the nigra to the striatum are dopaminergic.

Dr. Ungerstedt: Maybe Dr. Poirier and I could join each other and say that anybody who uses 6-hydroxydopamine has a responsibility to show good anatomy, and to show if there is degeneration. It is obvious that you can get unspecific as well as specific effects. And it is very important to use anatomical controls.

Dr. Poirier: I think we should establish a control with normal stains.

I'd like to add one word about the chemical basis of this. I think Achala and Cohen in New York have shown that when 6-hydroxydopamine is put in at a pH above 4.5, which is the case in brain, it is readily transformed to peroxide. As a matter of fact, Achala and Cohen claim that its specific effect is related to peroxide. So now we have to study the effect of peroxide in the brain.

Advances in Neurology, Vol. 5
Raven Press, New York © 1974

Catecholaminergic Control of Gonadotropin and Prolactin Secretion with Particular Reference to the Possible Participation of Dopamine

S. M. McCann, S. R. Ojeda, C. P. Fawcett, and L. Krulich

Department of Physiology, University of Texas Southwestern Medical School, Dallas, Texas 75235

In this chapter we briefly review the hypothalamic control system which regulates the secretion of gonadotropins and prolactin and then examine the evidence for the participation of monoamines in this system. Progress in this field has been facilitated by three primary advances: (a) the discovery of the hypothalamic hypophyseal releasing and inhibiting hormones which mediate the hypothalamic control over the anterior pituitary; (b) the development of sensitive, specific, and precise radioimmunoassays for adenohypophyseal hormones, which have aided greatly in the analysis of the control system; and (c) the development of the histochemical fluorescence technique, which has focused attention on the localization of monoamines within the hypothalamus in the very regions which are known to participate in the control of gonadotropin and prolactin release.

THE HYPOTHALAMIC CONTROLLER FOR GONADOTROPIN RELEASE

A variety of evidence has clearly established the important role of the hypothalamus in controlling the release of both gonadotropins, follicle-stimulating hormone (FSH), and luteinizing hormone (LH). Stimulation of a broad band of tissue extending from the medial preoptic area caudally and ventrally through the anterior hypothalamus to the median eminence-arcuate region evokes LH release as measured by an increase in plasma LH determined by radioimmunoassay (1). The increased release of LH results in ovulation. Stimulation slightly more caudally in an overlapping band of tissue extending from the anterior hypothalamic area to the median eminence-arcuate region results in the release of FSH as well. In two animals, a selective release of FSH was observed following anterior hypothalamic stimulation. These results suggest that the center controlling LH may be located slightly more rostrally than that controlling FSH release.

As expected, hypothalamic lesions produce a deficiency syndrome. Following lesions of the median eminence-arcuate region, there is an almost complete cessation of LH release and a marked impairment of FSH release (2). More rostral lesions in the suprachiasmatic region block ovulation and lead to a continuation of gonadotropin secretion at a relatively low level associated with development of large follicles in the ovary (3). Estrogen is secreted by the ovary, which leads to vaginal cornification; the condition is known as constant vaginal estrus. In the normal rat, the preovulatory surge of gonadotropins is thought to be due to the interaction of ovarian steroids with a cyclic clock mechanism (4). This clock apparently discharges every afternoon and, if plasma levels of estrogen and/or progesterone are adequate, there is a subsequent discharge of gonadotropins (principally LH, but to a lesser extent FSH). These suprachiasmatic lesions abolish the stimulatory effect of progesterone on LH release, but leave the stimulatory effect on FSH release unimpaired (5). This again suggests that the center controlling LH release is slightly more rostral than that controlling FSH release. The LH center would be destroyed by the suprachiasmatic lesions, leaving the FSH-controlling area more or less intact.

In these animals with suprachiasmatic lesions, the release of gonadotropins is not completely abolished, and, in fact, responses still occur to removal of the gonads. This eliminates the negative feedback of gonadal steroids and is followed even in these animals by an increase in gonadotropin release. Conversely, administration of gonadal steroids in animals with suprachiasmatic lesions can lower gonadotropin release (5).

Thus, the current concept is that LH release is controlled by a hypothalamic mechanism, possibly of two types (6). The rostral center, located in the preoptic-anterior hypothalamic area, is concerned with the cyclic discharge of LH and FSH which is triggered by estrogen and/or progesterone. The more caudal region in the arcuate nucleus-median eminence area is concerned with basal gonadotropin release, and the so-called negative feedback of gonadal steroids may be mediated primarily here. Evidence from implantation of gonadal steroids in various hypothalamic loci also supports this concept (7), as do the results from cuts made just behind the optic chiasm, which accomplish the same result as suprachiasmatic lesions and eliminate the cyclic center (8).

Hypothalamic control of gonadotropin release is mediated by hypothalamic peptides. Both FSH- and LH-releasing activities of hypothalamic extracts were reported (9, 10). The LH-releasing activity was purified and separated from other hypothalamic factors (11), and recently a decapeptide has been synthesized based on structural studies of the natural product which has a potent effect in releasing LH (12, 13). This decapeptide has a lesser effect in releasing FSH, leading some to postulate that there is only one gonadotropin-releasing hormone (14). Our own opinion is that there must also be a hypothalamic FSH-releasing factor, since FSH and LH release can be dissociated as indicated by hypothalamic stimulation and lesion experiments, and also are dissociated under a variety of physiological conditions (15).

THE HYPOTHALAMIC CONTROLLER OF PROLACTIN SECRETION

Less is known about the precise regions of the hypothalamus which control prolactin release; however, there is no doubt that the hypothalamus exercises a net inhibitory influence on prolactin release in contrast to its stimulatory effect on gonadotropin release. The evidence for this is the dramatic increase in prolactin release which follows lesions in the median eminence (2) or grafting of the pituitary to a distant site (16), so as to remove it from CNS control. A prolactin-inhibiting factor has been extracted from hypothalamic tissue (17) and has been partially purified (18); however, there is also suggestive evidence for the existence of a prolactin-releasing factor as well (19). This complicates the situation with regard to the hypothalamic control of prolactin. Changes in prolactin release could be due either to reciprocal increases or decreases in the release of both factors or to alteration in the release of only a single factor.

LOCALIZATION OF RELEASING AND INHIBITING FACTORS IN THE HYPOTHALAMUS

The FSH- and LH-releasing factors are localized to a medial band of tissue extending from the preoptic region ventrally and caudally through the anterior hypothalamus as far caudally as the arcuate-median eminence region and pituitary stalk (20). This is consistent, in general, with the results just reported with lesion and stimulation experiments, except that the FSH-releasing factor was found as far rostrally as the LH-releasing factor. This may be an artifact of the means of measurement of the gonadotropin-releasing factors. The tissue extracts were assayed by an *in vitro* assay which magnifies the FSH-releasing activity. Lesions in the suprachiasmatic region which result in constant estrus give a reduction in the stored LH-releasing factor in the median eminence-arcuate region (21). The activity is reduced by about 50%, suggesting that cell bodies of releasing-factor neurons in the suprachiasmatic region have been destroyed by these lesions, leading to a loss of stored material from the degenerating axon terminals which are postulated to extend to the median eminence. Since the activity does not disappear after these lesions, we postulate that there is a second population of LRF neurons whose cell bodies lie more caudally in anterior hypothalamic area or arcuate nucleus. The more rostral LRF neurons would presumably be concerned with the cyclic discharge of gonadotropins, whereas the more caudally located LRF neurons would be involved in mediating basal gonadotropin release and the negative feedback of gonadotropins.

These same studies (20) revealed prolactin-inhibiting activity in the lateral preoptic area and prolactin-releasing factor in the suprachiasmatic region. This is surprising and requires additional lesion and stimulation experiments for verification.

POSSIBLE ROLE OF CATECHOLAMINES IN THE CONTROL OF GONADOTROPIN AND PROLACTIN RELEASE

The discovery of the tubero-infundibular dopaminergic neurons with cell bodies in the arcuate nucleus and axon terminals in the external layer of the median eminence in juxtaposition with the portal vessels (22) raised the strong possibility that dopamine might be involved in control of anterior pituitary secretions. Several approaches have been used to evaluate this possibility. One of them has been to examine the effects of dopamine on pituitary hormone release using either *in vitro* or *in vivo* systems. Dopamine had no effect on gonadotropin release from pituitaries *in vitro* or when perfused through an isolated portal vessel. On the other hand, when it was incubated with hypothalamic fragments *in vitro* (23) or injected into the third ventricle of living animals (24, 25), it provoked a substantial increase in FSH and LH release. The greatest response of LH occurred in females near the time of ovulation or in females pretreated with large doses of gonadal steroids (24). A lesser response was observed in males, and recently there has been some difficulty in confirming the ability of dopamine to stimulate gonadotropin release in the male rat *in vivo* (26). In these experiments, norepinephrine also was capable of stimulating gonadotropin release, but it was less potent than dopamine, and epinephrine was even less active. Intraventricular dopamine acts via release of gonadotropin-releasing factors which then trigger gonadotropin release (27, 28).

In contrast to its stimulatory effect on gonadotropin release, dopamine can clearly inhibit prolactin release. It is active on the pituitary incubated *in vitro* to inhibit prolactin release (29, 30), but was reported not to be effective when perfused into a hypophyseal portal vessel (31). Dopamine can cause release of prolactin-inhibiting activity from hypothalami incubated *in vitro* (30) or when injected into the third ventricle (32). Again, norepinephrine and epinephrine, although sharing the activity of dopamine, were less active.

EFFECTS OF DRUGS BLOCKING CATECHOLAMINE RECEPTORS OR ALTERING CATECHOLAMINE SYNTHESIS ON GONADOTROPIN AND PROLACTIN RELEASE

Another approach was to evaluate the effect of these drugs on pituitary hormone release. Donoso, Bishop, Fawcett, Krulich, and McCann (33) observed an inverse correlation between the expected effects of various stimulators and inhibitors of catecholamine synthesis on brain dopamine levels, on the one hand, and plasma prolactin levels, on the other (Table 1). On the other hand, blockade of norepinephrine synthesis with diethyldithio-carbamate produced no effect on prolactin. Dihydroxyphenylserine, which augments central norepinephrine synthesis, produced an elevation of pro-lactin which raised the possibility that artificially elevated norepinephrine levels could promote prolactin release, possibly by releasing prolactin-releasing factor. Further evidence for the importance of dopamine as a transmitter to inhibit prolactin release comes from recent studies in which the dopamine receptor blocker, Pimozide®, has been shown to elevate plasma prolactin levels (Ojeda and Harms, *unpublished*). As would be expected, plasma prolactin was lowered by the administration of L-DOPA, and this lowering also takes place in man (34).

Rather surprisingly, when L-DOPA was administered to animals with median eminence lesions in which the CNS control of prolactin was elimi-nated, there was a decrease in prolactin (35), and this has also been observed in humans with stalk sections (34). It is possible that in this situation L-DOPA is taken up by the anterior pituitary and converted by DOPA decar-boxylase into dopamine, which acts directly on the gland to lower prolactin levels. This is in keeping with the ability of dopamine to decrease prolactin release when incubated with pituitaries *in vitro*. Whether or not dopamine may actually be released into hypophyseal portal vessels and exert an in-hibitory effect directly on the pituitary gland in normal animals remains to be determined; however, attempts so far to detect dopamine in portal

TABLE 1.

Drug	Expected effect on MA activity			Effect on plasma prolactin
	DA	NE	5-HT	
α-MT	—*	—	0	+
p-CPA	0	0	—	0
p-CPA + α-MT	—	—	—	+
Pargyline	+	+	+	—
α-MT + DOPA	0	0	0	0
DDC	0	—	0	0
DDC + DOPA	+	—	0	—
DDC + DOPS	0	—, 0**	0	0
DOPA	+	+	0	—
DOPS	0	+	0	+
Pimozide®	—	0	0	+

*— = decrease, + = increase, 0 = no change.
**= decrease followed by return toward normal.
(Modified from: Saxena, B., Beling, C., and Gandy, H., Eds., *Gonadotropins*, Wiley-Interscience, New York, 1972, p. 49.)

blood have failed (Porter and Crout, *unpublished*). Nonetheless, we should not lose sight of the possibility that dopamine may act directly on the pituitary to inhibit prolactin release.

Studies with receptor blockers and drugs which modify catecholamine synthesis have given little support to a possible role of dopamine in regulation of gonadotropin release. Rather, they support a possible role of norepinephrine. We have evaluated the effects of these drugs in several situations. The first of these is following removal of the gonads (36). In the normal animal, this results in a rise in FSH and LH release from the pituitary gland because of removal of the inhibitory influence of gonadal steroids. In this experimental model, drugs which block catecholamine synthesis and alpha receptor blockers were effective in blocking the postcastration rise in gonadotropins (Table 2). Although not conclusive, the blockade appeared to be more related to the inhibition of norepinephrine than dopamine synthesis, particularly in the case of LH. The dopamine receptor blocker, Pimozide®, did decrease somewhat the response of FSH to castration.

Several other models were also investigated. The effect of these drugs on the release of FSH and LH provoked by progesterone (37) or estrogen (38) in an estrogen-primed rat was studied. Their ability to interfere with the normal preovulatory discharge of gonadotropins was evaluated (Kalra, *unpublished*), and, lastly, the effects of these drugs on the LH release provoked by hypothalamic stimulation was examined (39). In these situations, all the evidence pointed to a possible role of norepinephrine in mediating the responses (Table 2). For example, diethyldithiocarbamate or U-14624 to block norepinephrine synthesis blocked the progesterone-induced release of FSH and LH, and the block could be reversed by the administration of dihydroxyphenylserine to bypass the block and reinitiate norepinephrine synthesis (Fig. 1). Similar results were obtained with estrogen-stimulated gonadotropin release and with the normal preovulatory release, both of which could be blocked by drugs which inhibit norepinephrine synthesis. In this situation, it was more difficult to reverse the blockade with the administration of precursors to reestablish norepinephrine synthesis.

In the case of hypothalamic stimulation, blockade of norepinephrine synthesis resulted in an abolition of the LH release provoked by preoptic stimulation (Fig. 2), whereas that provoked by median eminence-arcuate stimulation was unimpaired. We postulate that in the former case we were stimulating presynaptically, whereas in the latter case we were stimulating the axon terminals of the releasing-factor neurons directly. We speculate that a noradrenergic synapse may be localized to the preoptic region and that increased impulse traffic across this synapse on the afternoon of proestrus or following steroid treatment may mediate the gonadotropin discharge which ensues.

Consistent with this concept is the increased turnover of norepinephrine

TABLE 2.

Drug	Expected effect on MA activity			Effect on increase in gonadotropins in response to:							
				Castration (males)		Estrogen-primed				Preovulatory	Preoptic stimulation
	DA	NE	5-HT	FSH	LH	+ progesterone		+ estrogen		LH	LH
						FSH	LH	FSH	LH		
Phenoxybenzamine	C	−(α)	0	−	−	−	−	−	−	nt	nt
Haloperidol	−	−	0	nt	nt	−	−	−	−	nt	nt
Pronethalol or propranolol	0	−(β)	0	0	0	0	0	nt	nt	nt	nt
Pimozide®	−	0	0	−	0	nt	nt	nt	nt	nt	−
α-MT	−	−	0	−	−	r	−	r	r	−	R
α-MT + DOPA	r	r	0	r	r	R	r	r	r	−	R
α-MT + DOPS	−	r	0	r	r	−	−	−	−	−	−
DDC	0	−	0	0	−	R	−	r	−	−	r
DDC + DOPA	+	−	0	0	r	−	R	−	−	−	nt
DDC + DOPS	0	r	0	0	nt	R	R	r	r	−	nt
U-14624	0	−	0	nt	nt	−	R	−	−	nt	nt
U-14624 + DOPS	0	r	0	nt	nt	R	R	r	r	nt	nt
p-CPA	0	0	−	0	0	0	0	nt	nt	nt	nt

R = complete restoration; r = partial restoration; 0 = no effect; − = decrease; nt = not tested. Data of P. S. Kalra, S. P. Kalra, and S. R. Ojeda.

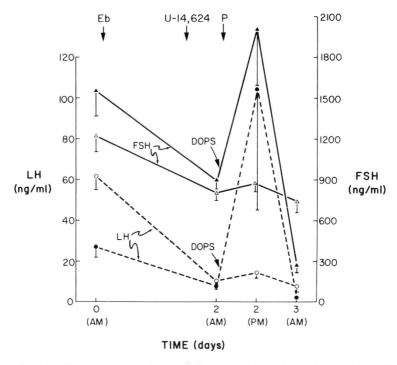

FIG. 1. The inhibition of plasma LH and FSH peaks of EB-P treated rats by U-14624 injected 18 hr prior to P (open circles and triangles – 10 rats); and recovery of the peaks by DOPS injected 1 hr prior to P (solid circles and triangles – 5 rats). (From Kalra, P. S., Kalra, S. P., Krulich, L., Fawcett, C. P., and McCann, S. M., *Endocrinology* 90; 1168, 1972.)

in the anterior hypothalamus on the afternoon of proestrus (40). On the other hand, a dopaminergic synapse located in the arcuate-median eminence region may trigger discharge of prolactin-inhibiting factor (Fig. 3). Dopaminergic synapses in this region may also trigger release of gonadotropin-releasing factors. These synapses may be involved in the mediation of the negative feedback of gonadal steroids, since estrogen can block the dopamine-induced release of LRF both *in vivo* and *in vitro* (41, 42) (Fig. 3). These postulated actions of dopamine and norepinephrine are consistent with the anatomical localization of the catecholamines (22).

CONCLUSIONS

1. Catecholamines can stimulate the release of gonadotropins and inhibit the release of prolactin. The response of gonadotropins appears to be mediated at the hypothalamic level, whereas it is possible that the response of prolactin is mediated both at the hypothalamic and pituitary levels.

2. Adrenergic receptor blockers can interfere with the release of gona-

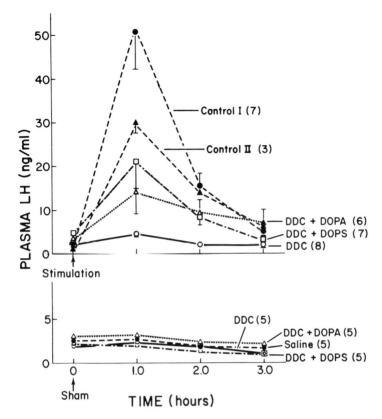

FIG. 2. Effects on plasma LH of EC (upper) or sham (lower) stimulation of medial preoptic area of proestrous rats pretreated with DDC or with DDC plus L-DOPA or DOPS. Control I = 50 μA for 30 sec; Control II = 25 μA for 30 sec; EC-stimulated rats injected with drugs were given 50 μA for 30 sec. (From Kalra, S. P., and McCann, S. M., *Endocrinology*, 93, 356, 1973.)

dotropins, on the one hand, and promote the release of prolactin, on the other. Alpha receptor blockers block gonadotropin release, whereas Pimozide ®, a dopamine receptor blocker, augments prolactin release.

3. Inhibition of catecholamine synthesis results in inhibition of gonadotropin release and augmented prolactin release.

4. Using drugs which selectively inhibit or augment either norepinephrine or dopamine synthesis, it appears that dopamine plays an important role as an inhibitory transmitter to lower prolactin levels, whereas norepinephrine appears to play a role in stimulating gonadotropin release.

5. We postulate that increased impulse traffic across noradrenergic synapses in the preoptic-anterior hypothalamic area may be involved in mediating the preovulatory discharge of gonadotropins.

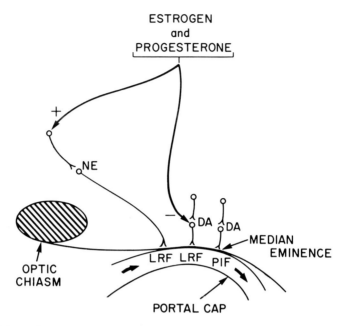

FIG. 3. Schematic representation of possible adrenergic synapses in the hypothalamus affecting discharge of LRF and PIF, and the effect of estrogen and progesterone at these sites. (From Saxena, B., Beling, C., and Gandy, H., Eds., *Gonadotropins*, p. 49, Wiley-Interscience, New York, 1972.)

6. On the other hand, a dopaminergic synapse located in the arcuate-median eminence region may be involved in inhibiting prolactin and possibly also in stimulating FSH and LH release via release of prolactin-inhibiting factor and gonadotropin-releasing factors.

ACKNOWLEDGMENTS

This work was supported by National Institutes of Health grants AM 10073 and HD 05151 and by grants from the Ford Foundation and the Texas Population Crisis Foundation.

REFERENCES

1. Kalra, S. P., Ajika, K., Krulich, L., Fawcett, C. P., Quijada, M., and S. M. McCann, *Endocrinology* 88, 1150 (1971).
2. Bishop, W., Krulich, L., Fawcett, C. P., and McCann, S. M., *Proc. Soc. Exp. Biol. Med.* 136, 925 (1971).
3. Bishop, W., Fawcett, C. P., Krulich, L., and McCann, S. M., *Endocrinology* 91, 643 (1972).
4. Schwartz, N. B., *Fed. Proc.* 29, 1907 (1970).
5. Bishop, W., Kalra, P. S., Fawcett, C. P., Krulich, L., and McCann, S. M., *Endocrinology* 91, 1404 (1972).

6. Barraclough, C. E., *Rec. Prog. in Hor. Res.* 22, 503 (1966).
7. Davidson, J. M., in: *Frontiers in Neuroendocrinology,* p. 47, Oxford University Press, New York (1969).
8. Halasz, B., in: *Frontiers in Neuroendocrinology,* p. 307, Oxford University Press, New York (1969).
9. McCann, S. M., *Am. J. Physiol.* 202, 395 (1962).
10. Igarashi, M., Nallar, R., and McCann, S. M., *Endocrinology* 75, 901 (1964).
11. Dhariwal, A. P. S., Antunes-Rodrigues, J., and McCann, S. M., *Proc. Soc. Exp. Biol. Med.* 118, 999 (1965).
12. Matsuo, H., Baba, Y., Nair, R. M. G., Arimura, A., and Schally, A. V., *Biochem. Biophys. Res. Commun.* 43, 1334 (1971).
13. Burgus, R., Butcher, M., Ling, N., Monahan, M., Rivier, J., Fellows, R., Amoss, M., Blackwell, R., Vale, W., and Guillemin, R., *C. R. Acad. Sci.* 273, 1611 (1971).
14. Schally, A. V., Arimura, A., Kastin, A. J., Matsuo, H., Baba, Y., Redding, T. W., Nair, R. M. G., and Debeljuk, L., *Science* 173, 1036 (1971).
15. McCann, S. M., Kalra, P. S., Kalra, S. P., Ajika, A., Libertun, C., Cooper, K. J., Fawcett, C. P., and Krulich, L., *Proceedings of the 4th International Congress of Endocrinology,* Washington, D.C., 1972 *(in press).*
16. Meites, J., and Clemens, J. A., *Vitamins and Hormones* 30, 166 (1972).
17. Talwalker, P. K., Ratner, A., and Meites, J., *Am. J. Physiol.* 205, 213 (1963).
18. Dhariwal, A. P. S., Antunes-Rodrigues, J., Grosvenor, C., and McCann, S. M., *Endocrinology* 82, 1236 (1968).
19. Nicoll, S. C., Fiorindo, R. P., McKennee, C. T., and Parsons, J. A., in: *Hypophysiotropic Hormones of the Hypothalamus: Assay and Chemistry,* p. 151, Williams & Wilkins, Baltimore (1970).
20. Krulich, L., Quijada, M., Illner, P., and McCann, S. M., *Proceedings of the 25th International Congress of Physiological Science,* Munich, 1971, p. 326.
21. Schneider, H. P. G., Crighton, D. B., and McCann, S. M., *Neuroendocrinology* 5, 271 (1969).
22. Fuxe, K., and Hökfelt, T., in: *Frontiers in Neuroendocrinology,* p. 47, Oxford University Press, New York (1969).
23. Schneider, H. P. G., and McCann, S. M., in: *Aspects of Neuroendocrinology,* p. 177, Springer-Verlag, Berlin (1970).
24. Schneider, H. P. G., and McCann, S. M., *Endocrinology* 86, 1127 (1970).
25. Kamberi, I. A., Schneider, H. P. G., and McCann, S. M., *Endocrinology* 86, 248 (1970).
26. Cramer, O., and Porter, J. C., in: *Progress in Brain Research: Drug Effects on Neuroendocrine Regulation,* Elsevier, New York, Vol. 39, 1973, p. 311.
27. Schneider, H. P. G., and McCann, S. M., *J. Endocrin.* 46, 401 (1970).
28. Kamberi, I. A., Mical, R. S., and Porter, J. C., *Science* 166, 388 (1969).
29. MacLeod, R. M., *Endocrinology* 85, 916 (1969).
30. Quijada, M., Illner, P., Krulich, L., and McCann, S. M., *Neuroendocrinology (in press).*
31. Kamberi, I. A., Mical, R. S., and Porter, J. C., *Endocrinology* 88, 1012 (1971).
32. Kamberi, I. A., Mical, R. S., and Porter, J. C., *Experientia* 26, 1150 (1970).
33. Donoso, A. O., Bishop, W., Fawcett, C. P., Krulich, L., and McCann, S. M., *Endocrinology* 89, 774 (1971).
34. Frantz, A. G., in: *Progress in Brain Research: Drug Effects on Neuroendocrine Regulation,* Elsevier, New York, Vol. 39, 1973, p. 311.
35. Donoso, A. O., Bishop, W., and McCann, S. M., *Proc. Soc. Exp. Biol. Med.* 143:360 (1973).
36. Ojeda, S. R., Krulich, L., and McCann, S. M., *Neuroendocrinology* 12:295 (1973).
37. Kalra, P. S., Kalra, S. P., Krulich, L., Fawcett, C. P., and McCann, S. M., *Endocrinology* 90, 1168 (1972).
38. Kalra, P. S., and McCann, S. M., in: *Progress in Brain Research: Drug Effects on Neuroendocrine Regulation,* Elsevier, New York, Vol. 39, 1973, p. 185.
39. Kalra, S. P., and McCann, S. M., *Endocrinology* 93, 356 (1973).
40. Donoso, A. O., and de Gutierrez Moyano, M. B., *Proc. Soc. Exp. Biol. Med.* 135, 633 (1970).
41. Schneider, H. P. G., and McCann, S. M., *Endocrinology* 87, 330 (1970).
42. Schneider, H. P. G., and McCann, S. M., *Endocrinology* 87, 249 (1970).

Advances in Neurology, Vol. 5
Raven Press, New York © 1974

L-DOPA and the Control of Prolactin Secretion

Andrew G. Frantz and Han K. Suh

Department of Medicine, Columbia University College of Physicians & Surgeons and the Presbyterian Hospital, New York, New York 10032

Prolactin is the most recent of pituitary hormones to come under active investigation in man, having only been definitely identified within the last few years in circulating human blood as a hormone distinct from growth hormone (1). The development of sensitive mammalian bioassays for prolactin in unextracted plasma (1–4) was followed rapidly by the isolation of the hormone from monkey and human pituitaries (5, 6), making possible the development of homologous human radioimmunoassays (7, 8). A heterologous radioimmunoassay, in which radioiodinated porcine prolactin is incubated with antiovine prolactin antibody, has also been developed which is sensitive to the human hormone (9). This chapter will briefly outline some of the recently identified factors affecting human prolactin secretion, based on data obtained in this and other laboratories, with particular emphasis on studies involving L-DOPA. A detailed review of the regulation of human prolactin has recently appeared (10).

MATERIALS AND METHODS

Plasma prolactin was measured by homologous radioimmunoassay by methods previously described (11), using human prolactin standards and antihuman prolactin antibody supplied by Dr. Henry Friesen. Many samples were also measured by mouse breast bioassay (2). Good agreement has been reported between these two assays when applied to human plasma (11).

PHYSIOLOGICAL FACTORS

Prolactin has been found to be measurable in the plasma of essentially all normal human subjects. Women tend to have slightly higher levels than men, although there is great overlap in the range of normal values, and to be more responsive than men, to most stimuli (10). Like human growth hormone, to which it is chemically related (12), prolactin is affected by many factors, although the two hormones appear to be regulated quite independently. Some of these factors are listed in Table 1.

TABLE 1. *Factors affecting prolactin secretion*

Factors	Effect on plasma prolactin
Physiological	
Nursing; breast stimulation	Increase
Sleep	Increase
Stress	Increase
Pregnancy	Increase
Estrogens	Increase
Sexual intercourse	Increase
Hypoglycemia	Increase
Pathological	
Hypothalamic lesions, pituitary stalk section	Increase, usually
Pituitary tumors	Increase or no change; less often decrease
Pharmacological	
L-DOPA	Decrease
Neuroleptic drugs	Increase
TRH	Increase
Ergot alkaloids	Decrease
Water load	Decrease
Hypertonic saline	Increase

Nursing and Breast Stimulation

One of the most specific as well as powerful stimuli for prolactin release is suckling in postpartum women (11, 13, 14). The effect is rapid, independent of milk letdown (an oxytocin-mediated phenomenon), and triggered by sensations arising from the breast and nipple. The majority of nonpostpartum, normally menstruating women do not have a significant response to breast stimulation, although about one-third of such subjects exhibit some prolactin rise (14). The factors that differentiate the responders from the nonresponders among normal women are not known at present.

Sleep

A pronounced diurnal variation in plasma prolactin has been identified, with peak of secretion occurring during the hours of sleep (15). As shown in Fig. 1, the timing of the prolactin peak is not coincident with that of growth hormone, and it has not as yet been possible to relate the increased prolactin secretion to a particular stage of the electroencephalogram. That nocturnal prolactin hypersecretion is related to sleep itself, and not to an intrinsic circadian rhythm, as is the case with ACTH, has been shown by studies involving abrupt shifts of the sleep-waking cycle (16).

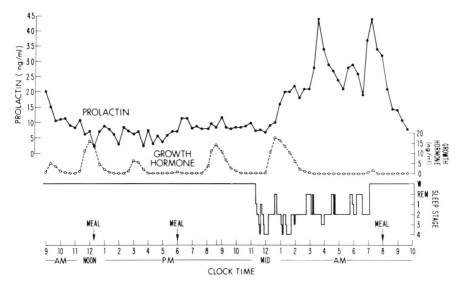

FIG. 1. Plasma prolactin and growth hormone in an adult male measured at 20-min intervals via indwelling intravenous catheter. Blood withdrawal did not interfere with normal sleep, which was monitored by EEG. A sleep-related peak of prolactin secretion has been seen in all normal subjects tested (15).

Stress

Stressful procedures of several kinds have been shown to result in increased plasma prolactin, the greatest rises having been noted in major surgery with general anesthesia (17).

Pregnancy

Plasma prolactin rises steadily throughout pregnancy in humans (7). It is possible that this phenomenon is related to the large estrogen rise which occurs during human pregnancy; in the monkey, which does not exhibit the same degree of hyperestrogenism during pregnancy as the human, there is no comparable prolactin rise (7).

Estrogens

A two- or threefold rise in baseline plasma prolactin has been observed in males given large doses of estrogens (11). Similar results in females have also been observed in unpublished studies from this laboratory. Preliminary evidence suggests that estrogens may sensitize the hypothalamic-pituitary axis to stimuli that release prolactin, in a manner similar to what has previously been demonstrated for growth hormone (18).

Sexual Intercourse

A minority of normal women have been found to exhibit a pronounced rise in plasma prolactin after sexual intercourse with orgasm (17). The phenomenon does not appear to be due to concomitant breast stimulation, and the mechanisms involved are as yet unclear.

Hypoglycemia

Acute hypoglycemia, such as that induced by intravenous insulin, can release prolactin as well as growth hormone (17). A greater degree of hypoglycemia appears to be necessary for prolactin release than is needed for growth hormone, and the phenomenon is probably chiefly of pharmacological rather than physiological significance.

PATHOLOGICAL FACTORS

Hypothalamic Lesions; Pituitary Stalk Section

The concept that prolactin is under predominantly inhibitory control from the hypothalamus via prolactin-inhibiting factor (PIF) has been established by extensive animal experimentation and appears to hold true for the human as well. Section of the pituitary stalk produces elevation of plasma prolactin in some patients (11, 19), and hypothalamic lesions of various kinds may be associated with high prolactin levels (10, 20).

Pituitary Tumors

Of all pituitary hormones, prolactin appears to be the one most commonly hypersecreted by tumors of the gland. Approximately one-third of all patients with pituitary tumors have elevated plasma prolactin, whether or not there is associated galactorrhea (10). These tumors are predominantly chromophobe adenomas; specific staining for intracytoplasmic hormone by the immunoperoxidase technique has shown large amounts of prolactin within the tumor cells, despite the absence of acidophilia by conventional stains (21). Although a nonsecreting pituitary tumor could conceivably induce hypersecretion of prolactin by adjacent, nontumorous cells through impingement on the stalk and interference with PIF transport, it appears likely from biological evidence that it is the tumor cells themselves that are the source of the excess prolactin secretion. The relatively high incidence of hyperprolactinemia in pituitary tumors makes the assay of plasma prolactin a useful test both for diagnostic purposes and for following the effects of therapy in cases where hypersecretion has been documented.

PHARMACOLOGICAL FACTORS

L-DOPA

An inhibitory effect of dopamine on prolactin secretion has been demonstrated in several animal studies. Direct incubation of pituitary glands with dopamine has resulted in suppression of prolactin release (22–24), although the doses employed have been relatively high and the physiological significance of this phenomenon has been uncertain. Kamberi, Mical, and Porter (25, 26) were unable to suppress prolactin in rats by direct injection of dopamine into the pituitary *in vivo,* but obtained lowered plasma prolactin and increased PIF activity in pituitary stalk blood when dopamine was injected into the third ventricle. These results are consistent with the hypothesis that dopamine or dopaminergic pathways acting on the hypothalamus can influence prolactin secretion through the stimulation of PIF, but that dopamine itself is not PIF.

In the human, transient lowering of plasma prolactin occurs after a single oral dose of L-DOPA both in normal individuals and in many of those with pathological elevations of the hormone (27–29). The effect of 500 mg of L-DOPA on plasma prolactin in six normal subjects (three men and three women, aged 22 to 28 years) is shown in Fig. 2. Suppression is maximal at 2 hr, after which there is a rise and in some subjects an apparent rebound above normal at 5 or 6 hr. Similar effects were obtained when a lower dose of L-DOPA, 100 mg, was given with 50 mg of the decarboxylase inhibitor MK-486 in the same six subjects on a separate occasion (Fig. 2).

Attempts at chronic suppression of plasma prolactin by L-DOPA have been made in patients with metastatic breast cancer (30, 31). Frequent administration of the drug in total doses averaging approximately 3.0 gm/day has resulted in a continued responsiveness to the acute suppressive effects of L-DOPA, although the effect of each dose is short-lived and administration every 3 to 4 hr appears necessary for optimum results. The sleep peak poses a special problem in this regard; we have not yet fully evaluated the effect of L-DOPA on prolactin during sleep. Objective evidence of remission of disease, including disappearance of metastatic skin nodules, has occurred in a minority of patients (31). We are further exploring the use of L-DOPA in breast cancer patients, both as a means of treatment and as a guide for selecting those patients with prolactin-dependent tumors who might be further benefited by the more complete suppression of prolactin achievable by hypophysectomy.

Neuroleptic Drugs

Earlier animal studies, reviewed by Sulman (32), indicated that chlorpromazine and other neuroleptic drugs could stimulate prolactin release,

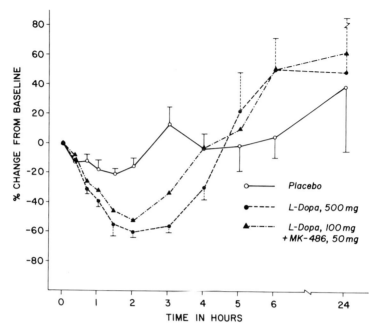

FIG. 2. Mean plasma prolactin as a percent of baseline values in six normal subjects (three men, three women). Each subject was tested during the morning on three separate occasions before and after receiving the following, in random order: L-DOPA, 500 mg; L-DOPA, 100 mg, plus MK-486, 50 mg; placebo. Vertical bars denote standard error of the mean.

and that the mechanism involved suppression of hypothalamic PIF. In humans, both chronic (2) and acute (27, 29) administration of chlorpromazine have been shown to raise plasma prolactin, and the acute administration of the drug appears to be a useful test of hypothalamic-pituitary function. The response of four normal subjects (three males and one female, aged 22 to 26 years) to 25 mg of chlorpromazine intramuscularly is shown by the solid line in Fig. 3. These same subjects were given the same dose of chlorpromazine on a subsequent occasion after pretreatment with oral L-DOPA, 500 mg 30 min beforehand. As shown by the dashed line, marked inhibition of the acute response is evident during the first 2 hr; after this the effect of the L-DOPA diminishes and the two curves come together. A slight rebound effect from L-DOPA at 4 hr may be adding to a persistence of chlorpromazine action to produce the elevation noted at 4 hr in subjects receiving both drugs. These results are consistent with the concept of antagonism between the two drugs at the level of the hypothalamus.

TRH

Thyrotropin-releasing hormone (TRH), the tripeptide pyroglutamyl-histidylprolinamide, has been found, unexpectedly, to release prolactin

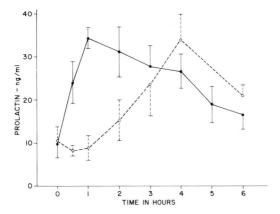

FIG. 3. Mean plasma prolactin in four normal subjects after receiving chlorpromazine, 25 mg intramuscularly, on two separate occasions. Solid line represents response to chlorpromazine alone; dashed line shows response to same dose after pretreatment with 500 mg of L-DOPA orally 30 min beforehand. Marked suppression of the chlorpromazine-induced rise is evident for the first 2 hr after L-DOPA.

as well as TSH. This effect was first observed in cloned pituitary cells in culture (33), and rapidly confirmed *in vivo* in humans (34, 35). Although studies in this laboratory as well as in others have shown that the threshold dose of TRH required to release prolactin is no greater than that required for TSH, there are many situations where the hormones vary quite independently, and it seems unlikely that TRH serves as a normal physiological releaser of prolactin in man. Evidence for another prolactin-releasing factor, different from TRH, has been obtained in animals (36, 37), although its physiological role and its presence or absence in the human have not as yet been determined. As shown by the solid lines in Fig. 4, the response to intravenous TRH in humans is rapid, reaching a peak at about 20 min, and is greater in women than in men. Pretreatment with L-DOPA, as shown by the dashed lines, markedly reduces the prolactin response in both sexes (38). These findings, although compatible with the concept that dopamine, acting on the hypothalamus, has stimulated sufficient PIF to antagonize TRH at a pituitary locus, have made us wonder about a possible direct antagonism between dopamine and TRH at the level of the pituitary. A third and less likely possibility is that TRH may act in part on the hypothalamus and be antagonized there by dopamine, since extrapituitary actions of TRH have recently been demonstrated (39, 40).

Ergot Alkaloids

Suppression of prolactin secretion by ergot derivatives has been shown in rats (41), and recently a new drug, 2-bromo-alpha-ergocryptine (CB-154),

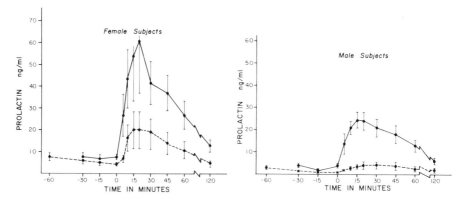

FIG. 4. Plasma prolactin after intravenous TRH in seven normal women (left) and seven normal men (right). Solid lines represent response to TRH alone; dashed lines show response to same dose of TRH in same subjects after pretreatment with L-DOPA. A suppressive effect of L-DOPA is clearly seen (38).

has been found to suppress prolactin and to stop both normal and abnormal lactation in humans (42). Its suppressive effect seems to be less marked but more prolonged than that of L-DOPA; its use as a physiologic and therapeutic tool will require further investigation.

Osmotic Changes

An osmoregulator role for prolactin in certain submammalian species has been known for a number of years. Recently evidence has been presented that prolactin secretion in man can be suppressed by the administration of water or hypotonic saline and increased by hypertonic saline (43). Further exploration of these observations will be necessary before their physiologic significance can be assessed.

CONCLUSIONS

Although it is still not possible to fit all of the diverse factors that have been found to affect prolactin secretion into a common unifying framework, human studies have reinforced the concept derived from animal experiments of a hormone whose dominant mode of control is that of tonic inhibition from the hypothalamus, mediated via prolactin-inhibiting factor. The hypothalamus in turn appears to be acted on primarily by dopaminergic impulses. The possible role of serotoninergic, as well as of cholinergic, pathways in the human is still a matter of speculation. The fact that prolactin is a relatively labile hormone, rapidly responsive to pharmacological and other stimuli, and readily measurable in humans as well as in animals, makes it a potentially useful indicator of the effects of L-DOPA and other drugs that may be important in the study or treatment of Parkinson's disease.

ACKNOWLEDGMENTS

This work was supported by U.S. Public Health Service grants AM-11294, TIAM-5397, CA-11704, and CA-13696, and American Heart Association grant 68–111. Mr. Robert Sundeen and Mrs. Irene Conwell provided expert technical assistance. We are grateful to Dr. Marvin E. Jaffe and the Merck Sharp and Dohme Research Laboratories for providing MK-486 and for assistance with the studies in which this drug was used.

REFERENCES

1. Frantz, A. G., and Kleinberg, D. L., *Science,* 170, 745 (1970).
2. Kleinberg, D. L., and Frantz, A. G., *J. Clin. Invest.,* 50, 1557 (1971).
3. Loewenstein, J. E., Mariz, I. K., Peake, G. I., and Daughaday, W. H., *J. Clin. Endocrinol. Metab.,* 33, 217 (1971).
4. Forsyth, I. A., and Myres, R. P., *J. Endocrinol.,* 51, 157 (1971).
5. Lewis, U. J., Singh, R. N. P., and Seavey, B. K., *Biochem. Biophys. Res. Commun.,* 44, 1169 (1971).
6. Hwang, P., Guyda, H., and Friesen, H., *J. Biol. Chem.,* 247, 1955 (1972).
7. Hwang, P., Guyda, H., and Friesen, H., *Proc. Nat. Acad. Sci.,* 68, 1902 (1971).
8. Sinha, Y. N., Selby, F. W., Lewis, U. J., and VanderLaan, W. P., *J. Clin. Endocrinol. Metab.,* 36, 509 (1973).
9. Jacobs, L. S., Mariz, I. K., and Daughaday, W. H., *J. Clin. Endocrinol. Metab.,* 34, 484 (1972).
10. Frantz, A. G., in: *Frontiers in Neuroendocrinology,* p. 337, Oxford University Press, New York (1973).
11. Frantz, A. G., Kleinberg, D. L., and Noel, G. L., *Recent Progr. Horm. Res.,* 28, 527 (1972).
12. Niall, H. D., Hogan, M. I.., Tregear, G. W., Segre, G. V., Hwang, P., and Friesen, H., *Recent Progr. Horm. Res.,* 29, 387 (1973).
13. Tyson, J. E., Friesen, H. G., and Anderson, M. S., *Science,* 177, 897 (1972).
14. Noel, G. L., Suh, H. K., and Frantz, A. G., *Program of Fourth International Congress of Endocrinology, Washington, D.C., Abstract No. 256, International Congress Series No. 256,* Excerpta Medica, Amsterdam (1972).
15. Sassin, J. F., Frantz, A. G., Weitzman, E. D., and Kapen, S., *Science,* 177, 1205 (1972).
16. Sassin, J. F., Frantz, A. G., Kapen, S., and Weitzman, E. D., *J. Clin. Endocrinol. Metab.* 37:436 (1973).
17. Noel, G. L., Suh, H. K., Stone, G., and Frantz, A. G., *J. Clin. Endocrinol. Metab.,* 35, 840 (1972).
18. Frantz, A. G., and Rabkin, M. T., *J. Clin. Endocrinol. Metab.,* 25, 1470 (1965).
19. Turkington, R. W., Underwood, L. E., and Van Wyk, J. J., *New Eng. J. Med.,* 285, 707 (1971).
20. Tolis, G., Goldstein, M., and Friesen, H. G., *J. Clin. Invest.,* 52, 783 (1973).
21. Zimmerman, E. A., Defendini, R., and Frantz, A. G., *Program of 55th Annual Meeting of Endocrine Society,* Abstract No. 474 (1973).
22. Birge, C. A., Jacobs, L. S., Hammer, C. T., and Daughaday, W. H., *Endocrinology,* 86, 120 (1970).
23. MacLeod, R. M., Fontham, E. H., and Lehmeyer, J. E., *Neuroendocrinology,* 6, 283 (1970).
24. Koch, Y., Lu, K. H., and Meites, J., *Endocrinology,* 87, 673 (1970).
25. Kamberi, I. A., Mical, R. S., and Porter, J. C., *Experientia,* 26, 1150 (1970).

26. Kamberi, I. A., Mical, R. S., and Porter, J. C., *Endocrinology,* 88, 1012 (1971).
27. Kleinberg, D. L., Noel, G. L., and Frantz, A. G., *J. Clin. Endocrinol. Metab.,* 33, 873 (1971).
28. Malarkey, W. B., Jacobs, L. S., and Daughaday, W. H., *New Eng. J. Med.,* 285, 1160 (1971).
29. Friesen, H., Guyda, H., Hwang, P., Tyson, J. E., and Barbeau, A., *J. Clin. Invest.,* 51, 706 (1972).
30. Frantz, A. G., Habif, D. V., Hyman, G. A., and Suh, H. K., *Clin. Res.,* 20, 864 (1972).
31. Frantz, A. G., Habif, D. V., Hyman, G. A., Suh, H. K., Sassin, J. F., Zimmerman, E. A., Noel, G. L., and Kleinberg, D. L., in: *International Symposium on Human Prolactin,* Excerpta Medica, Netherlands *(in press).*
32. Sulman, F. G., in: *Hypothalamic Control of Lactation,* Springer-Verlag, New York (1970).
33. Tashjian, A. H., Jr., Barowsky, N. J., and Jensen, D. K., *Biochem. Biophys. Res. Commun.,* 43, 516 (1971).
34. Bowers, C. Y., Friesen, H. G., Hwang, P., Guyda, H. J., and Folkers, K., *Biochem. Biophys. Res. Commun.,* 45, 1033 (1971).
35. Jacobs, L. S., Snyder, P. J., Wilber, J. F., Utiger, R. D., and Daughaday, W. H., *J. Clin. Endocrinol. Metab.,* 33, 996 (1971).
36. Nicoll, C. S., Fiorindo, R. P., McKenee, C. T., and Parsons, J. A., in: *Hypophysiotropic Hormones of the Hypothalamus: Assay and Chemistry,* p. 115, Williams & Wilkins Co., Baltimore (1970).
37. Krulich, L., Quijada, M., and Illner, P., *Program of the 53rd Meeting of the Endocrine Society,* Abstract No. 82 (1971).
38. Noel, G. L., Suh, H. K., and Frantz, A. G., *J. Clin. Endocrinol. Metab.,* 36, 1255 (1973).
39. Plotnikoff, N. P., Prange, A. J., Jr., Breese, G. R., Anderson, M. S., and Wilson, I. C., *Science,* 178, 417 (1972).
40. Kastin, A. B., Ehrensing, R. H., Schalch, D. S., and Anderson, M. S., *Lancet,* 2, 740 (1972).
41. Meites, J., Lu, K. H., Wuttke, W., Welsch, C. W., Nagasawa, H., and Quadri, S. K., *Recent Progr. Horm. Res.,* 28, 471 (1972).
42. del Pozo, E., del Re, R. B., Varga, L., and Friesen, H., *J. Clin. Endocrinol. Metab.,* 35, 768 (1972).
43. Buckman, M. T., and Peake, G. T., *Program of 55th Annual Meeting of the Endocrine Society,* Abstract No. 2 (1973).

DISCUSSION

Dr. Smith: Dr. McCann, don't you have evidence *in vitro* to demonstrate that releasing and inhibiting factors could, in fact, interact at the pituitary level?

Dr. McCann: I think it is quite reasonable to assume that in Dr. Franz's experiment where he gave TRH and then L-DOPA he released PIF and that counteracts the action of the TRH. That is consistent with an effect of L-DOPA through dopamine-releasing PIF at the hypothalamic level. There is the possibility that dopamine or L-DOPA may act also at the pituitary level. Actually it has been shown by other groups that if you give L-DOPA, it is actually converted into dopamine which then shows its effect in the glycoprotein hormone cell. Dopamine released there can act directly as well. In favor of that hypothesis is the ability of dopamine to inhibit prolactin at the pituitary level *in vitro*, and the ability of L-DOPA to lower prolactin in animals with hypothalamic lesions which presumably knock out PIF. Opposed to the hypothesis is the fact that Canberry and Porter when they used dopamine in the portal vessels were unable to show any effect on prolactin. My current position would be that there is an effect at the hypothalamic level with PIF being released, but I wouldn't want to rule out an effect at the pituitary level as well. What is needed now is to find out whether there is really any dopamine in the portal blood. Ruff and Harris have looked for this, and also Kraut and Porter, and they have not found it. But that does not mean it is not there; it might just have been degraded before they measured.

Dr. Fuxe: Dr. McCann's group and our group in Stockholm have had some agreement and disagreement as the years have passed. We certainly have agreed that the dopamine system in the median eminence is involved in gonadotropin secretion. We have agreed that dopamine could inhibit the secretion of prolactin. I would like to point out that there is a very impressive increase of dopamine turnover after the injection of prolactin, directly suggesting that there is an action at the hypothalamic level. The disagreement had been that we have interpreted our data to indicate that dopamine inhibits LRF secretion, whereas the others have given data that dopamine should stimulate LRF secretion. I have wondered, in view of our recent findings with DPH, dopamine beta hydroxylase immunofluorescence, demonstrating in a particular part of the median eminence a zone of noradrenaline buttons lying in a crucial position close to the capillary plexus, if it is possible to conceive or interpret the data that you have obtained, as being due to a stimulation involving noradrenaline instead of dopamine.

Dr. McCann: I appreciate Dr. Fuxe's comments: he is very kind; we came up with diametrically opposite views at one point. Actually the views have changed over the years, and they are closer now than they have been at any time since we started working. But most of his work has been based on attempts to measure the turnover of dopamine by histochemical fluorescence techniques, and we have done a different type of experiment. Namely, either injecting catecholamine or using drugs to try to block either catecholamine synthesis or action. Using blocking drugs, we have not got too much evidence for a role of dopamine in control of gonadotropins. Dopamine seems to be more potent than norepinephrine. It is always possible when you do the injection experiment that the dopamine could be taken up, converted into norepinephrine, which could then be re-released and exert the action. I think it is not settled yet. We need more information. The turnover studies have criticisms leveled at them, too. The main problem with them, I think, is that you are looking at the whole dopaminergic system, and that you are perhaps influencing the release of 10 different hypothalamic hormones controlling the pituitary. If you look at the total activity in that system, you could get misleading results. It is quite clear, I think, from all the work that there is a catecholaminergic role. The only question is how much of it is due to norepinephrine and how much due to dopamine.

Dr. Fuxe: I certainly agree with you, of course, but I would like to mention that we have developed new types of dopamine receptor stimulating agents, for instance, ET-495, which have the interesting property of blocking ovulation.

Dr. Vogt: Could either of you give us any indication as to what the physiological role of prolactin is, for instance, in sleep?

Dr. Frantz: I think that is really impossible to say at the present time. The only major physiological action of prolactin that has been demonstrated so far that seems applicable in the human is its role in promoting lactogenesis. It also probably is important in breast development. It has a mammotropic action, in other words. But the various other actions that have been described in lower animals which include growth hormone-like actions, behavior-regulating actions, particularly parental behavior, and so forth, have not as yet really been demonstrated in mammals.

In man we do not know because there is not enough human prolactin as yet to test. I think the various animal prolactins may have somewhat different actions because they are significantly different chemically.

Dr. Carlsson: Have you tried a peripheral decarboxylase inhibitor and DOPA, and studied these things?

Dr. Frantz: Yes. We have tried that and it markedly potentiates the effect of L-DOPA in prolactin suppression.

Dr. Carlsson: Then it cannot be the pituitary in that case.

Dr. Mars: We studied a group of normal patients for plasma DOPA levels, prolactin levels, and growth hormone levels, with concurrent determinations of each. We found that it required at least 400 nanograms of DOPA per milliliter plasma to evoke an unequivocal growth hormone response, which means a level at least twice that obtained at base line. The second thing we found was that there was a delay in the growth hormone peak of about 30 to 45 minutes following the plasma DOPA peak. We also found that following a decarboxylase inhibitor, there was a potentiation of growth hormone release over what was obtained with DOPA alone. What is the current status regarding prolactin and breast cancer and modification by DOPA?

Dr. Frantz: Very briefly, we reported it at the Eastern Federation Section meetings last January that at that time, I think, some 21 patients with metastatic breast cancer had been treated with chronic L-DOPA therapy for periods of 1 to 7 months. Objective remissions of generally short duration had been observed in four of these. In one it lasted 7 months with disappearance of skin metastases. I think the agent does have promise in the treatment of breast cancer.

Advances in Neurology, Vol. 5
Raven Press, New York © 1974

L-DOPA and Growth Hormone Secretion in Man

Harold E. Lebovitz, Jay S. Skyler, and A. E. Boyd, III*

Division of Endocrinology, Departments of Medicine and Physiology, Duke University Medical Center, Durham, North Carolina 27710

The mechanisms involved in the control of growth hormone secretion are extremely complex. Animal studies have shown that growth hormone secretion is regulated by both peptidergic and monoaminergic systems. How these systems interact is unknown.

The peptidergic system consists of both a hypothalamic releasing factor (1) and an inhibitory factor. The exact nature of the releasing factor is still questionable, but the structure of a hypothalamic peptide that inhibits growth hormone secretion in the rat has been elucidated recently and its synthesis achieved (2).

Much experimental evidence indicates that hypothalamic monoamines also play a role in the regulation of growth hormone secretion. Data in rats and baboons have been presented to suggest that hypothalamic norepinephrine and serotonin stimulate and dopamine inhibits growth hormone secretion (3, 4). Several years ago, we became interested in the possibility that dopamine might be involved in the control of anterior pituitary hormone secretion in man. Our interest was kindled by the histochemical demonstrations of very high concentrations of dopamine in the median eminence, and the many animal studies implicating hypothalamic monoamines in the control of gonadotropin secretion (5). The administration of L-DOPA to patients with Parkinson's disease presented a unique opportunity to study the effect of alterations in hypothalamic monoamines on endocrine function and glucose metabolism in man. Our initial studies demonstrated that L-DOPA administration stimulates growth hormone secretion (6).

This paper reviews the current status of our knowledge about the effects of L-DOPA on growth hormone secretion in man.

EFFECT OF L-DOPA ON PLASMA GROWTH HORMONE LEVELS IN PATIENTS WITH PARKINSON'S DISEASE

In our original observations on the effects of L-DOPA administration to patients with Parkinson's disease, we found that doses as small as 0.5 g

---

*Present address: U.S. Army Research Institute of Environmental Medicine, Natick, Massachusetts 01760.

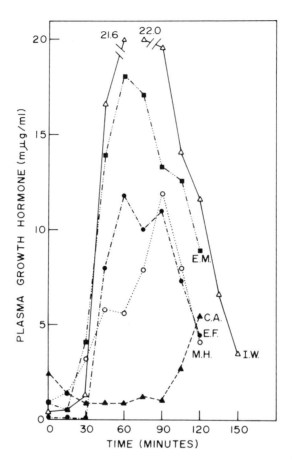

FIG. 1. Effect of L-DOPA (0.5 g) on plasma growth hormone in five patients with Parkinson's disease during the initial therapy with the drug (i.e., acute therapy). For details see text. [From *New Engl. J. Med.* 283, 1425 (1970).]

orally caused a dramatic and rapid rise in plasma growth hormone levels (6). Figure 1 illustrates this rise in plasma growth hormone in five patients. Each patient received 0.5 g of L-DOPA at time 0. They had been fasting overnight, were kept at bedrest, and had an indwelling scalp vein needle inserted in the antecubital vein 30 min prior to the L-DOPA administration. Each of the patients had received L-DOPA, 0.25 g, three times a day with meals for 2 days prior to the study. Four of the five patients had a striking rise in plasma growth hormone beginning at 45 min and peaking between 60 and 90 min. The fifth patient had a rise beginning at 105 min, and her highest level was reached at 120 min, the time the last sample was taken.

The most striking characteristic of L-DOPA-stimulated growth hormone secretion in the patients with Parkinson's disease is the failure of oral or

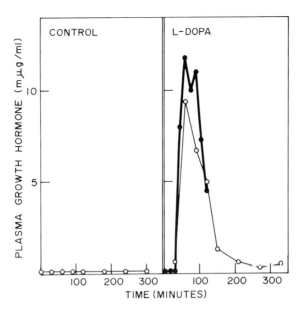

FIG. 2. Failure of oral glucose to suppress L-DOPA-stimulated growth hormone release in a patient with Parkinson's disease. For details see text.

intravenous glucose to suppress it (6). This is illustrated in Fig. 2. The panel marked "control" shows the plasma growth hormone levels in a patient following 100 g of oral glucose. The heavy black line in the panel marked "L-DOPA" is the plasma growth hormone following 1 g of oral L-DOPA in this patient. The thin black line in the L-DOPA panel depicts the plasma growth hormone in the same patient following 1 g L-DOPA and 100 g oral glucose 30 min later. The glucose had no effect on the growth hormone secretion stimulated by L-DOPA. Figure 3 shows the mean results of oral glucose and L-DOPA administration, compared to oral glucose alone, in seven patients with Parkinson's disease. These data show that the failure of oral glucose to suppress L-DOPA-stimulated growth hormone secretion occurred uniformly in all the patients (7).

Another important characteristic of L-DOPA-stimulated growth hormone secretion in patients with Parkinson's disease is that the effect occurs in patients who have been on chronic L-DOPA therapy (6). Figure 4 shows the effect of 0.5 g of L-DOPA given in the morning to patients who had been taking L-DOPA in doses of 3.5 to 6.0 g daily for from 6 to 11 months. Each of the four patients showed a significant rise in plasma growth hormone. The magnitude of the growth hormone rise was comparable to that seen in patients who had never before received the drug. These observations indicated that L-DOPA probably stimulates growth hormone secretion each time a dose is given.

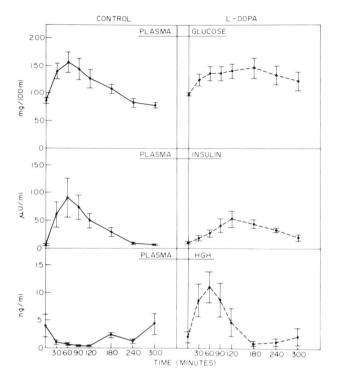

FIG. 3. Plasma glucose, insulin, and growth hormone response to 100 g oral glucose in seven patients with Parkinson's disease. The control studies were done prior to, and the L-DOPA studies during, the third week of L-DOPA therapy (6.0 g/day). For the L-DOPA studies, 1.0 g L-DOPA was given 30 min prior to the oral glucose. The data are given as the mean ± SE for each time. Oral glucose failed to suppress the L-DOPA-stimulated increase in plasma growth hormone.

These two observations, that is, the lack of glucose suppressibility and the repetitive stimulation of secretion on chronic therapy, suggested that patients on chronic L-DOPA therapy might develop some of the signs and symptoms of a growth hormone hypersecretory state, such as acromegaly.

EFFECT OF L-DOPA ON PLASMA GROWTH HORMONE SECRETION IN NORMAL INDIVIDUALS

Many subsequent studies have shown that L-DOPA stimulates the secretion of growth hormone in normal individuals (8, 9). The dose of L-DOPA required to stimulate growth hormone secretion and the magnitude of this response appears to be the same in normal subjects as in patients with Parkinson's disease. The stimulatory effect of L-DOPA on growth hormone secretion is diminished by treatment with phentolamine, suggesting that the action of L-DOPA may be mediated through an alpha adrenergic receptor mechanism (9). One recent study has suggested that the growth hormone

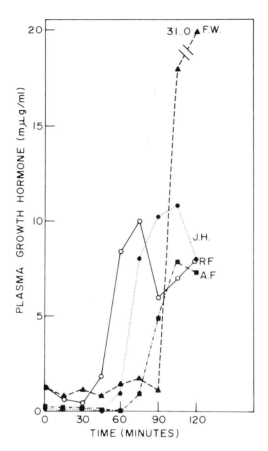

FIG. 4. Effect of L-DOPA on plasma growth hormone in four patients with Parkinson's disease who had been taking the drug for 6 to 11 months (i.e., chronic therapy). For details see text. [From *New Engl. J. Med.* 283, 1425 (1970).]

response to L-DOPA is decreased in older individuals (ages 48 to 68) as compared to younger individuals (ages 20 to 32) (10). The oral administration of L-DOPA stimulates growth hormone secretion in children with normal pituitary function, as well as insulin-induced hypoglycemia or intravenous arginine (11, 12). Several studies have indicated that L-DOPA can be used to diagnose growth hormone deficiency states (11, 12).

ARE SOME DISEASE STATES WITH ABNORMAL GROWTH HORMONE SECRETION RELATED TO ABNORMALITIES OF HYPOTHALAMIC MONOAMINES?

Since L-DOPA is such a potent stimulator of growth hormone secretion in man, it seems reasonable to hypothesize that it is exerting its action through a dopaminergic or noradrenergic mechanism in the hypothalamus.

One might then raise the question as to whether abnormalities in endogenous norepinephrine or dopamine in the hypothalamus could lead to alterations of growth hormone secretion. If diminished growth hormone secretion were due to such a mechanism, one might expect the administration of L-DOPA to correct the abnormality.

One disease state in which hypothalamic dopamine might be deficient is Parkinson's disease itself. We studied the growth hormone response to insulin-induced hypoglycemia in nine patients with Parkinson's disease (7). Two had markedly deficient, and one borderline, growth hormone secretory response to the stimulus. The study was repeated in one of the two deficient patients after administration of 1 g of L-DOPA, and the growth hormone secretion corrected to normal. These data suggest the possibility that some patients with Parkinson's disease may have impaired growth hormone secretion due to deficient hypothalamic monoamines. Clearly, this problem needs to be studied systematically in a large group of patients with Parkinson's disease.

A second group of patients with decreased growth hormone secretion that we studied were patients with marked obesity. It is well known that obesity is associated with decreased growth hormone secretion. Table 1 gives the results of our studies in seven obese patients. Two of the seven patients exhibited a normal growth hormone secretory response to a 30 to 40 min intravenous infusion of 30 g of arginine. The other five had a markedly deficient

TABLE 1. *Failure of L-DOPA to correct abnormal growth hormone secretion in patients with obesity or isolated growth hormone deficiency*

No.	Sex	Age (years)	Weight (lb)	L-DOPA 0.5 g orally	Arginine 30 g i.v.	L-DOPA 0.5 g orally followed by arginine 30 g i.v.
A. Obese patients						
1	F	25	236	712	1734	1617
2	M	36	462	368	384	253
3	F	33	264	555	222	400
4	F	38	192	401	783	852
5	F	24	218	237	555	318
6	M	41	417	206	216	156
7	F	54	220	100	375	241
B. Isolated growth hormone-deficient patients						
1	F	13	106	0*	0	
2	F	28	96	0	0	
3	M	14	107	0	0	

Growth hormone secretion is calculated by the area under the plasma growth hormone curve (L-DOPA, 0 to 180 min, and arginine, 0 to 120 min) and is expressed as ng-min/ml.
*All plasma values < 0.50 ng/ml.

response. The administration of L-DOPA alone failed to stimulate growth hormone secretion in four of the five patients with the deficient response to arginine. Pretreatment of the patients with 1.0 g of L-DOPA 30 min prior to arginine infusion had no effect on the growth hormone secretory response in any of the seven obese patients. Thus, it appears that the defect in growth hormone secretion in obesity is not correctable by L-DOPA administration.

A third group of patients that we studied were children with isolated growth hormone deficiency. These children had statural growth retardation due to lack of growth hormone secretion. As seen in Table 1, L-DOPA had no effect on growth hormone secretion in these children. Thus, the possibility that isolated growth hormone deficiency is related to disturbances of hypothalamic monoamines seems unlikely.

An intriguing observation that L-DOPA administered to patients with acromegaly causes a striking decrease in plasma growth hormone levels has recently been reported (13). The significance of this finding is not clear, but it raises many perplexing and interesting questions.

WILL CHRONIC L-DOPA THERAPY LEAD TO ACROMEGALY?

Since the acute administration of L-DOPA to chronically treated parkinsonian patients still causes growth hormone secretion, it is evident that patients treated four times a day will have elevated plasma growth hormone levels for at least 8 hr each day. Additionally, since the L-DOPA-stimulated growth hormone secretion is not suppressed by glucose, one would expect patients treated with this drug to have elevated growth hormone levels during meals. Acromegaly is characterized by excessive growth hormone secretion that is not suppressed by glucose. One might then expect that chronic L-DOPA therapy in patients would lead to the development of an acromegalic syndrome. Such findings have not been reported, but conceivably they could take many years to develop.

Growth hormone itself has no effect on skeletal growth. Many studies indicate that skeletal growth is controlled by a growth hormone-dependent serum factor called sulfation factor or, more recently, somatomedin (14). Serum from normal individuals contains somatomedin, but it is diminished, or absent, from the serum of hypophysectomized individuals. Treatment of hypophysectomized individuals with growth hormone restores serum somatomedin activity to normal. The origin of somatomedin is not known, but some have suggested that it is made in the liver or kidney. Somatomedin stimulates cartilage growth and therefore leads to enlargement of the skeletal system. In patients with acromegaly, serum somatomedin levels are elevated (15).

One might suspect that chronic L-DOPA therapy, with its increased growth hormone secretion, would lead to elevated plasma levels of somatomedin. Utilizing an assay system which employs pelvic rudiments from 10-

to 11-day-old chick embryos (16), we assayed the serum somatomedin levels in three of the four patients studied who had been on 3.5 to 6.0 g of L-DOPA daily for between 6 and 11 months (Fig. 4). Table 2 shows the results of these studies. The plasma assayed for each patient was an aliquot of a pool of all samples collected during the first 120 min after a morning dose of 1.0 g of L-DOPA. In all three patients, the somatomedin level was within the range of our normal pool. Thus, in spite of the continuous elevation of plasma growth hormone, there was no rise in serum somatomedin levels. From our data we are unable to determine whether the growth hormone secretion stimulated by L-DOPA is insufficient to increase somatomedin production or whether L-DOPA itself, or some metabolic consequence of its administration, interferes with somatomedin generation. In any event, the normal serum somatomedin levels in patients on chronic L-DOPA therapy suggest that the patients will not develop the skeletal abnormalities of acromegaly. However, the possibility that chronically elevated growth hormone levels may affect carbohydrate and lipid metabolism is not precluded.

TABLE 2. *Serum sulfation factor activity in the plasma of patients with Parkinson's disease who had been chronically treated with L-DOPA for 6 to 11 months*

Patient	Age (years)	Peak plasma HGH following L-DOPA 1 g orally (ng/ml)	HGH secretion for the 120 min following L-DOPA 1 g orally (ng-min/ml)	Plasma Sulfation factor			
				Mean potency (%)	95% fiducial limits	λ	g*
J. H.	58	13.9	769	59.9	35.0 to 102.7	0.32	0.044
A. F.	52	8.6	439	88.6	52.5 to 149.3	0.34	0.050
F. W.	58	23.5	1480	103.1	56.1 to 187.2	0.40	0.067

Data are expressed as a mean potency and 95% confidence limits compared to a serum pool from 10 normal adults.
*Finney g.

SUMMARY

The administration of 0.5 g of L-DOPA stimulates growth hormone secretion in patients with Parkinson's syndrome, as well as normal volunteers. The mechanism by which L-DOPA stimulates growth hormone secretion is unknown, but may be through noradrenergic or dopaminergic mechanisms in the hypothalamus. Growth hormone secretion stimulated by L-DOPA administration is not suppressed by glucose administration and occurs in patients on chronic therapy. Patients with Parkinson's disease may have decreased growth hormone secretion due to diminished hypothalamic monoamines. Further studies are necessary to clarify this possibility. The impaired growth hormone secretion in obesity and solitary growth hormone deficiency are not corrected by L-DOPA. Chronic L-DOPA therapy in patients with Parkinson's syndrome does not lead to elevated serum somatomedin levels in spite of the elevated plasma growth hormone levels. The mechanism for this is not known. The normal somatomedin levels in patients on chronic L-DOPA therapy suggest that they will not develop the abnormalities of acromegaly.

ACKNOWLEDGMENTS

These studies were supported by grants from the National Institutes of Arthritis, Metabolic and Digestive Diseases (AM 01324, 5T1 AM 5074, and K3 AM 17954), grant MO 1 RR-30 from the Clinical Research Center Branch Division of Research Facilities and Resources, U.S. Public Health Service, and by Hoffmann-LaRoche Company.

The authors would like to express their appreciation to Dr. Walter Kempner and his staff for their assistance and encouragement in the studies of the obese patients. Miss Sylvia White and Mrs. Stella Cook provided excellent technical assistance.

REFERENCES

1. Daughaday, W. H., Peake, G. T., and Machlin, L. J., in: *Hypophysiotropic Hormones of the Hypothalamus: Assay and Chemistry*, Williams & Wilkins, Baltimore, 1970, p. 208.
2. Brazeau, P., Valle, W., Burgu, R., Ling, N., Butcher, M., Rivier, J., and Guillemin, R., *Science* 179, 77 (1973).
3. Collu, R., Fraschini, F., Visconti, P., and Martini, I.., *Endocrinology* 90, 1231 (1972).
4. Toivola, P., and Gale, C. C., *Neuroendocrinology* 6, 210 (1970).
5. Lebovitz, H. E., Boyd, A. E., III, and Feldman, J. M., *Proc. IV Intern. Cong. of Endocrinology*, Excerpta Medica *(in press)*.
6. Boyd, A. E., III, Lebovitz, H. E., and Pfeiffer, J. B., *New Engl. J. Med.* 283, 1429 (1970).
7. Boyd, A. F., III, Lebovitz, II. E., and Feldman, J. M., *J. Clin. Endocrinol. Metab.* 33, 829 (1971).
8. Eddy, R. L., Jones, A. L., Chakmakjian, Z. H., and Silverthorne, M. C., *J. Clin. Endocrinol. Metab.* 33, 709 (1971).
9. Kansal, P. C., Buse, J., Talbert, O. R., and Buse, M. G., *J. Clin. Endocrinol. Metab.* 34, 99 (1972).
10. Sachar, E. J., Mushrush, G., Perlow, M., Weitzman, E. D., and Sassin, J., *Science* 178, 1304 (1972).
11. Root, A. W., and Russ, R. D., *Pediatrics* 81, 808 (1972).
12. Weldon, V. V., Gupta, S. K., Haymond, M. W., Pagliara, A. S., Jacobs, L. S., and Daughaday, W. H., *J. Clin. Endocrinol. Metab.* 36, 42 (1973).
13. Liuzzi, A., Chiodini, P. G., Botalla, L., Cremascoli, G., and Silvestrini, F., *J. Clin. Endocrinol. Metab.* 35, 941 (1972).
14. Daughaday, W. H., *Am. J. Med.* 50, 277 (1971).
15. Hall, K., *Acta Endocrinol.* Supp. 163, 1 (1972).
16. Hall, K., *Acta Endocrinol.* 63, 338 (1970).

Advances in Neurology, Vol. 5
Raven Press, New York © 1974

Chronic Treatment with L-DOPA and Growth Hormone Release

Ismael Mena, George C. Cotzias, Paul S. Papavasiliou,
Jorge Mendez, and Frances C. Brown

Medical Research Center, Brookhaven National Laboratory, Upton, New York 11973

INTRODUCTION

We are pleased to follow Dr. Lebovitz, since Boyd, Lebovitz, and their colleagues (1, 2) discovered the release of growth hormone by L-DOPA after administering a single dose of 0.5 to 1.0 g to normal subjects and to patients with parkinsonism. On the basis of similar experiments, others have warned that chronic treatment with L-DOPA might induce both acromegaly and diabetes mellitus (3). From our observations on the multiple daily doses of L-DOPA necessary for therapy, we found evidence that led us to dispute the morbid potential of the hormone's release by this drug (4, 5).

We wish to report that the increases in circulating growth hormone brought about by single fixed doses of L-DOPA in fasting subjects do not necessarily reflect the behavior of the hormone in nonfasting patients with parkinsonism under actual treatment with L-DOPA. Sufficient assessments of the total serum levels of growth hormone and of the patterns which these levels assume could be obtained only by frequent sampling over 24 hr, since only then were we able to compare the serum hormone levels of untreated versus L-DOPA-treated patients with parkinsonism.

PROTOCOLS

Twenty patients with parkinsonism under optimal treatment with L-DOPA either given alone or in combination with MK-486 were studied on a metabolic ward for periods ranging from 3 to 12 months. Serum growth hormone levels were assessed with a radioimmunoassay (Abbott Laboratories) at intervals of 30 min. Blood was obtained via an inlying catheter and a three-way stopcock so as not to awaken the patients at night. The blood samples were immediately refrigerated and the serum was separated, frozen in liquid nitrogen, and kept at −20°C until analysis could be performed at the completion of each run. In 14 patients runs lasting 8 hr were secured, and in another 14 the runs were continued for 24 hr. Both types of runs included untreated patients as well as those under therapy. During these runs, all patients remained in their rooms. During the night, sleep was graded by observing snoring, turning, and respiratory rate. Two of these patients displayed involuntary adventitious movements while asleep, but none displayed tremor. During the day, the patient's symptoms were scored with a system discussed elsewhere (6).

The growth hormone measurements, obtained as nanograms per milliliter, were expressed thereafter as follows: (a) the sum of all measurements conducted each 30 min for 8 or 24 hr; (b) the sum of all values remaining after subtracting the basal levels [to reflect only the rises (peaks) of the hormone]; and (c) the basal levels themselves, obtained by calculating the means of the lowest five values in the 8-hr runs and of the lowest 10 values in the 24-hr runs. All these calculated values were intercompared from one group to the next, and correlations were sought with the neurological scores.

OBSERVATIONS

In eight untreated parkinsonian patients, the basal levels were not statistically different from those of the treated patients, although the mean concentration was higher in the untreated group (mean $\pm$ SE, 2.84 $\pm$ 0.43 ng/ml versus 1.78 $\pm$ 0.34; $p < 0.09$). However, the 24-hr records from all eight untreated patients were flat, except for a few short-lived rises above the basal level occurring mostly at night (Fig. 1). These contrasted with the

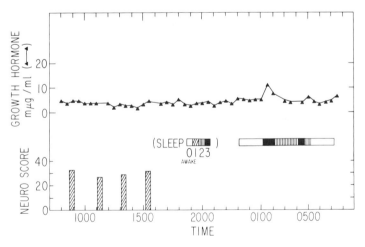

FIG. 1. Serum growth hormone concentrations (ng/ml) during 24 hr in untreated parkinsonian patient. Note steady low concentrations during most of the 24-hr period.

periodic releases of growth hormone reported for normal individuals, in whom several pulses of growth hormone, lasting from 1 to 2 hr, have elevated the concentration of the hormone beyond 20 ng/ml (7). The rises found in nine parkinsonian patients (six studied for 8 hr and three for 24 hr) treated with optimal doses of L-DOPA (400 to 700 mg, six times a day) were roughly similar to those reported for normals. Similar 24-hr records were obtained from three patients receiving L-DOPA in combination with MK-486 (Fig. 2).

In the nonfasting patients, the morning dose of L-DOPA often increased the levels of growth hormone by 10 to 50 ng/ml above the basal ones. Several subsequent doses also evoked intermittent rises, but these were usually smaller than the first. Although all these rises were drug dependent, their duration and numbers were often similar to those reported for normal subjects (Fig. 2).

The differences between untreated and L-DOPA-treated patients with parkinsonism were reflected in the calculations shown in Tables 1 and 2. While the sum of the 8-hr measurements remaining after subtracting basal levels was significantly different between these two groups (Table 1), it was not significantly different when 24-hr measurements were performed (Table 2). The rises (net concentration), however, showed highly significant differ-

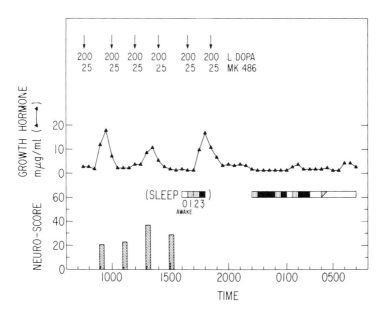

FIG. 2. Serum growth hormone concentrations (ng/ml) during 24 hr in a parkinsonian patient treated with L-DOPA and MK-486. After 30 to 60 min of L-DOPA, there are rises after three of six doses. Basal level is lower than that of Fig. 1. No correlation between rises and neuro scores is evident.

ences both in the 8-hr and the 24-hr runs ($p < 0.001$ and < 0.01, respectively). This indicated that the 24-hr output was not affected by L-DOPA in these parkinsonian patients, suggesting that L-DOPA does not affect the hormone's rate of synthesis. The drug, however, modified profoundly the patterns of release of the somatotropic hormone: from a continuous, slow release in the untreated patient, L-DOPA produced a pattern of pulses with rises above the basal level of at least one order of magnitude. These resembled those seen after exercise, during some phases of sleep, or during hypoglycemia in normal subjects. This is in sharp contrast to acromegaly, in which increased synthesis and increased release of this hormone are essential features.

TABLE 1. Eight-hour growth hormone release. Parkinsonism-integrated concentrations (ng/ml per 8 hr)

	Total	p <	Net rises	p <
Untreated (8)	67 ± 8		13 ± 4	
L-DOPA (6)	102 ± 16	0.05	70 ± 15	0.001

Sum of all measurements conducted each 30 min for 8 hr, and sum of all values remaining after subtracting the basal levels (net rises).

TABLE 2. Twenty-four-hour growth hormone release. Parkinsonism-integrated concentrations (ng/ml per 24 hr)

	Total	p	Net rises	p <
Untreated (8)	201 ± 26		67 ± 7	
L-DOPA (6)	223 ± 25	0.5	138 ± 23	0.01

Sum of all measurements conducted each 30 min for 24 hr, and sum of all values remaining after subtracting the basal levels (net rises).

That L-DOPA affects the pattern of release and not the total output of growth hormone was evident from a comparison between the 8-hr sampling (8 A.M. to 4 P.M., Table 1) and the 24-hr sampling (Table 2). With 8 hr of sampling, the sum of all measurements was slightly different between the treated and untreated patients, but it was not significant with 24 hr of sampling because the untreated patients had higher basal levels and small rises at night. Conversely, the treated patients had lower basal levels and released their hormone in pulses during the day, with minimal releases during the night. The responses to isolated fixed doses of L-DOPA appeared to be misleading and depended, among other factors, on the time elapsed between doses. This is evident in Fig. 2, where only three of six equal doses of L-DOPA were followed by increases of growth hormone levels.

This intermittent effect of L-DOPA was responsible for the great individuality among individual records of growth hormone release. This individual variance might be a consequence of variations in the doses of L-DOPA required for treatment of parkinsonism. Modification of the response to L-DOPA by manipulating the patient's protein intake (8–10) did affect the release of growth hormone determined over 8 hr. Six patients on high protein intake (2 g of protein/kg of body weight per day) had a significant diminution of the sum of all measurements when compared with the measurements performed while on 1 g of protein/kg of body weight per day (mean $\pm$ SE, 55 ± 12 ng/ml versus 102 ± 16 ng/ml; $p < 0.04$). Since L-DOPA was more effective for the symptomatic control on the lower protein intake, correlations were sought between neurological scores and (a) the sum of all measurements of growth hormone for 24 hr, and (b) the values corresponding to the hormonal rises. Thus far, statistically significant correlations were not found.

While the restoration in parkinsonian patients of seemingly normal patterns of growth hormone by L-DOPA might have some metabolic advantages, there remained a possibility that release of the hormone could change the response of the parkinsonian symptoms to the drug. This was suggested by experiments in mice which were pretreated with growth hormone intraperitoneally or intracerebrally prior to being treated with L-DOPA (11). The hormone itself failed to change the behavior of these mice, whereas L-DOPA administration caused the widely known behavioral effects. When the hormone and L-DOPA were given together, there was no effect of the former on the behavior induced by the latter. Two to 4 hr after intraperitoneal injection of bovine growth hormone (30 μg/g), there occurred more rapid onset, longer duration, and potentiation of the effects of L-DOPA, which was not the case with intracerebral injections of the hormone. The major differences observed with pretreatment via the intraperitoneal route were the following. First, the initial period of hypoactivity which generally followed the administration of L-DOPA was almost abolished by the pretreatment with growth hormone; instead, there emerged rapid onset of hyperactivity. Second, the period of hyperactivity was significantly extended, so that the hormone-treated animals remained hyperactive after those treated only with L-DOPA had resumed normal or subnormal motor activities. Third, the intensity of hyperactivity and of the other behavioral effects induced by L-DOPA was increased as measured by either a scoring system or by the Animex activity meter.

Measurements of brain dopamine levels after L-DOPA in growth hormone-pretreated mice showed a significant increase 30 min after L-DOPA or $2\frac{1}{2}$ hr after growth hormone (mean $\pm$ SE, 2.55 ± 0.08 μg/brain versus 2.06 ± 0.11 μg/brain; $p < 0.01$).

SUMMARY

The sum of this evidence suggests that L-DOPA tends to change the pattern by which growth hormone is released from the pituitary, without significantly affecting the total output of hormone per 24 hr. Since not all patients were compared in both the treated and the untreated states, this conclusion is subject to confirmation. Despite the fact that we found no evidence that the release of growth hormone changed the control of parkinsonism, this possibility must be reinvestigated with protocols differing from those used here, in view of our animal experiments.

ACKNOWLEDGMENTS

This work was supported by the U.S. Atomic Energy Commission; the National Institutes of Health (grant NS 09492–03 and grant OH 00313–08, coordinated by Pan American Health Organization, Project AMRO-4618); by the Charles E. Merrill Trust, and by Mrs. Katherine Rodgers Denckla.

REFERENCES

1. Boyd, A. E., Lebovitz, H. E., and Pfeiffer, J. B., *New Engl. J. Med.* 283, 1425 (1970).
2. Boyd, A. E., Lebovitz, H. E., and Feldman, J. M., *J. Clin. Endocrinol.* 33(5), 829 (1971).
3. Sirtori, C. R., Bolme, P., and Azarnoff, D. L., *New Engl. J. Med.* 287, 729 (1972).
4. Cotzias, G. C., *New Engl. J. Med.* 287, 1302 (1972).
5. Mena, I., Cotzias, G. C., Brown, F. C., Papavasiliou, P. S., Miller, S. T., *New Engl. J. Med.* 288, 320 (1973).
6. Cotzias, G. C., Papavasiliou, P. S., Fehling, C., Kaufman, B., and Mena, I., *New Engl. J. Med.* 282, 31 (1970).
7. Sassin, J. F., Frantz, A. G., Weitzman, E. D., and Kapen, S., *Science* 177, 1205 (1972).
8. Gillespie, N. G., Mena, I., Cotzias, G. C., and Bell, M. A., *J. Am. Dietetic Assoc. (in press).*
9. Mena, I., and Cotzias, G. C., Abstract FASEB (1973).
10. Cotzias, G. C., Mena, I., and Papavasiliou, P. S., in: *The Treatment of Parkinson's Disease — The Role of Dopa Decarboxylase Inhibitors,* p. 265, M. D. Yahr, Ed., Raven Press, New York (1973).
11. Cotzias, G. C., Tang, L. C., and Mena, I., in: *Neuroscience Research,* Vol. 6, I. J. Kopin and S. Ehrenpreis, Eds., Academic Press, New York *(in press).*

DISCUSSION

Dr. Lebovitz: I think one of the features which must be pointed out is that we really do not know what the relationship is between plasma growth hormone levels and growth. We cannot say that a child who has a mean growth hormone level of 1.5 will grow at half the rate of a child who has a level of 3. In fact, the only practical value that we have found for growth hormone levels in our group has been in the diagnosis of either acromegaly, where the levels are clearly very high, or hypopituitarism where they are very low. In the widely fluctuating range during sleep and the other things that have been shown, there is absolutely no information that I know of that correlates how or why, or if indeed, growth hormone does change growth.

The point I tried to emphasize is that growth hormone levels ordinarily go up during fasting, and they are suppressed every time you eat, if you eat a carbohydrate meal. If you eat a protein meal, there is a rise in growth hormone, but much less than with insulin-induced hypoglycemia. People have reflected about what it is about growth hormone secretion that may cause growth and there have been at least two major theories that I am aware of. One is that growth occurs during sleep—that the spike in growth hormone during sleep is what causes growth. If this is so, everybody should tell their children to go to bed early so they can get a good growth hormone spike. I do not really believe that, but I do not have any evidence to say that it is not true. The other idea, proposed a number of years ago by Dave Rabinowitz and a number of other people is that it is the coordinated action of several hormones which causes growth. For instance, when you eat, what ordinarily happens is that you raise insulin levels; if insulin levels go up and you are eating carbohydrate, your growth hormone levels go down. It turns out that insulin and growth hormone have many actions in unison and many competitive actions. But they both affect amino acid transport and protein synthesis. If they act together, then, as Rabinowitz and many others have said, maybe that is the time that you grow. I think the fact that growth hormone levels are ordinarily suppressed or low after meals is very important. It concerns me that the growth hormone levels seem to be going up at the same time the patients may be eating. This would mean that these levels may be more significant than the mean value taken over a 24-hour period. We have seen some acromegalic patients whose plasma growth hormone level in a fasting state may be 6 or 7, but in response to a meal it may jump up to 30 or 40. This paradoxical rise may be of more physiologic significance. I am not sure that one can use mean values and say that this correlates with growth. I think this is the reason why we were concerned with serum sulfation as being more definitive in terms of assessing this growth pattern.

Dr. Van Loon: I would like to insert a word of caution in the interpretation of data which relate the administration of adrenergic agents in man to the regulation of growth hormone secretion. In almost every paper which has been written by an investigator in this field, inferences are made about mediation by a central adrenergic mechanism. There are no data I am aware of to demonstrate that this is centrally mediated in man. And I think the onus remains on the investigators in this area to demonstrate that these effects are not mediated by a peripheral adrenergic mechanism.

Dr. Mena: Concerning Dr. Lebovitz's point about the possible influence of diet on the release of growth hormone by DOPA, I would like to comment that a high protein diet, as Dr. Papavasiliou has reported, tends to block the effect of L-DOPA, and it does block the releasing capacity of growth hormone by L-DOPA. The pulses that we have shown in patients receiving a normal house diet are absent, and their curves more nearly resemble the curves of the untreated patients.

Advances in Neurology, Vol. 5
Raven Press, New York © 1974

The Role of Brain Catecholamines in the Regulation of ACTH Secretion

Glen R. Van Loon

Departments of Medicine and Physiology, University of Toronto, Toronto, Ontario, Canada

The role of the central nervous system in the regulation of secretion of adrenocorticotropic hormone (ACTH) has been well documented (1–3). The neuroanatomical substrate for this regulation appears to involve pathways from several brain areas including brainstem, amygdala, hippocampus, and others, which converge in the hypothalamus, probably on the neurons secreting corticotropin-releasing factor (CRF). Neurophysiological studies have provided evidence for both stimulatory and inhibitory mechanisms in this regulation, but the neurotransmitters in these pathways remain to be defined.

The substances which have been suggested as having transmitting function at central synapses include acetylcholine and three monoamines, dopamine, norepinephrine, and serotonin. All of these substances have been implicated in some way in the regulation of ACTH secretion. Acetylcholine may function in excitatory pathways regulating ACTH secretion (4–6). The role of serotonin in regulation of ACTH secretory mechanisms appears complex and remains unclear (7–9). The nature of the possible role of catecholamines in these mechanisms will be discussed in this chapter.

A considerable body of experimental data has been described relating studies of catecholamine metabolism and ACTH secretion. Until recently, however, there have been no unifying hypotheses presented concerning such a relationship. The catecholamines are apparently not in themselves CRFs (10), but there is abundant evidence that they are involved in the control of ACTH secretion (11).

Central catecholamine-containing neuronal pathways have been described (12), and are discussed in greater detail elsewhere in this volume. A dopaminergic pathway, with cell bodies in the arcuate nucleus of the floor of the third ventricle and nerve endings in the median eminence adjacent to portal vessels and to neurons which are perhaps "peptidergic," appears important in the regulation of luteinizing hormone, follicle-stimulating hormone, and prolactin secretion. The median eminence also contains noradrenergic nerve endings, but these fiber systems are not well understood. The primary noradrenergic pathways have cell bodies in the brainstem and nerve endings in various nuclei of hypothalamus as well as the hippocampus and amygdala.

Early attempts to elucidate the role played by biogenic amines in the central regulation of the hypothalamic-pituitary-adrenal axis involved the use of pharmacological agents known to alter amine metabolism; reserpine was the most commonly employed drug. Reserpine stimulates ACTH secretion in several species (13–16) when the dose is sufficient to decrease brain monoamine content by greater than 50%. The effects of reserpine and other stresses on ACTH secretion can be prevented by monoamine oxidase inhibitors (17, 18).

The literature relating the effects of chlorpromazine on ACTH secretion is confusing and has been reviewed by DeWied (19). Release of ACTH and, in contrast, inhibition of stress-induced ACTH release by chlorpromazine have been observed in laboratory animals and man.

Many stressful stimuli that increase ACTH secretion are associated also with a decrease in brain norepinephrine content (10). Stressful agents and situations vary considerably in their effectiveness to produce brain norepinephrine depletion (20–22). Increased turnover of brain norepinephrine has been reported in response to stressful stimuli (23–25). The effects of stress on central dopaminergic neurons have been less well documented. Both change (24) and failure to find change (10, 25) in dopamine depletion after α-methyl-p-tyrosine have been reported in animals exposed to stress.

Various changes in brain catecholamine metabolism have been reported after adrenalectomy or steroid administration. Conflicting results of the effects of adrenalectomy on catecholamine fluorescence of the tuberoinfundibular neurons of the median eminence have been reported (26, 27). Although Fuxe and co-workers (28) failed to find changes in dopamine turnover in the median eminence and neostriatum following adrenalectomy, they did find an increase in norepinephrine turnover in both the hypothalamus and cerebral cortex. Others have reported similar results with no change in brain norepinephrine concentration but increased norepinephrine turnover following adrenalectomy (29–31). Hypophysectomy was associated with a decrease in amine turnover in central norepinephrine neurons, but there was no change in neostriatal dopamine neurons (28). Corticosteroid administration has, in general, failed to produce consistent effects on brain norepinephrine concentration and turnover (28, 32, 33). However, exogenous corticosteroids appeared to counteract the increase in norepinephrine turnover found after adrenalectomy (28). Corticosteroids also increased dopamine turnover in nigroneostriatal and mesolimbic dopamine neurons in adrenalectomized but not in normal rats. Administration of ACTH increased norepinephrine turnover in brain of normal male rats, but failed to reverse the decreased norepinephrine turnover of hypophysectomized rats (28). In hypophysectomized rats, ACTH decreased dopamine turnover in neostriatum and limbic forebrain. A single hypothesis of the effects of experimental manipulation of the pituitary-adrenal axis on brain catecholamine metabolism has not yet emerged from these data.

The preceding paragraphs have dealt with the effects of drug administration, stress, and hormonal manipulation on brain catecholamine metabolism. Although in many of the experiments a correlation between change in brain catecholamine activity and change in ACTH secretion was demonstrated, these studies failed to provide a unifying hypothesis formulating a role of brain norepinephrine and dopamine in the regulation of ACTH secretion. In subsequent paragraphs I shall review several studies which have failed to find a correlation between catecholamines and ACTH secretion, and others which appear to provide evidence for either excitatory or inhibitory roles of catecholamines in the regulation of ACTH secretion.

Based on a study in which the ACTH responses to various stressors remained unchanged in rats in which median eminence fluorescence was depleted by reserpine implants, Smelik (34) concluded that under both normal and stressful conditions hypothalamic monoamines are not involved in stimulatory or inhibitory mechanisms affecting ACTH secretion. It must be remembered, however, that depletion of catecholamine fluorescence from brain tissue does not mean that the catecholamines have been removed entirely. Also, depletion of median eminence catecholamines does not exclude an adrenergic effect at another brain site. Moore and co-workers (35, 36) found that depletion of brain catecholamines with a combination of reserpine and α-methyl-p-tyrosine failed to alter the plasma corticosterone response to various stressors or to a subsequent injection of reserpine. Bhattacharya and Marks (37) failed to demonstrate a change in hypothalamic CRF content, pituitary ACTH content, or plasma corticosterone after administration of the catecholamine synthesis inhibitor, α-methyl-p-tyrosine. Also, these rats responded normally to stress with elevations in plasma corticosterone.

Most investigators have sought a role for catecholamines as excitatory neurotransmitters in central mechanisms regulating ACTH secretion. This concept has been discussed in considerable depth in an earlier review (11). Release of ACTH following injection of catecholamines directly into the brain has been reported by several workers (5, 6, 38). Naumenko (38) has proposed that norepinephrine implanted in the hypothalamus activated an efferent pathway via the brainstem to the spinal cord; this in turn activated peripheral mechanisms that were relayed back to the hypothalamus and the CRF neuron.

Several possible mechanisms by which catecholamines stimulate ACTH secretion have been suggested. The possibility that catecholamines may act as neurotransmitters in central pathways affecting ACTH secretion has been discussed. Neurohumors liberated into the hypothalamic-hypophyseal portal blood might affect anterior pituitary secretion by altering the caliber of portal vessels, thus changing adenohypophyseal blood flow (10,

11). The possibility that catecholamines may stimulate ACTH secretion via a peripheral neural mechanism has been discussed by several authors (11, 38–40). It is difficult to draw firm conclusions in summarizing a possible excitatory role of catecholamines in the regulation of ACTH secretion. Although exogenous catecholamines do stimulate ACTH secretion, these substances do not seem to be necessary mediators of the stimulation of ACTH secretion (11).

Examination of the literature relating catecholamines to ACTH secretion has suggested the possibility of an inverse relationship (11). Reserpine, a drug that decreases brain catecholamine activity, increases ACTH secretion. Chlorpromazine may act in the brain to decrease catecholamine activity by blocking catecholamine receptor sites and is also associated with stimulation of ACTH secretion. The monoamine oxidase inhibitor iproniazid potentiated the effect of dexamethasone in blocking the plasma corticosterone response to stress (41, 42). Depletion of median eminence CRF in association with increased plasma and adrenal corticosterone and decreased pituitary ACTH has been reported in rats treated with reserpine or chlorpromazine (16). The systemic administration of pargyline and amphetamine, drugs which increase central catecholaminergic activity, produced decreased resting levels of plasma corticosterone and decreased response to stress (43). In other studies from the same laboratory, the intraventricular administration of norepinephrine or dopamine, which are ineffective in normal animals, caused a depression of reserpine-induced increases in adrenal corticosterone (44). Using a microelectrophoretic technique, it has been demonstrated that the action potentials of some hypothalamic and midbrain neurons are depressed by both dexamethasone and norepinephrine.

The remainder of this chapter will summarize studies carried out by the author and various colleagues (see references) supporting a hypothesis of a central adrenergic neural system which inhibits ACTH secretion. The catecholamine precursor L-DOPA, administered intravenously, inhibited the adrenal venous 17-hydroxycorticosteroid (17-OHCS) response to laparotomy in dogs (45). On the other hand, the catecholamines norepinephrine and dopamine, which do not cross the blood-brain barrier to any extent and do not alter brain catecholamine concentration, were ineffective in preventing the 17-OHCS response to surgical stress. Furthermore, the time course of inhibition of the 17-OHCS response to surgical stress produced by L-DOPA in dogs (45) coincides with both the alteration in motor activity produced by L-DOPA in mice (46) and the increase in brain catecholamine content following administration of L-DOPA (47).

The minimum effective dose of L-DOPA necessary to inhibit the 17-OHCS response was increased by a drug (α-methyl-p-tyrosine) that decreases adrenergic activity and decreased by a drug (pargyline) that increases adrenergic activity (45). These data provide further support for the concept that L-DOPA inhibits ACTH secretion via an increase in adrenergic activity.

The adrenal venous 17-OHCS response to surgical stress was studied in response to the administration of large doses of several adrenergic agents directly into the third ventricle in dogs (48). L-DOPA, L-norepinephrine, L-isoproterenol, dopamine, tyramine, and α-ethyltryptamine inhibited the 17-OHCS response to stress, whereas D-norepinephrine and vanillylmandelic acid failed to inhibit the 17-OHCS response.

Intraventricular administration of the α-adrenergic blocking agent phenoxybenzamine counteracted the inhibition of ACTH secretion induced by intravenous L-DOPA (49, 50). Another α-adrenergic blocking agent, phentolamine, and the β-adrenergic blocking agent propranolol did not affect this inhibition.

Adrenergic inhibition was studied with regard to different parameters of ACTH secretion in the rat. Thus, the effects of alterations in brain catecholamine metabolism on plasma corticosterone resting level and circadian variation rather than stress response were investigated. The soluble methyl ester of α-methyl-p-tyrosine administered intraperitoneally increased plasma corticosterone, and this increase was inhibited by the simultaneous administration of L-DOPA but not by norepinephrine (51). Thus, the catecholamine precursor which freely crosses the blood-brain barrier prevented the effect of α-methyl-p-tyrosine, whereas norepinephrine, which fails to penetrate the blood-brain barrier, also failed to prevent the effect of α-methyl-p-tyrosine on plasma corticosterone.

α-Methyl-p-tyrosine did not produce its effect on plasma corticosterone by acting directly on the adrenal, since it did not increase plasma corticosterone concentration in the acutely hypophysectomized rat (G. R. Van Loon, W. E. Nicholson, and G. W. Liddle, *unpublished observations*). Additional evidence that the effect of α-methyl-p-tyrosine on plasma corticosterone is mediated through the brain is provided by the finding that the intraventricular administration of a systemically ineffective dose of α-methyl-p-tyrosine increased plasma corticosterone concentration (51). Also, guanethidine, a drug that depletes catecholamines from neurons but fails to cross the blood-brain barrier to any significant extent, increased plasma corticosterone concentration after intraventricular but not systemic administration (52).

Intraventricular administration of a systemically ineffective dose of phentolamine, an α-adrenergic blocking agent, increased plasma corticosterone (53). These data in the rat support the study described above showing inhibition by intraventricular phenoxybenzamine of the effect of L-DOPA on the ACTH response to stress (49, 50). The potentiation by iproniazid of the suppressive effect of dexamethasone on plasma corticosterone response to stress is blocked by phentolamine, but not by propranolol (53).

All of these data suggest the possibility of α-adrenergic receptor mediation of catecholamine inhibition of ACTH secretion.

Evidence that norepinephrine is the catecholamine-mediating inhibitor of ACTH secretion has been reported. The dopamine-β-oxidase inhibitor FLA-63 produced decreased hypothalamic norepinephrine concentration and increased plasma corticosterone with no change in hypothalamic dopamine concentration (52). Also, dihydroxyphenylserine prevents both the depletion of hypothalamic norepinephrine and the increase in plasma corticosterone induced by α-methyl-p-tyrosine without altering the depletion of hypothalamic dopamine (49).

The effect of catecholamines on ACTH secretion does not appear to be mediated by a direct action on the pituitary, since dopamine failed to alter the release of ACTH from rat anterior pituitaries incubated in vitro (54).

Some support for the hypothesis of central adrenergic neural inhibition of ACTH secretion has been provided in man. In three of five patients studied, chronic treatment with L-DOPA for 1 month decreased the plasma 11-hydroxycorticosteroid (11-OHCS) response to insulin-induced hypoglycemia; one of these patients failed completely to show a rise in 11-OHCS after treatment with L-DOPA (55). Resting levels of plasma 11-OHCS and urinary 17-OHCS and 17-ketosteroids were unaffected by treatment with L-DOPA. It is possible that some patients treated with L-DOPA may not be able to respond adequately to stress with an appropriate rise in plasma corticosteroids.

In the preceding paragraphs evidence has been presented in support of a hypothesis of a central adrenergic neural system that inhibits ACTH secretion. If such an inhibitory system regulating ACTH secretion were absent, increased secretion of ACTH might be expected. Increased secretion of ACTH in man manifests as Cushing's disease. Could Cushing's disease be somewhat analogous to Parkinson's disease with functional loss of a catecholaminergic system in a different brain area? In an attempt to provide a possible model for further investigation of the pathophysiology of human Cushing's disease, the effect of catecholamine depletion with α-methyl-p-tyrosine on various parameters of ACTH secretion was studied in the rat. Acute treatment with α-methyl-p-tyrosine is associated with increased plasma corticosterone levels, abolishment of diurnal rhythm of plasma corticosterone, resistance to suppression of plasma corticosterone with dexamethasone, enhanced response of plasma corticosterone to ACTH, and enhanced response of plasma deoxycorticosterone to metyrapone (11, 56). All of these abnormalities in pituitary-adrenal function are present in patients with Cushing's disease. Furthermore, in the rat the simultaneous administration of L-DOPA with α-methyl-p-tyrosine returns the abnormal function tests toward normal. It is possible that the hyperadrenocortisolism induced in animals may not be relevant to human disease, and these studies may simply represent the pituitary-adrenal response to stress. Preliminary studies with administration of L-DOPA to patients with Cushing's disease have not provided consistent correction of pituitary-adrenal hyperfunction (Van Loon, *unpublished observations;* 57). This mode of treatment may not provide a suitable means of increasing norepinephrine concentration in the relevant brain areas, or alternatively this animal model may not be a valid model of the human disease.

Much of the evidence relating a possible role of catecholamines in the regulation of ACTH secretion is conflicting, and the data could support several different hypotheses regarding such a possible interaction. Considerable experimentation will be necessary before the possible neurotransmitter roles of brain catecholamines in the regulation of ACTH secretion are clearly understood.

REFERENCES

1. Mangili, G., Motta, M., and Martini, L., *Neuroendocrinology* 1, 297 (1966).
2. McCann, S. M., and Porter, J. C., *Physiol. Rev.* 49, 240 (1969).
3. Van Loon, G. R., and Kragt, C. L., *Progr. Neurol. Psychiat.* 26, 261 (1971).
4. Hedge, G. A., and Smelik, P. G., *Science* 159, 891 (1968).
5. Endroczi, E., Schreiberg, G., and Lissak, K., *Acta Physiol. Acad. Sci. Hung.* 24, 211 (1963).
6. Krieger, D. T., and Krieger, H. P., *Proceedings of the 2nd International Congress of Endocrinology,* Vol. 1, pp. 640–645 (1965).
7. Krieger, D. T., and Rizzo, F., *Am. J. Physiol.* 217, 1703 (1969).
8. Scapagnini, U., Moberg, G. P., Van Loon, G. R., De Groot, J., and Ganong, W. F., *Neuroendocrinology* 7, 90 (1971).
9. Vermes, I., Telegdy, G., and Lissak, K. *Acta Physiol. Acad. Sci. Hung.* 41, 95 (1972).
10. Ganong, W. F., and Lorenzen, L. C., in: *Neuroendocrinology,* Vol. 2, pp. 583–640, Academic Press, New York (1967).
11. Van Loon, G. R., in: *Frontiers in Neuroendocrinology, 1973,* Oxford University Press, New York (1973).
12. Fuxe, K., and Hokfelt, T., in: *Frontiers in Neuroendocrinology, 1969,* pp. 47–96, Oxford University Press, New York. (1969).
13. Maickel, R. P., Westermann, E. O., and Brodie, B. B., *J. Pharmacol. Exp. Ther.* 134, 167 (1961).
14. Harwood, C. T., and Mason, J. W., *Endocrinology* 60, 239 (1957).
15. Khazan, H., Sulman, F. G., and Winnik, H. Z., *Proc. Soc. Exp. Biol. Med.* 106, 579 (1961).
16. Bhattacharya, A. N., and Marks, B. H., *J. Pharmacol. Exp. Ther.* 165, 108 (1969).
17. De Schaepdryver, A. F., and Preziosi, P., *Arch. Int. Pharmacodyn. Ther.* 119, 506 (1959).
18. Gaunt, R., Renzi, A. A., and Chart, J. J., *Endocrinology* 71, 527 (1962).
19. De Wied, D., *Pharmacol. Rev.* 19, 251 (1967).
20. Maynert, E. W., and Levi, R., *J. Pharmacol. Exp. Ther.* 143, 90 (1964).
21. Bliss, E. L., and Zwanziger, J., *J. Psychiat. Res.* 4, 189 (1966).
22. Thierry, A. M., Javoy, F., Glowinski, J., and Kety, S. S., *J. Pharmacol. Exp. Ther.* 163, 163 (1968).
23. Gordon, R., Spector, S., Sjoerdsma, A., and Udenfriend, S., *J. Pharmacol. Exp. Ther.* 153, 440 (1966).
24. Bliss, E. L., Ailion, J., and Zwanziger, J., *J. Pharmacol. Exp. Ther.* 164, 122 (1968).
25. Corrodi, H., Fuxe, K., and Hokfelt, T., *Life Sci. (1)* 7, 107 (1968).
26. Akmayev, I. G., and Donath, T., *Z. Mikrosk. Anat. Forsch.* 74, 83 (1966).
27. Fuxe, K., and Hokfelt, T., *Neurosecretion* 165 (1967).
28. Fuxe, K., Hokfelt, T., Jonsson, G., and Lidbrink, P., in: *Proceedings of the 2nd Congress of the International Society of Psychoneuroendocrinology (in press)* (1972).
29. Javoy, F., Glowinski, J., and Kordon, C., *Eur. J. Pharmacol.* 4, 103 (1968).
30. Pfeifer, A. K., Vizi, E., Satory, E., and Galambos, E., *Experientia* 19, 482 (1963).

31. Utevskii, A. M., Gaisinskaya, M. Y., Raisin, M. S., and Braude, I. Y., *Bull. Exp. Biol. Med.* 70, 1388 (1971).
32. De Schaepdryver, A. F., Preziosi, P., and Scapagnini, U., *Br. J. Pharmacol.* 35, 460 (1969).
33. Petrovic, V. M., and Davidovic, V., *J. Physiol. (Paris)* 62, Suppl. 3, 427 (1970).
34. Smelik, P. G., *Neuroendocrinology* 2, 247 (1967).
35. Carr, L. A., and Moore, K. E., *Neuroendocrinology* 3, 285 (1968).
36. Hirsch, G. H. and Moore, K. E., *Neuroendocrinology* 3, 398 (1968).
37. Bhattacharya, A. N., and Marks, B. H., *Neuroendocrinology* 6, 49 (1970).
38. Naumenko, E. V., *Brain Res.*, 11, 1 (1968).
39. Naumenko, E. V., Maslova, L. N., and Popova, N. K., *Bull. Exp. Biol. Med. U.S.S.R. (in press)*.
40. Vernikos-Danellis, J., in: *Pharmacology of Hormonal Polypeptides and Proteins*, pp. 175–189, Plenum Press, New York (1968).
41. Dallman, M. F., and Yates, F. E., *Mem. Soc. Endocrinol.* 17, 39 (1968).
42. Gann, D., Schoeffler, J. D., and Ostrander, L., in: *Systems Symposium*, pp. 62–93, Springer-Verlag, New York (1968).
43. Bhattacharya, A. N., and Marks, B. H., *Proc. Soc. Exp. Biol. Med.* 130, 1194–1198 (1969).
44. Marks, B. H., Hall, M. M., and Bhattacharya, A. N., *Progr. Brain Res.* 32, 57 (1970).
45. Van Loon, G. R., Hilger, L., King, A. B., Boryczka, A. T., and Ganong, W. F., *Endocrinology* 88, 1404 (1971).
46. Boissier, J. R., and Simon, P., *Psychopharmacologia*, 8, 428 (1966).
47. Bertler, A., and Rosengren, E., *Experientia*, 15, 10 (1959).
48. Van Loon, G. R., Scapagnini, U., Cohen, E., and Ganong, W. F., *Neuroendocrinology* 8, 257 (1971).
49. Ganong, W. F., *Progr. Brain. Res. (in press)*.
50. Ganong, W. F., in: *Brain-Endocrine Interaction*, Knigge, K. M., Scott, J. E., and Weindl, A., p. 254, Karger, Basel and New York, 1972.
51. Van Loon, G. R., Scapagnini, U., Moberg, G. P., and Ganong, W. F., *Endocrinology* 89, 1464 (1971).
52. Scapagnini, U., Van Loon, G. R., Moberg, G. P., Preziosi, P., and Ganong, W. F., *Neuroendocrinology* 10, 155 (1972).
53. Scapagnini, U., and Preziosi, P., *Arch. Int. Pharmacodyn. Ther.* 196 (Suppl.), 205 (1972).
54. Van Loon, G. R., and Kragt, C. L., *Proc. Soc. Exp. Biol. Med.* 133, 1137 (1970).
55. Von Werder, K., Van Loon, G. R., Yatsu, F., and Forsham, P. H., *Klin. Wochenschr.* 48, 1454 (1970).
56. Van Loon, G. R., Nicholson, W., and Brown, R., *Program of the 53rd Meeting of the Endocrine Society*, p. 129 (1971).
57. Krieger, D. T., *J. Clin. Endocrinol. Metab.* 36, 277 (1973).

DISCUSSION

Dr. Goldberg: I'm worried a little bit about that large dose of L-DOPA in the dog, particularly when you're dealing with stress. Fifty milligrams per kilogram of L-DOPA would probably give you a blood pressure of 250 millimeters, a heart rate of maybe 280, and perhaps ventricular tachycardia. If you give 10 milligrams of pargyline I think you would do about the same. So, I just wondered if you measured cardiovascular functions. If you did, and it produced these effects, did you try dopamine which does not cross the blood-brain barrier, and see if it does the same things with stress?

Dr. Van Loon: This is a very important control to be done in these studies. Prior to this, some investigators had suggested that one mechanism by which ACTH secretion might be inhibited was via an increase in blood pressure, and obviously the amounts of L-DOPA which were used did increase blood pressure. However, there were two pieces of data which still supported our hypothesis. (1) Administration of either norepinephrine or dopamine intravenously produced the same degree of blood pressure increase and did not inhibit ACTH secretion. (2) We pretreated dogs with phenoxybenzamine in amounts sufficient to inhibit the blood pressure rise induced by L-DOPA, but we did not inhibit the response of ACTH secretion.

Dr. Lebovitz: We looked at adrenocortical function in a very crude way in people receiving 6 grams of L-DOPA a day, and neither their basal 24-hour urinary 17-hydroxysteroids nor their steroid response to metapyrone changed. So we have doubts that, at these dose levels, one sees any significant effect.

Dr. Van Loon: In response to that point, we investigated five patients with Parkinson's disease before and 1 month after the administration of L-DOPA. We found that similarly there were no changes in the resting levels of plasma or urinary corticoids, but in one of the patients there was complete obliteration of the response to insulin-induced hypoglycemia. You might just keep that in mind when you send your parkinsonian patients on L-DOPA to surgery.

Dr. Mena: Dr. Van Loon, Dr. Lebovitz reported that L-DOPA in acromegalic patients could have some paradoxic effect. Do you have information about the effect of L-DOPA in Cushing's syndrome?

Dr. Van Loon: We have looked at about four patients with Cushing's disease, after administering L-DOPA in the same sorts of doses which you used treating your parkinsonians for 1 month, and we did not find any consistent return toward normal of the abnormal pituitary adrenal function tests. One thing we have found, which may be purely coincidental, is that these patients were treated by irradiation. In two of the first three patients we studied, their diurnal rhythms and their pituitary function tests were normal before the end of their pituitary irradiation. Usually these patients do not return to normal until at least 3 months after treatment. Dorothy Krieger has just published some data on several patients with Cushing's disease treated with L-DOPA, and she found no improvement.

Dr. Smith: Dr. Van Loon, do you know the response in the steroid system to amphetamine injection?

Dr. Van Loon: Besser, Reese, and colleagues at Bart's Hospital in London did some studies in which they looked at both dexamphetamine and methamphetamine and found increases in plasma ACTH and plasma steroids in response to the administration of these agents. I think that the data are sound, but I do not know how they fit in. I'm bothered most because I think that at the times at which they demonstrated increases in steroids you could not correlate a decrease in brain amines resulting from amphetamine.

Dr. Carlsson: You say that phenoxybenzamine did not block the effect of DOPA on ACTH secretion.

Dr. Van Loon: In the dog we found that phenoxybenzamine was ineffective. I don't know if there was sufficient phenoxybenzamine used to produce central blockade, so I would not say from this evidence that this is not an alpha-adrenergic phenomenon. Ganong has demonstrated that the effect of intravenous L-DOPA is inhibited by the intraventricular administration of phenoxybenzamine, and it is not inhibited by the intraventricular administration of either propranolol or phentolamine.

Dr. McCann: Just a possible explanation for some of the discrepancies that Dr. Van Loon has pointed out. Namely, you can under certain conditions by giving catecholamines stimulate ACTH, and in other conditions you seem to be able to inhibit it. Perhaps the circulating catecholamines may act in the brainstem on the general alerting mechanism which could then trigger ACTH release, whereas the intrahypothalamic mechanism may well serve as an inhibitor. This may explain why you can get divergent results depending on how you administer the drug.

Dr. Van Loon: I think this is a very important point. Central and peripheral adrenergic mechanisms may have different effects; norepinephrine and dopamine centrally may have different effects.

Advances in Neurology, Vol. 5
Raven Press, New York © 1974

The Effect of L-DOPA on the Hypothalamic-Pituitary-Thyroid Axis

Gerard N. Burrow, Stephen W. Spaulding, Richard Donabedian, Melvin Van Woert, and Lalit Ambani

Departments of Medicine, Laboratory Medicine, and Pharmacology, Yale University School of Medicine, New Haven, Connecticut 06510

The identification of the chemical structure of thyrotropin-releasing hormone (TRH) (1, 2) and the subsequent synthesis of this peptide have provided an important tool for the study of thyroid-hypothalamic relationships. The elucidation of the chemical structure of TRH has made it possible to study the synthesis of endogenous TRH by incubating hypothalamic fragments with radioactive amino acid precursors and measuring TRH synthetase activity (3). With this technique Reichlin and co-workers found that reserpine-treated animals had a reduced concentration of TRH synthetase activity compared to nontreated animals. Furthermore, the addition of norepinephrine, or dopamine, to hypothalami *in vitro* enhanced the rate of discharge of labeled TRH. They proposed that the total function of the TRH peptidergic neuron is subject to control by noradrenergic neurons.

Dopamine granules have been found in proximity to the pituitary portal system, and dopamine levels are increased in the hypothalamus and median eminence (4). The acute administration of L-DOPA lowers plasma prolactin and elevates plasma growth hormone (5, 6) but has no effect on serum TSH (7). Long-term therapy with L-DOPA suppresses plasma prolactin (8) but does not result in chronically elevated growth hormone levels (9).

With the availability of synthetic TRH, it seemed pertinent to study the effect of long-term L-DOPA therapy on the response of the pituitary to TRH stimulation. Nine males and four females with Parkinson's disease who were between 46 and 71 years of age, were studied (10). The five control subjects had not received L-DOPA for more than 3 months, whereas eight experimental subjects had been on 2.5 to 5 g of L-DOPA per day for 1 to 4 years prior to the study. The last dose of L-DOPA (0.75 to 1.0 g) was given 1 hr prior to TRH injection. Some of the patients in both groups were taking other antiparkinsonian medications, such as trihexyphenidyl or benztropine. After two fasting blood samples were drawn, 500 µg of synthetic TRH was injected as a bolus through an indwelling venous Cournand needle. Serum samples were then collected every 15 min for at least 1 hr following the in-

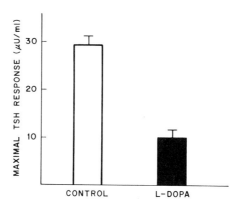

FIG. 1. Effect of L-DOPA on the maximal TSH response to TRH. The bars represent the mean maximal TSH response ± 1.0 SD in μU/ml.

jection. Serum TSH levels were determined by the double-antibody radioimmunoassay technique. Serum thyroxine was determined by displacement analysis, and serum triiodothyronine was determined by immunoprecipitation.

There was no significant difference between the two groups with regard to age or serum thyroxine values, both of which may affect the TSH response to TRH. Following the injection of TRH, there was a two- to threefold rise above normal serum TSH levels in all the control (untreated parkinsonian) patients. The mean value for the maximal TSH concentration obtained following TRH injection in the control patients was 28.8 ± 3.0 (SD) μU/ml, and in patients on L-DOPA it was 10.1 ± 3.0 μU/ml ($p < 0.001$) (Fig. 1). Only three patients on L-DOPA reached TSH levels above the normal range (11, 11, and 17 μU/ml), and these values did not approach the control response. It is conceivable that L-DOPA could merely alter the time of the TSH response to TRH. Accordingly, TSH levels were monitored for 3 hr in three subjects receiving L-DOPA and, after reaching a diminished peak value 20 to 30 min after injection, TSH levels fell steadily. To ascertain whether L-DOPA had an effect on unstimulated TSH values, serum TSH determinations were obtained before and during chronic L-DOPA therapy in nine patients with Parkinson's disease. Serum TSH levels were normal in all of the patients and did not change during L-DOPA treatment.

We also examined the dosage and duration of L-DOPA treatment required to suppress the TSH response to TRH. The acute administration of L-DOPA does not appear to inhibit the TSH response in normal patients, although it has been reported to do so in hypothyroid patients (11). One patient whom we studied received 1 g of L-DOPA daily for 3 weeks and had no inhibition of the TSH response to TRH. Figure 2 shows the TSH response at different

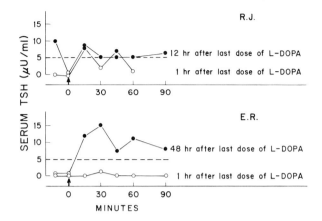

FIG. 2. TSH response to TRH after cessation of L-DOPA therapy. Open circles represent values below 5 μU/ml of serum TSH.

intervals after the withdrawal of L-DOPA in two patients. In both patients there was a smaller response when the last dose of L-DOPA was given 1 hr before injecting TRH. In another patient studied 72 hr after the withdrawal of L-DOPA, the response to TRH appeared normal. It would appear from this indirect evidence that there is a relatively long induction period for L-DOPA and a disappearance of the inhibitory effect within several days of the cessation of therapy.

To determine whether other agents which alter brain dopamine affect the TSH response to TRH, six parkinsonian patients were tested with TRH before and during γ-hydroxybutyrate (GHB) therapy. GHB causes a marked increase in brain dopamine, perhaps by preventing release by dopaminergic neurons (12). The patients were taking 5 to 14 g of GHB daily and received their last dose 1 hr before the TRH test. The maximal TSH response to TRH before and during GHB therapy is shown in Fig. 3. There was greater variation in TSH maximal responses after GHB therapy. However, although individual responses differed between the control and GHB testing, there was no consistent difference among the group as a whole, with a mean maximal TSH response to TRH of 23 μU/ml during the control period and 20 μU/ml during GHB therapy.

The failure of TRH to elevate TSH levels in patients receiving L-DOPA could be explained by chronic L-DOPA stimulation of TSH release at the pituitary level with a consequent inability of the pituitary to respond to TRH. However, the inability to detect a rise in serum TSH concentrations during chronic L-DOPA therapy makes this explanation less likely.

Alternatively, L-DOPA or its metabolites might act directly on the pituitary to inhibit TSH release or depress its response to TRH. Dopamine does

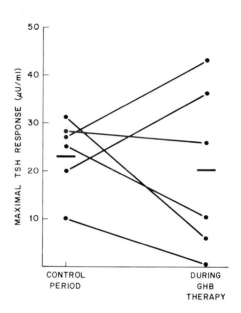

FIG. 3. Effect of γ-hydroxybutyrate on the maximal TSH response to TRH. The maximal TSH response to TRH in μU/ml is recorded for six subjects before and during GHB therapy.

inhibit prolactin secretion from pituitaries incubated *in vitro,* but this may be a pharmacologic effect (13).

If L-DOPA acted directly on the thyroid gland to increase serum thyroxine, this would in turn decrease pituitary responsiveness to TRH through the negative feedback mechanism. Although dopamine has been reported to have a direct effect on thyroid hormone release (14), the data in the present study and that of Boyd, Lebovitz, and Feldman (15) did not reveal significantly different serum thyroxine values between L-DOPA and control groups. Snyder and Utiger (16) have reported that TSH responsiveness to TRH may be inhibited without any alteration in serum thyroxine if the serum triiodothyronine concentration is increased. Serum triiodothyronine (T3) determinations were obtained before and at various intervals after starting L-DOPA therapy in seven patients with parkinsonism. No consistent alterations in serum T3 concentrations were found. It therefore seems unlikely that the suppressive effects of L-DOPA on the TSH response to TRH can be explained by a direct effect on the thyroid.

Finally, it is possible that the catecholamines might stimulate the release of a hypothalamic TSH inhibitory factor (TSH-IF) in a manner similar to the stimulation of TRH. L-DOPA might thus inhibit TRH-induced release of TSH by mechanisms similar to those regulating TRH-induced prolactin release (17). Such an inhibitory factor has been reported in teleosts, where it is apparently the major regulator (18). Although TSH-IF has not yet been reported in mammals, areas have been found in the rat brain which appear to inhibit TSH release.

In summary, dopamine apparently both increases endogenous TRH levels and inhibits the TSH response to synthetic TRH. Despite these diverse catecholamine effects on the hypothalamic-pituitary-thyroid axis, or perhaps because of them, patients receiving L-DOPA remain euthyroid.

ACKNOWLEDGMENTS

This work was supported by U.S. Public Health Service, National Institutes of Health, grants Am 19273, Am 5015, CA 08341, and NS 07542. TRH was generously provided by Dr. Michael S. Anderson, Abbott Laboratories. We thank Dr. Bert Malkis for the serum T3 determinations.

REFERENCES

1. Burgus, R., Dunn, T. F., Desiderio, D., Vale, W., and Guillemin, R., *C.R. Acad. Sci. Ser.* D, 269 (1970).
2. Boler, J., Enzmann, F., Folkers, K., Bowers, C. Y., and Schally, A. V., *Biochem. Biophys. Res. Commun.* 37, 705 (1969).
3. Reichlin, S., Martin, J. B., Mitnick, M., Boshans, R. L., Grimm, Y., Bollinger, J., Gordon, J., and Malacara, J., *Rec. Prog. Hormone Res.* 28, 229 (1972).
4. Fuxe, K., and Hokfelt, T., *Acta. Physiol. Scand.* 66, 235 (1966).
5. Kleinberg, D. L., Noel, G. L., and Frantz, A. G., *J. Clin. Endocrinol.* 33, 873 (1971).
6. Kansal, P. C., Buse, J., Talbert, O. R., and Buse, M. G., *J. Clin. Endocrinol.* 34, 99 (1972).
7. Eddy, R. L., Jones, A. L., Chakmakjian, E. H., and Silverthorne, M. C., *J. Clin. Endocrinol.* 33, 709 (1971).
8. Turkington, R. W., *J. Clin. Endocrinol.* 34, 306 (1972).
9. Van Woert, M. II., and Mueller, P. S., *Clin. Pharmacol. and Therapy* 12, 360 (1971).
10. Spaulding, S. W., Burrow, G. N., Donabedian, R. A., and Van Woert, M., *J. Clin. Endocrinol.* 35, 182 (1972).
11. Rapoport, B., Refetoff, S., Fang, U. S., and Friesen, H. G., *J. Clin. Endocrinol.* 36, 256 (1973).
12. Busto, J., and Roth, R., *Brit. J. Pharmacol.* 44, 816 (1972).
13. Koch, Y., Lu, K. H., and Meites, J., *Endocrinology* 87, 673 (1970).
14. Maayan, M. L., Shapiro, R., and Ingbar, S. H., *Endocrinology* 92, 912 (1973).
15. Boyd, A. E., Lebovitz, H. E., and Feldman, J. M., *J. Clin. Endocrinol.* 33, 829 (1971).
16. Snyder, P. J., and Utiger, R. D., *J. Clin. Invest.* 51, 2077 (1972).
17. Kamberi, I. A., Mical, R. S., and Porter, J. C., *Endocrinology* 88, 1012 (1971).
18. Peter, R. E., *J. Endocrinol.* 51, 31 (1971).

Advances in Neurology, Vol. 5
Raven Press, New York © 1974

Dopamine Receptor Site Sensitivity in Hyperthyroid and Hypothyroid Guinea Pigs

Harold L. Klawans, Jr., Christopher Goetz, and William J. Weiner

Department of Neurological Sciences, Rush-Presbyterian–St. Luke's Medical Center, Chicago, Illinois 60612

Several sets of observations suggest that the level of thyroid function influences the sensitivity or responsiveness of catecholamine receptor sites to the appropriate neurotransmitter. Although this phenomenon is best documented in the peripheral noradrenergic system (1–3), some evidence suggests that the sensitivity of dopamine receptor sites within the central nervous system may be influenced by alterations in thyroid function (3). This possibility is suggested by the occurrence of chorea during hyperthyroidism (4–6), the responsiveness of such hyperthyroid chorea to dopamine antagonists (6), and the influence of thyroid status on dopamine metabolism as measured by cerebrospinal fluid homovanillic acid levels (6).

To study the effect of thyroid function on dopamine receptor-site responsiveness, amphetamine- and apomorphine-induced stereotyped behavior were studied in hypothyroid, euthyroid, and hyperthyroid guinea pigs. Both amphetamine and apomorphine-induced stereotyped behavior are due to an effect on striatal dopamine receptors (7, 8). Amphetamine acts by releasing endogenous dopamine onto the receptors, while apomorphine acts directly on the receptors. Amphetamine-induced stereotyped behavior has proven to be a useful model in studying the physiology and pharmacology of tardive dyskinesia (9, 10), a movement disorder which is often felt to involve the activity of dopamine at striatal dopamine receptors (10, 11).

MATERIALS, METHODS, AND RESULTS

All studies were initiated with 1-month-old male guinea pigs with an average initial weight of 250 to 275 g. The handling of the animals and the grading of behavior were done as described previously (9).

Ten guinea pigs were made hypothyroid by the injection of 40 μC of radioactive iodine (^{131}I). Two months later, 4.5 mg/kg amphetamine given subcutaneously elicited sustained stereotyped behavior in only 2 of 10 animals (see Table 1). This dose of amphetamine elicited stereotyped behavior in 100% of normal control animals (see Table 1). At the time these euthyroid animals were tested, the average weight and age of these animals was approximately midway between the age and weight of the hypothyroid animals at the two times of testing. Four months after the injection of ^{131}I, 4.5 mg/kg amphetamine elicited stereotyped behavior in three of seven guinea pigs (see Table 1).

TABLE 1. *Effect of amphetamine in hypothyroid and euthyroid guinea pigs*

Previous treatment	Time since treatment (days)	Number	Age (months)	Weight (g)	Stereotyped behavior	Percent with stereotyped behavior
None		7	4	550	7	100
[131]I	60	10	3	450	2	20
[131]I	120	7	5	700	3	41

In a second experiment, a group of 30 guinea pigs was given 500 g/kg thyroxine subcutaneously daily for 10 days. The hyperthyroid state was demonstrated by weight loss, increased heart rate, and mortality. At the end of 10 days, 20 animals and 60 age-matched controls were given apomorphine. Apomorphine was used because amphetamine in doses studied here is associated with 100% mortality in hyperthyroid guinea pigs (12). The results are shown in Table 2. While 0.30 mg/kg apomorphine regularly induced stereotyped behavior in euthyroid guinea pigs, 0.25 mg/kg apomorphine induced stereotypy only occasionally (three of 36 guinea pigs tested, or 8%). This same dose resulted in stereotyped behavior in 90% (18 of 20) of hyperthyroid guinea pigs.

TABLE 2. *Effect of apomorphine in hyperthyroid and euthyroid guinea pigs*

Previous treatment	Dosage of apomorphine (mg/kg)	Number	Stereotyped behavior	Percent with stereotyped behavior
None	0.30	24	24	100
	0.25	36	3	8
Thyroxine	0.25	20	18	90

DISCUSSION

Stereotyped behavior is felt to be due to excessive activation of striatal dopamine receptors (7, 8, 10). This conclusion is based on several observations. Intrastriatal injection of dopamine and several other agents capable of acting on dopamine receptors elicits stereotyped behavior, while injection of these same agents into other areas of the brain does not elicit stereotyped behavior (13, 14). Intrastriatal injections of dopamine antagonists prevent stereotyped behavior, while injections of the same agents elsewhere in the brain do not block this behavior (15). Destruction of the striatum also prevents stereotyped behavior (7). Since its activity is blocked by alpha-methylparatyrosine, amphetamine is considered to be an indirect dopamine agonist which acts by releasing dopamine onto dopamine receptors (16). Since the ability of apomorphine to elicit stereotyped behavior is not blocked by alpha-methylparatyrosine, which blocks dopamine synthesis, apomorphine is considered to be a direct dopamine agonist which acts directly on dopamine receptors (8).

The results presented above suggest that significant alterations in thyroid status alter the responsiveness of striatal dopamine receptors to dopamine and apomorphine. In hyperthyroid animals, amounts of apomorphine which can elicit stereotyped behavior in only 8% (three of 36) of euthyroid guinea pigs elicit this behavior in 90% (18 of 20) of hyperthyroid guinea pigs. This difference is significant ($p < 0.01\%$). Since apomorphine acts directly on striatal dopamine receptors to produce stereotyped behavior, these observations suggest that hyperthyroidism is associated with increased responsiveness of striatal dopamine receptor sites to dopamine agonists.

The results of the studies in hypothyroid guinea pigs suggest that hypothyroidism is associated with decreased striatal dopamine receptor-site sensitivity. Amounts of amphetamine which produced stereotyped behavior in 100% (seven of seven) of euthyroid guinea pigs produced these movements in only 20% (two of 10) and 41% (three of seven) of hypothyroid guinea pigs when tested at two separate times. This difference is also significant ($p < 0.05\%$). Since amphetamine is an indirect agonist, these results could suggest that amphetamine might release decreased amounts of dopamine in hypothyroid animals or that striatal dopamine receptors could be less responsive to normal amounts of dopamine. Since hypothyroid animals have been shown to have increased activity of tyrosine hydroxylase (17), which is felt to be the rate-limiting step in dopamine synthesis (18), it is unlikely that decreased amounts of releasable dopamine are present in hypothyroid animals.

The concept that dopamine receptor-site sensitivity is directly related to level of thyroid function is supported by similar observations on the relationship of norepinephrine receptor-site sensitivity to thyroid status. Lipton et al. (2) studied norepinephrine synthesis in hypothyroid rats. These rats appeared to be markedly hypoadrenergic. These investigators found that the rats showed a marked increase in the synthesis of norepinephrine in the heart, with a similar increase in the synthesis of norepinephrine in the brain. Despite the increased synthesis of norepinephrine, these animals were markedly hypoadrenergic. Prange et al. (3) found that despite the excessive sympathetic activity in hyperthyroid rats these rats manifested decreased catecholamine turnover in the heart and brain. This was attributed to hyperthyroid-induced hypersensitivity of the catecholamine receptors. Conversely, in hypothyroidism, receptor-site sensitivity seemed to be decreased. Prange et al. (3) hypothesize that in hyperthyroid animals the increased sensitivity of the receptors produces an increase in sympathetic response. This, in turn, leads to a decrease in sympathetic neuronal activity, including catecholamine synthesis. In hypothyroidism, decreased receptor sensitivity leads to a decreased sympathetic response and a consequent increased catecholamine turnover in order to increase sympathetic neuronal activity. There appears to be a negative feedback system in operation here. The activity of a catecholamine at postsynaptic receptor sites is inversely related to the rate of synthesis of the catecholamine within the presynaptic neuron.

Prange et al. (3) demonstrated that thyroid hormones could sensitize central aminergic receptors in man. They demonstrated that the antidepressant effect of imipramine was increased by thyroid hormone. Imipramine appears to function by increasing the effect of norepinephrine at norepinephrine receptors. They felt that the enhancement of imipramine's antidepressant effect in these patients was due to increased sensitivity of norepinephrine receptors due to exogenous thyroid hormone.

It has also been shown that hypothyroid rats demonstrate decreased spontaneous motor activity, a measure of central norepinephrine activity, while at the same time these animals have increased tyrosine hydroxylase activity (17). Hyperthyroid rats demonstrated increased spontaneous motor activity and showed increased sensitivity to the effects of intraventricular norepinephrine. These results suggest that central norepinephrine receptor-site responsiveness, as manifested by motor activity, is directly related to thyroid status. The results presented here extend these observations to dopamine receptor-site responsiveness as manifested by stereotyped behavior.

There are two possible clinical implications of these observations. The first of these is the relationship of hyperthyroidism and chorea. If hyperthyroidism increases the sensitivity of receptor sites in the striatum to dopamine, this should produce two results. Patients with hyperthyroidism could have chorea, since choreatic movements are felt to be related to the activity of dopamine at striatal dopamine receptors (19–21). These patients may also manifest decreased cerebral dopamine turnover. In 1952, a review of the German literature listed 28 instances of chorea associated with hyperthyroidism (22). More recently, patients with this association have been described by Syner, Fancher, and Kemble (23); Heffron and Eaton (4); and Fidler et al. (5). In terms of possible dopaminergic mechanisms, the best-studied patient was the one presented by Klawans and Shenker (6). In this patient, the chorea was relieved by the dopamine antagonist haloperidol. These authors also found an inverse relationship between thyroid status and brain dopamine turnover as estimated by CSF HVA levels. Taken as a whole, this evidence suggests that hyperthyroidism in man increased the sensitivity of striatal dopamine receptor sites to dopamine, with the decrease in dopamine turnover being secondary to the increased receptor-site response. The observations reported here support this proposal.

The other clinical state in which the pathophysiology is even more clearly related to the activity of dopamine at striatal dopamine receptors is parkinsonism (24, 25). If altered thyroid function alters dopamine receptor-site responsiveness, hypothyroidism might worsen parkinsonism or decrease responsiveness to L-DOPA or both. There are scant data that hypothyroidism has any effect on parkinsonism. We have had experience with only one patient with both parkinsonism and untreated hypothyroidism. A 62-year-old woman had severe parkinsonism, with a disability of 28 on the scale of Canter, de la Torre, and Mier (26). An initial trial of L-DOPA of 5.0 g/day for 10 weeks resulted in no improvement. After this patient was placed on replacement therapy and was felt to be euthyroid, a similar trial of L-DOPA resulted in a decrease in disability from 28 to 15, an improvement of 46%. This suggests that hypothyroidism can decrease clinical response to L-DOPA.

This raises the possibility that exogenous thyroid might increase the therapeutic effect of L-DOPA. The possibility is further supported by numerous observations that exogenous thyroid in small doses increased the clinical efficacy of tricyclic antidepressants (27, 28). The efficacy of the latter drugs is thought to be related to increasing the activity of either norepinephrine (29) or serotonin (30) at their respective receptors within the brain. One study of this possibility has been carried out using small doses of liothyronine similar to the doses which do potentiate the effect of tricyclic antidepressants (31). In the doses used, liothyronine did not increase the response to L-DOPA. While it is possible that larger doses might increase L-DOPA response, it is also possible that this might increase peripheral side effects by increasing peripheral norepinephrine receptor-site responsiveness. In this regard it is also of interest that liothyronine does not potentiate the antidepressant effect of L-tryptophan (28).

SUMMARY

Hyperthyroidism increases the responsiveness of guinea pigs to apomorphine, as manifested by the production of stereotyped behavior. Hypothyroidism decreases the responsiveness of guinea pigs to amphetamine, as measured by the production of stereotyped behavior. These observations suggest that striatal dopamine receptor-site responsiveness varies with thyroid status, being increased in hyperthyroidism and decreased in hypothyroidism. These observations support the hypothesis that increased receptor-site sensitivity plays a role in the pathophysiology of hyperthyroid chorea.

ACKNOWLEDGMENT

This work was supported by a grant from the United Parkinson Foundation, Chicago, Illinois. Mr. Goetz's work was supported by a Parkinson's Disease Foundation Student Research Fellowship.

REFERENCES

1. Krishna, G., Hynie, S., and Brodie, B. B., *Proc. Nat. Acad. Sci.* 59, 884 (1968).
2. Lipton, M. A., Prange, A. J., Diarman, W., and Udenfriend, S., *Fed. Proc.* 27, 399 (1968).
3. Prange, A. J., Meek, J. L., and Lipton, M. A., *Life Sci.* 9, 901 (1970).
4. Heffron, W., and Eaton, R. P., *Ann. Intern. Med.* 73, 425 (1970).
5. Fidler, S. M., O'Rourke, R. A., and Buchsbaum, H. W., *Neurology* 21, 55 (1971).
6. Klawans, H. L., Jr., and Shenker, D. M., *J. Neural Trans.* 33, 73 (1972).
7. Munkvad, I., Pakkenberg, H., and Randrup, A., *Brain Behav. Evol.* 1, 89 (1968).
8. Ernst, A. M., *Psychopharmacology* 10, 316 (1967).
9. Klawans, H. L., Jr., and Rubovits, R., *J. Neural Trans.* 33, 235 (1972).
10. Rubovits, R., and Klawans, H. L., Jr., *Arch. Gen. Psychiat.* 27, 502 (1972).
11. Klawans, H. L., Jr., *Am. J. Psychiat.* 130, 82 (1972).
12. Weiner, W. J., and Klawans, H. L., Jr., unpublished observation.
13. Cools, A. R., and Van Rossum, J. M., *Arch. Int. Pharmacodyn. Ther.* 187, 163 (1970).
14. Fog, R. L., Randrup, A., and Pakkenberg, H., *Psychopharmacology* 11, 179 (1967).
15. Fog, R. L., Randrup, A., and Pakkenberg, H., *Psychopharmacology* 12, 428 (1968).
16. Randrup, A., and Munkvad, I., *Nature* 211, 540 (1966).
17. Emlen, W., Segal, D. S., and Mandell, A. T., *Science* 175, 79 (1972).
18. Nagatsu, T., Levitt, S., and Udenfriend, S., *J. Biol. Chem.* 239, 2910 (1964).
19. Birkmayer, W., *Wein Klin. Wschr.* 81, 10 (1969).
20. Klawans, H. L., Jr., *Europ. Neurol.* 4, 148 (1970).
21. Klawans, H. L., Jr., Paulson, G. W., Ringel, S. P., and Barbeau, A., *New Engl. J. Med.* 286, 1332 (1972).
22. Sattler, H., in: *Basedow's Disease*, p. 143, Grune & Stratton, New York (1952).
23. Syner, J. C., Fancher, P. S., and Kemble, J. W., *U.S. Armed Forces Med. J.* 5, 61 (1954).
24. Hornykiewicz, O., *Pharmacol. Rev.* 18, 925 (1966).
25. Klawans, H. L., Jr., Ilahi, M. M., and Shenker, D. M., *Acta Neurol. Scand.* 46, 409 (1970).
26. Canter, G. J., de la Torre, R., and Mier, M., *J. Nerv. Ment. Dis.* 133, 143 (1961).
27. Wilson, I. C., Prange, A. J., McClane, T. K., Rabon, A. M., and Lipton, M. A., *New Engl. J. Med.* 282, 1063 (1970).
28. Coppen, A., Whybrow, P. C., Naguera, R., Maggo, R., and Prange, A. J., *Arch. Gen. Psychiat.* 26, 234 (1972).
29. Glowinski, J., and Axelrod, J., *Nature* 204, 1318 (1964).
30. Coppen, A., *Brit. J. Psychiat.* 113, 237 (1967).
31. Prange, A. J., Morris, C. E., Hall, C. D., and Weiss, E. A., *J. Am. Med. Ass.* 217, 1393 (1971).

DISCUSSION

Dr. Burrow: Regarding the use of thyroid with antidepressants in treating Parkinson's disease, there is a negative feedback control, and if you give a quarter of a grain of thyroid, you are simply going to decrease the response.

Dr. Klawans: I am very skeptical about the use of thyroid hormone to potentiate tricyclic antidepressants. A number of studies have supported this, including double-blind studies. The investigators themselves are at a loss to explain the response. I think the clinical implications of the kind of receptor site sensitivity are more related to hyperthyroidism, perhaps in relation to chorea, than in really potentiating L-DOPA.

Dr. Burrow: Gerald Levy in Miami has done a great deal of work looking at the question of catecholamine sensitivity. He concluded that he was not sure he can really demonstrate any change in sensitivity.

Dr. Klawans: In our animals that had 100% mortality, we could prevent the mortality from amphetamine in hyperthyroid guinea pigs by giving propranolol. It was purely a cardiac arrhythmia, norepinephrine-mediated mortality, and regardless of whether the animals were hypersensitive, they died.

Dr. McCann: I would like to comment on Dr. Burrow's interesting postulate about the existence of a TIF which is under the influence of L-DOPA. The way to solve this, of course, is to do the experiment in patients who have a hypothalamic lesion, or, easier than that, simply to test this in the *in vitro* pituitary incubation system to see if L-DOPA will block the response to TRF in the rat. I wonder if you have done any of those experiments.

Dr. Burrow: I have.

Dr. Frantz: I would like to suggest, in relation to Dr. Carlsson's comment on my talk, that if it can be shown that the L-DOPA effect is potentiated by an inhibitor, this might indicate a hypothalamic rather than a pituitary locus of action.

SUBJECT INDEX

A

Acetylcholine
  atropine and, 15
  dopamine and, 12-13
  5-hydroxytryptamine and, 3-4
  parkinsonism and, 1-2
  release of, 2-4, 11-13
  in striatum, 1-4, 15
  turnover rate, 108
S-Adenosylmethionine, polysome aggregation and, 89
Adenylate cyclase as dopamine receptor,
  83-84
α-Adrenergic receptors, 161-167
Adrenochrome, 288-289
Adrenocorticotrophic hormone (ACTH)
  secretion
    acetylcholine and, 479
    α-adrenergic receptor and, 484-485
    catecholamines and, 479-485
    Cushing's disease and, 484-485
    17-hydroxycorticosteroid and, 482-483
    hypophysectomy and, 480
    parkinsonism and, 484
    stress and, 480
Age, Parkinson's disease and, 187-190
Akinesia
  catecholamines and, 350
  definition of, 348
  diurnal oscillations in, 354-357
  dopamine deficiency and, 348
  dopamine receptors and, 12-13
  "on-off" response and, 350-351
Akinesia paradoxica
  DOPA and, 351-352
Alzheimer's tangles,
  neuromelanin and, 195-202
  parkinsonism and, 175-193
γ-Aminobutyric acid (GABA),
  basal ganglia and, 137-140
  DOPA and, 163
  dopamine and, 362, 377
  functional site, 132-133
  globus pallidus and, 153-157
  hippocampus and, 132-133
  inhibitory neurons and, 129-130
  membranes and, 131-132
  metabolism of, 130-131
  regulation of, 131-132
  release of, 131
  spinal cord and, 133
  in substantia nigra, 4, 153-157

γ-Aminobutyric acid-α-ketoglutarate transaminase, 131
Amphetamine
  action of, 206
  dopamine receptor and, 495-497
  dopamine release, 72-73
  thyroid function and, 495-497, 501
Antergrade reaction, 51-52, 57
Apomorphine
  derivatives of, 307
  DOPA and, 295-297
  dopamine and, 298
  dopamine receptors and, 80-81, 495-497
  dopamine synthesis and, 80-81
  dopaminergic activity of, 307
  monoamine oxidase and, 299
  "on-off" response and, 380-381
  in parkinsonism, 295-297
  pharmacology of, 298-299
  polysomes and, 92, 97
  side effects of, 297
  striatal function and, 322-323
  vascular effects, 166
Artane, 312-313
Atropine
  acetylcholine release and, 15
  dopamine release and, 74-75
  dopamine turnover and, 3-4
  tranquilizers and, 3
  tremor and, 5
Axoplasmic flow
  dopamine-β-hydroxylase, 47
  norepinephrine and, 47, 52-53
  tyrosine hydroxylase, 47
Axonal injury
  norepinephrine and, 50-51

B

Basil ganglia, GABA and, 137-140
  See also: specific nuclei
Basket cells, GABA and, 129, 132, 133
Benztropine
  dopamine release and, 74-75
  dopamine uptake, 74
  tremor and, 5
Brainstem, norepinephrine and, 135
Breast cancer, DOPA and, 459
2-bromo-α-ergocryptine (CB 154), tremor
  and, 79-80
Brocresine, histamine metabolism and, 103, 107
Bulbospinal system, norepinephrine in, 45-46